Third Edition

Guide to Clinical Laboratory Diagnosis

Third Edition

Guide to Clinical Laboratory Diagnosis

John A. Koepke, M.D.
Professor of Pathology
Associate Professor of Medicine
Duke University Medical Center
Durham, North Carolina

John F. Koepke, M.D.
Resident in Pathology
North Carolina Memorial Hospital
Chapel Hill, North Carolina

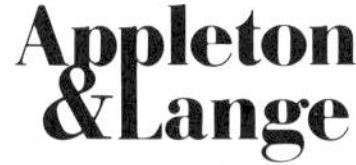
Appleton & Lange
Norwalk, Connecticut / Los Altos, California

0-8385-3519-4

87 88 89 90 91 / 10 9 8 7 6 5 4 3

Prentice-Hall of Australia, Pty. Ltd., Sydney
Prentice-Hall Canada, Inc.
Prentice-Hall Hispanoamericana, S.A., Mexico
Prentice-Hall of India Private Limited, New Delhi
Prentice-Hall International (UK) Limited, London
Prentice-Hall of Japan, Inc., Tokyo
Prentice-Hall of Southeast Asia (Pte.) Ltd., Singapore
Whitehall Books Ltd., Wellington, New Zealand
Editora Prentice-Hall do Brasil Ltda., Rio de Janeiro

Library of Congress Cataloging-in-Publication Data

Koepke, John A., 1929–
   Guide to clinical laboratory diagnosis

   Includes bibliographies and index.
   1. Diagnosis, Laboratory.   I. Koepke, John F.
II. Title. [*DNLM:* 1. Diagnosis, Laboratory.   QY 4 K78g]
RB37.K715   1987   616.07'5   86-32248
ISBN 0-8385-3519-4

Design: Cindy Lee Lombardo

PRINTED IN THE UNITED STATES OF AMERICA

CONTENTS

PREFACE

Laboratory medicine or clinical pathology can be defined as the application of laboratory techniques to the study of the blood, urine, other fluids, excretions and secretions from the patient for the purpose of medical diagnosis and treatment.

The laboratory is an important part of medical diagnostic procedure, adding its objective information to the more subjective history and physical examination of the patient. Clinical laboratory studies have immeasurably advanced the medical diagnostic process. Definitive diagnoses are now made earlier as well as more correctly than in the past. Take, for example, the measurement of those erythrocyte enzymes, which, if deficient, can precipitate episodes of acute hemolysis when the patient is inadvertently exposed to certain drugs or chemicals.

The physician is faced with a host of tests and measurements which can be done on the patient's blood, serum, plasma, urine, stool, exudates, transudates, secretions, or other fluids. The problem is to choose those tests which will give the greatest amount of information in the most efficient manner and for the least possible cost. It is the aim of this book to give some guidelines to students, house officers, and practitioners for a better and more efficient use of the clinical laboratory so that when they hear hoofbeats they will think first of horses rather than zebras.

This book is an expansion of a seminar entitled The Hospital Clinical Laboratory given to medical students in the early sixties. This aspect of medical school teaching has been neglected in many medical schools; in its stead there has been a reliance on learning by experience, a method which may be very expensive in both time and money. It is therefore heartening to see the increasing interest in laboratory medicine courses which are becoming increasingly popular.

During the middle years of the medical school curriculum the student reorients his thinking from the subject-oriented approach of the basic sciences to patient-oriented clinical science. In an effort to help in this reorientation, the book is arranged into sections and chapters according to the tentative clinical diagnosis assigned to the patient after the initial history, physical examination, and routine blood count and urinalysis. It is somewhat akin to the problem-oriented medical record, popularized some years ago. For instance, in the chapter entitled "Anemia", a logical rather than haphazard laboratory investigation of anemia is outlined. It is hoped that this approach will be useful to the clinician. In this way many common clinical conditions are discussed and unnecessary minutiae are avoided, unless they are of value for teaching certain principles of laboratory medicine.

Following the publication of the first edition of this book, much of this material was validated by extensive chart reviews as well as in the peer review of medical care. It was found that almost eighty percent of chief complaints of inpatients are covered in the chapters which follow. The twenty percent of admissions not discussed includes trauma, such as fractures and lacerations, elective surgical procedures (e.g., herniorrhaphy, hysterectomy), dermatologic complaints and, finally, psychosomatic and psychiatric problems.

After the second edition was published, significant changes were made in the methods of reimbursement to hospitals for the care of patients. The development and implementation of the so-called Diagnostic Related Groups (DRGs) has given impetus to cost-effective patient care, including laboratory testing. We believe the schemes advanced in these pages help to achieve the twin goals of efficiency and cost-effectiveness in testing.

It is our hope that through education medical laboratories will be used in such a manner so as to result in optimal care for all patients.

John A. Koepke

John F. Koepke

Third Edition

Guide to Clinical Laboratory Diagnosis

1
GUIDELINES TO THE INTERPRETATION OF LABORATORY DATA

THE EVOLUTION OF LABORATORY MEDICINE

In the past the science and art of clinical diagnosis has been primarily dependent on an exhaustive patient history coupled with a complete physical examination of the patient. Within the past few years, however, there has been a phenomenal growth in the use of the clinical laboratory, which has greatly increased the data base of the clinician. Many laboratories report a 10 to 15 percent increase in tests per year, at least until recent cost controls. The use of automated and semiautomated laboratory equipment, capable of doing multiple analyses on microliter quantities of serum or whole blood, has played a key role in this growth. This has resulted in a plethora of data that threatens to bury the physician in a mass of unnecessary and extraneous information and may even result in pertinent information being overlooked.

It is the responsibility of the clinical pathologist to control and direct this phenomenon by studying and improving the technical aspects of laboratory data acquisition. He or she also must promote the proper use of the laboratory, with the interpretation of laboratory data based on a thorough knowledge of the disease processes in humans as well as an intimate acquaintance with the technical details, failings, and strengths of the many available laboratory tests. Any laboratory data must be interpreted in the context of the clinical condition and treatment of the patient. This does not mean, however, that data that do not agree with the tentative diagnosis are laboratory errors and should, therefore, be disregarded. But such an inconsistency should alert the physician to the possibility that the diagnosis may require modification or that unusual complications are becoming manifest. The clinical pathologist should also be aware of such problems so that the test can be re-checked and he or she will be conscious of this apparent false-positive or false-negative result in the interpretation of future data.

The clinician should also point out to the pathologist conditions in which the history, the physical examination, and the laboratory studies presently available are not adequate for optimal patient care. Perhaps innovative studies would improve the sometimes less than optimal status quo.

THE LABORATORY TEST

Functions of Laboratory Testing

The various laboratory tests available today can be grouped into several categories according to their clinical application. The first group, comprised of the so-called diagnostic or pathognomonic tests, is not very large because only a few tests are so specific. Examples of such tests include pregnancy tests, many bacteriologic culture procedures, tests for a low hormone level, a low serum iron level, or the specific identification of toxic substances. Such tests are usually quite sensitive as well as specific.

Most laboratory tests are more nonspecific in that abnormalities detected by the test may be seen in several or even a wide spectrum of clinical conditions. The results support the clinical diagnosis, but not necessarily to the exclusion of other diagnoses. Singly, such results might be consistent with, but not diagnostic of, a certain diagnosis. A pattern of reactions in a panel of tests may make the several laboratory determinations considerably more specific or even diagnostic of a single clinical entity. For example, the occurrence of hypokalemic hypernatremic alkalosis strongly points to primary aldosteronism.

The appropriate use of the laboratory to corroborate certain normal factors can also be of considerable assistance in clinical diagnosis. A normal test result may dismiss groups of diseases from further consideration. Refer, for example, to a normal 2-hour post-prandial blood glucose; this finding essentially rules out diabetes mellitus as a consideration.

Laboratory studies are frequently used to follow the progress of a disease or to monitor the results of therapy. Serial white blood cell counts done on a patient undergoing chemotherapy are an example of this use of the laboratory.

Recently, the laboratory has been asked to provide monitoring data for drugs, particularly antibiotics, cardiac drugs and more specifically theophylline and lithium. This is probably the most persuasive argument for laboratory medicine because the data have such a direct bearing on clinical care.

Ordering

The physician may request more laboratory measurements than are necessary or, more frequently, desirable. He or she may fail to realize the discomfort to the patient (or their pocketbook). Likewise, the physician may not understand exactly what variable he or she is attempting to measure, or the importance of time relationships. For example, in monitoring the blood count of a patient receiving potentially toxic drugs, the order of a daily CBC may be erroneously substituted for a daily WBC and possibly a weekly hemoglobin with the option of pursuing any abnormalities if indicated by these single procedures. In addition to the above sins of commission, the omission of needed laboratory studies is also potentially detrimental to the patient. One objective of this book is to provide some guidelines to a more beneficial use of laboratory testing.

The concept of panels of laboratory tests is basically an extension of the first panels that were used for many years. The two most common laboratory procedures, the complete blood count (hemoglobin/hematocrit, total white blood cell and differential count, and platelet count) and the complete urinalysis (pH, specific gravity, reducing substances, protein and microscopic examination of the sediment), are essentially panels of single tests. It is often helpful to have related laboratory studies to interpret certain information more properly, for example the use of coagulation panels. Multitest automated analysis has made this a reality. Multitest screening (see Chap. 2) has been an application of this principle.

Reference or Normal Values

The result of any laboratory test is judged as being normal or abnormal, usually either described as elevated or decreased. How does one determine the limits of normal, which is basic to making such a judgment? Probably the most commonly used method has been to determine the normal range after calculating the mean and standard deviation (SD) of a series of measurements done on a presumably healthy population. Statisticians define the normal range as the mean value ± 2 SD.

TABLE 1–1. REFERENCE INTERVALS FOR COMMON LABORATORY TESTS WITH CONVERSIONS TO SI UNITS

A. Chemistry

System	Component	Present Reference Intervals	Present Unit	Conversion Factor	SI Reference Intervals	SI Unit Symbol
S	Alanine aminotransferase (ALT)	0–35 (37C)	units/L	1.00	0–35	U/L
S	Albumin	4.0–6.0	g/dl	10.0	40–60	g/L
S	Aldolase	0–6 (37C)	units/L	1.00	0–6	U/L
P	Ammonia	10–80	μg/dl	0.05871	5–50	μmol/L
S	Amylase, enzymatic	0–130 (37C)	units/L	1.00	0–130	U/L
S	Aspartate aminotransferase (AST)	0–35 (37C)	units/L	1.00	0–35	U/L
S	Bilirubin					
	Total	0.1–1.0	mg/dl	17.10	2–18	μmol/L
	Conjugated	0–0.2	mg/dl	17.10	0–4	μmol/L
S	Calcium	8.8–10.3	mg/dl	0.2495	2.20–2.58	mmol/L
		4.4–5.2	mEq/L	0.500	2.20–2.58	mmol/L
S	Calcium, ionized	2.00–2.30	mEq/L	0.500	1.00–1.15	mmol/L
B,P,S	Carbon dioxide content (bicarbonate + CO_2)	22–28	mEq/L	1.00	22–28	mmol/L
S	Chloride	95–105	mEq/L	1.00	95–105	mmol/L
P	Cholesterol					
	<29 yr	<200	mg/dl	0.02586	<5.20	mmol/L
	30–39 yr	<225	mg/dl	0.02586	<5.85	mmol/L
	40–49 yr	<245	mg/dl	0.02586	<6.35	mmol/L
	>50 yr	<265	mg/dl	0.02586	<6.65	mmol/L
S	Creatine					
	Male	0.17–0.50	mg/dl	76.25	10–40	μmol/L

	Female	0.35–0.93	mg/dl	76.25	30–70	μmol/L
S	Creatine kinase (CK)	0–130 (37C)	units/L	1.00	0–130	U/L
S	Creatine kinase isoenzymes MB fraction	>5 in myocardial infarction	percent	0.01	>0.05	1
S	Creatinine	0.6–1.2	mg/dl	88.40	50–110	μmol/L
B	Gases (arterial)					
	PO_2	75–105	mm Hg	0.1333	10.0–14.0	kPa
	PCO_2	33–44	mm Hg	0.1333	4.4–5.9	kPa
P	Glucose	70–110	mg/dl	0.05551	3.9–6.1	mmol/L
S	γ-Glutamyltransferase (GGT)	0–30 (30C)	units/L	1.00	0–30	U/L
S	Iron					
	Male	80–180	μg/dl	0.1791	14–32	μmol/L
	Female	60–160	μg/dl	0.1791	11–29	μmol/L
S	Iron-binding capacity	250–460	μg/dl	0.1791	45–82	μmol/L
P	Lactate (as lactic acid)	0.5–2.0	mEq/L	1.00	0.5–2.0	mmol/L
		5–20	mg/dl	0.1110	0.5–2.0	mmol/L
S	Lactate dehydrogenase (L P)	50–150 (37C)	units/L	1.00	50–150	U/L
S	Lactate dehydrogenase isoenzymes					
	LD_1	10–60	units/L	1	10–60	U/L
	LD_2	20–70	units/L	1	20–70	U/L
	LD_3	10–45	units/L	1	10–45	U/L
	LD_4	5–30	units/L	1	5–30	U/L
	LD_5	5–30	units/L	1	5–30	U/L
S	Lipase	0–160 (30C)	units/L	1.00	0–160	U/L
P	Lipids, total	400–850	mg/dl	0.01	4.0–8.5	g/L
P	Lipoproteins					
	Low-density (LDL), as cholesterol	50–190	mg/dl	0.02586	1.30–4.90	mmol/L

TABLE 1–1. (*Cont.*)
A. Chemistry

System	Component	Present Reference Intervals	Present Unit	Conversion Factor	SI Reference Intervals	SI Unit Symbol
	High-density (HDL), as cholesterol					
	Male	30–70	mg/dl	0.02586	0.80–1.80	mmol/L
	Female	30–90	mg/dl	0.02586	0.80–2.35	mmol/L
S	Magnesium	1.8–3.0	mg/dl	0.4114	0.80–1.20	mmol/L
		1.6–2.4	mEq/L	0.500	0.80–1.20	mmol/L
P	Phosphatase, acid (prostatic)	0–5.5	units/L	1.00	0–5.5	U/L
S	Phosphate (as phosphorus, inorganic)	2.5–5.0	mg/dl	0.3229	0.80–1.60	mmol/L
S	Phosphatase, alkaline	30–120	units/L	1.00	30–120	U/L
S	Potassium	3.5–5.0	mEq/L	1.00	3.5–5.0	mmol/L
			mg/dl	0.2558	—	mmol/L
S	Protein, total	6–8	g/dl	10.0	60–80	g/L
S	Protein, electrophoresis					
	Albumin	3.6–5.2	g/dl	10.0	36–52	g/L
	Alpha 1	0.1–0.4	g/dl	10.0	1–4	g/L
	Alpha 2	0.4–1.0	g/dl	10.0	4–10	g/L
	Beta	0.5–1.2	g/dl	10.0	5–12	g/L
	Gamma	0.6–1.6	g/dl	10.0	6–16	g/L
B	Pyruvate (as pyruvic acid)	0.3–0.9	mg/dl	113.6	35–100	μmol/L
S	Sodium	135–147	mEq/L	1.00	135–147	mmol/L
S	Transferrin (β_1-siderophilin)	170–370	mg/dl	0.01	1.70–3.70	g/L
P	Triglycerides (as triolein)	<160	mg/dl	0.01129	<1.80	mmol/L
S	Urate (as uric acid)	2.0–6.0	mg/dl	59.48	120–360	μmol/L
S	Urea nitrogen	8–18	mg/dl	0.3570	3.0–6.5	mmol/L of urea

B. Hematology

System	Component	Present Reference Intervals	Present Unit	SI Reference Intervals	SI Unit Symbol
B	Erythrocytes				
	Hematocrit				
	Males	40–50	vol%	0.40–0.50	L/L
	Females	38–47	vol%	0.38–0.47	L/L
	Hemoglobin				
	Males	14–18	g/dl	140–180	g/L
	Females	12–16	g/dl	120–160	g/L
	Red blood cells (RBC)				
	Males	4.5–6.2	million/μ^3	4.5–6.2	$\times 10^{12}$/L
	Females	4.2–5.4	million/μ^3	4.2–5.4	$\times 10^{12}$/L
B	Erythrocyte indices				
	Mean corpuscular volume (MCV)	82–97	femtoliter	92–97	femtoliter
	Mean corpuscular Hb (MCH)	27–32	femtomole	27–32	femtomole
	Mean corpuscular Hb concentration (MCHC)	32–36	g/dL	32–36	g/dl
B	Reticulocytes				
	Males	1.2–2.0	percent	0.06–0.11	$\times 10^9$/L
	Females	1.6–3.2	percent	0.07–0.15	$\times 10^9$/L
B	Platelets	180–450	thousand/μ^3	180–450	$\times 10^9$/L
B	Leukocytes				
	Total	4.6–10.2	thousand/μ^3	4.6–10.2	$\times 10^9$/L
	Differential	Proportional		Absolute	
	Segmented neutrophil	37–80	percent	2.0–6.93	$\times 10^9$/L

TABLE 1–1. (*Cont.*)

B. Hematology

System	Component	Present Reference Intervals	Present Unit	Reference Intervals	SI Unit Symbol
	Band neutrophil	0–6	percent	0–0.87	× 10⁹/L
	Normal lymphocyte	10–50	percent	0.6–3.44	× 10⁹/L
	Variant lymphocyte	0–6	percent	0–0.66	× 10⁹/L
	Monocyte	0–12	percent	0.03–0.90	× 10⁹/L
	Eosinophil	0–9.5	percent	0–0.67	× 10⁹/L
	Basophil	0–2.5	percent	0–0.20	× 10⁹/L
	or				
	Granulocytes	43–85	percent		
	Monocytes	0–12	percent		
	Lymphocytes	12–51	percent		
	or				
	Granulocytes	43–85	percent		
	Mononuclears	12–57	percent		

C. Urine and Other Fluids

	Value	Units
Routine urinalysis		
Physicochemical		
Specific gravity	1.010–1.035	
pH	4.5–8.0	pH Units
Protein	negative	mg/dl or tr to 4+
Glucose	negative	mg/dl or tr to 4+
Hemoglobin	negative	mg/dl or tr to large amount
Bilirubin	negative	mg/dL or tr to large amount

Routine urinalysis (*cont.*)
  Physicochemical (*cont.*)

Ketones	negative	negative or positive
Leukocyte esterase	negative	trace to large amount
Microscopic		
White cells	<10	per high–power field
Red cells	<3	per high–power field
Casts	<3 hyaline no others	per low–power field

Semen

Volume	3–5	ml
pH	7–9	pH U
Sperm count	100–150	$\times 10^6$
Viability	>75	percent in 4 hours
Abnormal forms	<20	percent

Gastric analysis

Basal acid output (BAO)	2.5	mmol/hr
Maximal acid output (MAO)	12	mmol/hr

Cerebrospinal fluid

Cell count (all lymphocytes)	0–5	$\times 10^6$/L
Glucose	40–80	mg/dl
Protein, total	15–45	mg/dl

B, blood; P, plasma; S, serum.

Lundberg GD, Iverson C, Raduleseu G: Now read this: The SI units are here (editiorial). JAMA 255:2329, 1986.

Ninety-five percent of the healthy population are included in this so-called normal range, but 5 percent are, by definition, excluded. Although this system has worked reasonably well in the past, there are several serious problems. The 95 percent range presupposes that the population studied is normally distributed and assumes a Gaussian distribution. This may not always be true, however, and skewed distributions of normals do occur frequently. Refer, for example, to the normal distributions of eosinophils or basophils. This phenomenon will significantly affect the calculation of the normal range if the presence of a skewed population is not appreciated. The construction of distribution plots helps to uncover this phenomenon. Table 1–1 is a table of normal values showing both conventional and the upcoming SI units which are in the process of being implemented.

Another serious flaw in the determination of normal ranges lies in the selection of the normal population. Does normal mean young, healthy men, acceptable blood donors, outpatients in apparent good health, laboratory personnel, or other hospitalized patients?

These difficulties have not been satisfactorily resolved as yet. By repeated studies one can define the normal values and variation for the individual patient and then note any significant deviation from this baseline with the passage of time. The determination of baseline values for an individual during times of health provides a data base against which future measurements are compared. Individuals frequently show minimal variability within themselves, and subsequent illnesses may show significant trends but still be within the normal range as determined for the whole normal population.

Significant Changes in Laboratory Data

What constitutes a significant change in a laboratory determination? Here again, we have become somewhat arbitrary in our interpretation of what constitutes a significant change. A significant change is defined as a change from a previous measurement that is greater than 3 SD. This deviation is determined by replicate analyses done in the laboratory on multiple aliquots of a single pool. It is the quality control standard deviation that is used in the laboratory and it must not be confused with the standard deviation as determined by single measurements done on a large population sample. Changes from any previous determination greater than 3 SD constitute a significant change. If, for example, the laboratory can mea-

TABLE 1–2. LABORATORY QUALITY CONTROL DATA

Test	Control Material Mean	SD of Method	Quality Control Limits (±2 SD)	Significant Change (3 SD)	Units
Glucose	99	3.0	93–105	9.0	mg/dl
Urea nitrogen	22	0.6	21–23	1.8	mg/dl
Creatinine	1.6	0.1	1.4–1.8	0.3	mg/dl
Sodium	132	2.0	128–136	6.0	mmol/L
Potassium	3.7	0.1	3.5–3.9	0.3	mmol/L
Carbon dioxide	18	1.0	16–20	3.0	mmol/L
Chloride	95	1.0	93–97	3.0	mmol/L
Calcium	8.2	0.2	7.8–8.6	0.6	mg/dl
Phosphorus	3.2	0.1	3.0–3.4	0.3	mg/dl
Transaminase (AST)	25	3.0	17–23	9.0	IU/L
Alkaline phosphatase	94	3.5	87–101	11.0	IU/L
Protein, total	6.1	0.1	5.9–6.3	0.3	g/dl
Bilirubin, total	19.8	0.6	18.6–21.0	1.8	mg/dl
Cholesterol	180	4.5	171–189	14.0	mg/dl
Uric acid	4.8	0.1	4.6–5.0	0.3	mg/dl
Hemoglobin	16.5	0.3	15.9–17.1	0.9	g/dl
Hematocrit	0.45	0.012	0.435–0.475	0.037	v/v
Red cell count	4.64	0.06	4.52–4.76	0.18	x 10^9/L
White cell count	47	1.2	44.6–49.4	3.6	x 10^9/L

sure hemoglobin with a single quality control standard deviation of ± 0.3 g/L (± 1 SD), a change in the hemoglobin level greater than 0.9 g/L would be considered significant in, for example, a patient with gastrointestinal bleeding.

The significant changes for some common chemical and hematologic studies are found in Table 1–2. Obviously such changes will vary from one laboratory to another because of variations in methodology and technique. However, some appreciation of these values is very helpful in the interpretation of repeated laboratory studies.

Predictive Value of Laboratory Tests

The value of a laboratory test lies in its efficiency in predicting or confirming the presence of a disease (or the absence of disease). The predictive value of a laboratory test is the interaction of the two important attributes of the test, i.e., its sensitivity and specificity. A mathematical formula allows us to interrelate sensitivity and specificity so that the predictive value of the test can be determined.

Before proceeding further, it is useful to define our terms. The interrelationships of true and false results are better appreciated by arranging data in a table as follows:

	Test Result		
Clinical Cases	*Positive*	*Negative*	*Total*
Sick	TP	FN	TP + FN
Not sick	FP	TN	FP + TN
Total	TP + FP	FN + TN	TP + FP + FN + TN

In this tabulation, TP (true positives) is the number of sick patients who are correctly classified by the test; FP (false positives) is the number of persons free of the disease who are misclassified by the test; TN (true negatives) is the number of persons free of the disease who are correctly classified by the test; and FN (false-negatives) is the number of patients who are misclassified by the test.

Finally, it must be appreciated that the usual method of expressing normal values of a quantitative test is to include the central 95 percent of results obtained on a so-called normal population. Therefore, 5 percent of healthy persons will have an abnormal result for any particular test.

Sensitivity refers to the percentage of positive test results in patients with a particular disease. A sensitivity of 95 percent means that 95 percent of patients with the disease will be detected by the test whereas 5 percent of patients with the disease will have false negative results. Sensitivity is calculated as follows:

$$\text{Sensitivity} = \frac{\text{True positives}}{\text{All sick patients}} \times 100 = \frac{\text{TP}}{\text{TP} + \text{FN}} \times 100$$

where TP is true-positive results and FN are false-negative results.

Specificity refers to the percentage of negative test results in persons without the disease. A specificity of 95 percent means that 95 percent of persons without the disease will have a negative test, whereas 5 percent of patients without the disease will have false-positive results. Specificity is calculated as follows:

$$\text{Specificity} = \frac{\text{True negatives}}{\substack{\text{All persons free} \\ \text{of the disease}}} \times 100 = \frac{\text{TN}}{\text{TN} + \text{FP}} \times 100$$

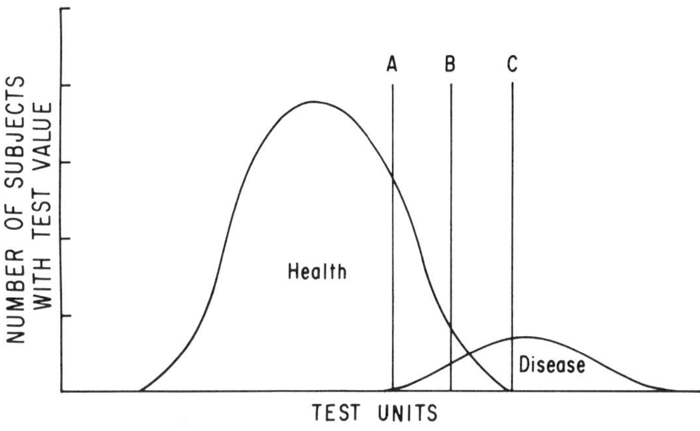

Figure 1–1. Frequency distributions for a hypothetical test performance in health and disease. Limits A, B and C result in significantly different performance of the test. See text for a more complete discussion.

where TN are true-negative results and FP are false-positive results.

Because there is usually a degree of overlap between the ranges of quantitative test values found in patients with and without a particular disease, the choice of a cutoff point beyond which the test is taken to be abnormal defines the diagnostic sensitivity and specificity (Fig. 1–1). If the cutoff point between health and disease is at point A, there is 100 percent sensitivity (i.e., all patients with disease will be detected) but the specificity will be low as there will be many normal individuals with an abnormal result. If point C is chosen as the dividing line between normal and abnormal the specificity will rise to 100 percent but the sensitivity will greatly decrease because of many false negatives. The cutoff Point B is an example of a compromise where neither the sensitivity nor specificity is 100 percent, but both are relatively high. Figure 1–1 illustrates that it is usually not possible to achieve both high sensitivity and high specificity at the same time. Sensitivity can only be increased at the sacrifice of specificity and specificity can only be increased at the expense of sensitivity.

The predictive value of a laboratory study includes two categories. The predictive value of a positive result is the probability that the disease is present when the test is positive. The predictive value of a negative test is the probability that the disease is absent when the test is negative. These can be expressed mathematically as follows:

$$\text{Predictive value of a positive test} = \frac{TP}{TP + FP} \times 100$$

$$\text{Predictive value of a negative test} = \frac{TN}{FN + TN} \times 100$$

Finally, the efficiency of a laboratory test is the percentage of true-positive and true-negative results as compared with the total number of tests done.

$$\text{Efficiency} = \frac{TP + TN}{TP + FP + FN + TN} \times 100$$

Effect of Disease Prevalence on Predictive Value

Taking the above discussion into account, it is of utmost importance for the clinician to appreciate the effect of disease prevalence on the predictive value of a positive test. This concept has special importance when screening programs for occult disease are being carried out. Galen and Gambino have carefully demonstrated these effects, and the interested reader is referred to their writings.

In recent years the use of the carcinoembryonic antigen (CEA) for the detection of patients with adenocarcinoma, particularly of the large bowel, has been touted. Let us apply the above principle to see how this test actually performs. The sensitivity of the test is reported to be 72 percent in patients with colon cancer. The specificity was determined to be 80 percent, i.e., 80 percent of normal persons had a negative test. But interestingly, many false positives were related to cigarette smoking.

If we complete the 2 × 2 table presuming that the incidence of colon cancer is 1 percent, we obtain the following:

	Test Result		
Patient's Condition	*Positive*	*Negative*	*Total*
Colon cancer	720	280	1,000
No colon cancer	19,800	79,200	99,000
Total	20,520	79,480	100,000

The researchers who promoted the procedure studied a highly selected group, probably similar to the 1000 patients in the top line of the above table. However, when the study group was expanded, disenchantment with the test was inevitable. Observe that the predictive value of a positive test is only 720/20,520 (3.5 percent). The predictive value of a negative test is somewhat better (79,200/79,480, or 99.6 percent), but one of four patients (280/1000) with cancer is missed. The clinician's problem of dealing with the false positives is evident.

What can the physician do to improve this rather dismal situation? He or she can, and indeed must, work to improve the odds. The physician's most important function is to carefully choose which patients should be studied. Thus, by testing only older patients possibly with anemia and/or a family history of cancer, the incidence of colon cancer is artificially increased. In doing so, let us say that the incidence is increased to 10 percent. Again completing the table:

	Test Result		
Patient's Condition	*Positive*	*Negative*	*Total*
Colon cancer	7,200	2,800	10,000
No colon cancer	18,000	72,000	90,000
Total	25,200	74,800	100,000

Now the predictive value of a positive test becomes 7,200/25,200 (29 percent). The predictive value of the negative test falls to 96 percent, however, and 2,800 patients out of 10,000 with the disease are not discovered by this test.

It is only when both the sensitivity and specificity of the test approach 95 percent and the disease in question is present in 50 percent of patients that the predictive value becomes 95 percent. The immunologic test for pregnancy is one of the all too few laboratory tests in this class. Most tests are much less sensitive or specific.

Interferences in Laboratory Testing

Several different factors may interfere with laboratory testing, and the physician should be aware of them, especially when laboratory data seem to be at variance with clinical impression.

Biologic Interferences

This type of interference may result from immunologic, pharmacologic, or toxic actions of medications or other chemicals in the patient. For example, diuretics alter blood electrolyte concentrations; probenecid decreases urate levels in patients receiving this medication; methyldopa and cephalothin may cause a positive direct anti-human globulin (Coombs) test. Examples are legion, and a number of listings have been published that catalogue such interferences.

Physicochemical Interferences

Colorimetric or spectrophotometric determinations may be altered by physical factors in the specimen itself. Certain urinary analgesics impart an orange color to the urine, which may interfere with testing. Lipemic specimens may yield artifactually elevated blood chemistries. The failure of red cells to completely lyse when hemoglobin is being measured (e.g., in sickle cell disease) may lead to an apparent hemoglobin level higher than it actually is.

Literally hundreds of examples of drug interferences with laboratory tests have been found. The mode of interference includes interfering chelators, enzyme inactivators, and drug metabolites being measured. Although many of these problems may be minor, occasionally major problems occur which lead to serious problems in the interpretation of laboratory tests.

Cost of Laboratory Tests

Laboratories based in hospitals usually provide about 15 to 20 percent of all hospital revenue. This fraction has grown because of the great increase in the use of laboratory tests. Laboratories have been able to meet the demand by using automated batch processing.

The actual costs of laboratory work are not well appreciated by many medical students and physicians. It is only when they themselves receive a substantial bill for a few common tests that the patient charges become more meaningful. Charges vary from one locality to another, but the tests are always expensive. If they are ordered indiscriminately, their cost drives up the overall cost of medical care unnecessarily.

Portent of Things to Come: SI Units

The international system of units (systeme international d'unites, SI) is the culmination of many years of international effort to develop a universally acceptable system of units of measure. This system has received additional impetus in medicine from the increasing exchange of scientific information. Already many European countries as well as Canada have converted to SI units in clinical medicine. A program to change to SI units in American medicine is in place and by 1989 we should be converted if all goes as planned.

Although the number of new units involved in the change to SI units in medical practice is small, several important factors are involved in their application. The SI recommends that molar units be used for those substances whose relative molecular mass is known. Thus, molality is expressed in moles or millimoles or micromoles per liter, the liter being the only volume unit used.

Some substances in body fluids cannot yet be measured in terms of amount of substance because of the uncertainty regarding their relative molecular mass. All proteins, including immunoglobulins are presently reported in mass concentrations, i.e., in grams per liter (g/L). The molecular masses of many proteins are, of course, known, but it is felt that all proteins should be reported in a similar manner. One significant difference will be that hemoglobin will be reported in grams per *liter* rather than the present grams per deciliter. The present 14.5 grams per deciliter will become 145 grams per liter with the new system of reporting in SI. Regarding enzymes, no definitive recommendations beyond the use of international units (IU) have yet been made. Finally, the partial pressures of blood gases (PO_2 and PCO_2) are expressed in terms of kilopascals (kPa) rather than millimeters of mercury (mm Hg).

Although the American Medical Association has indicated its endorsement of the SI, the system is relatively unknown to the majority of American medical practitioners. Where appropriate, SI units will be given in parentheses in this book. The SI prefixes are listed in Table 1–3, and conventional and SI units are compared in Table 1–1.

TABLE 1–3. SI PREFIXES

Factor	Prefix	Symbol
10^3	kilo	K
10^0	—	—
10^{-3}	milli	m
10^{-6}	micro	μ
10^{-9}	nano	n
10^{-12}	pico	p

SUGGESTED READINGS

Galen RS, Gambino SR: Beyond Normality. New York, Wiley, 1975.

Krieg A, et al.: Why are clinical laboratory tests performed? When are they valid? JAMA 233:76, 1975.

Ladenson J: Nonanalytic sources of variation in clinical chemistry results. In Sonnewirth A, Jarett L (eds): Gradwohl's Clinical Laboratory Methods and Diagnosis, 8th ed. St. Louis, C. V. Mosby, 1980.

Lundberg GD, Iverson C, and Raduleseu G: Now read this: The SI units are here (editorial). JAMA 255:2329, 1986.

Statland B, Winkel P: Pre-instrumental sources of variation. In Henry J (ed): Clinical Diagnosis and Management by Laboratory Methods, 17th ed. Philadelphia, Saunders, 1984.

Sunderman F: Current concepts of "normal values", "reference values" and "discrimination values" in clinical chemistry. Clin Chem 21:1873, 1973.

The SI for the Health Professions. Geneva, World Health Organizations, 1977.

SCREENING TESTS

BASIC INFORMATION

It is the hope of health professionals that certain laboratory analyses or procedures will indicate significant abnormalities before there is any other manifestation of disease. This is one of the most important goals of today's medicine. In contrast to acute diseases, chronic diseases are gradual in onset and are often confused with the minor aches and pains of growing old. Although acute illness is characterized by the sudden onset of fever and chills, nausea and vomiting, or severe pain, the large group of chronic illnesses is largely unnoticed by the patient until the disease is in an advanced stage and often beyond cure.

The development of automated techniques in chemistry and hematology has made screening of large numbers of persons possible. The automated methods have several distinct advantages. They are accurate and precise and are designed to use small amounts of serum for many different determinations. Finally, the cost per test is considerably less than that of manual procedures, therefore it is now economically feasible to do large numbers of laboratory tests at a fraction of previous costs. Even the initial large outlay of funds for instrumentation becomes reasonable if the instruments are used for a significant proportion of their maximum production time.

MULTIPHASIC HEALTH SCREENING

A panel of biochemical tests was done at the VA hospital in Durham, North Carolina, when a patient was admitted to the hospital. Of all the tests with abnormal results, only half had been requested by the patient's physician. A value judgment of the abnormal results in the unordered tests was made to determine if the unexpected findings were medically significant. Nineteen percent of the 288 patients studied were felt to have a significant abnormality that would have remained undiscovered in the ordinary mode of practice.

A much larger study was done on 58,000 persons in Sweden. About 14 percent of the persons screened had markedly abnormal results in at least one of the chemical tests. The follow-up group showed that in more than one third, 5 percent of the entire group of 58,000, a previously unknown disease had been discovered. As screening procedures for unsuspected disease, the chemical determinations yielded a much greater number of abnormalities than either urinalysis or measurement of the blood pressure.

Value of Screening

All of the studies mentioned (as well as the many studies undertaken and completed since then) indicate that with such methods it is quite possible to detect the presence of unsuspected chronic disease. There are, however, a number of questions that will have to be answered in the future to determine if these methods of detection of disease are truly worthwhile.

Does the early detection of a disease prevent the complications of the disease? For many illnesses this can be answered positively. For example, the early discovery and treatment of syphilis will prevent the progression to the tertiary stages of the disease. Likewise, the discovery of glaucoma coupled with appropriate treatment will prevent the blindness that is the final result of increased intraocular pressure. The lowering of the hematocrit in the polycythemic patient will avoid the complicating thromboses so often seen in this condition, and early treatment of urinary tract infections undoubtedly prevents the onset of renal failure secondary to pyelonephritis.

Does the early treatment of the disease with the purpose of normalizing the abnormal parameter prevent progression of the disease? This question is somewhat similar to the previous one but more complex. It also highlights how little we actually know about many diseases. Sometimes one can say positively that normalizing the parameter prevents progression of disease. The best example is the treatment of carcinoma of the cervix in situ. With other diseases the answer is not quite so clear-cut, as, for example, diabetes mellitus. The treatment of diabetes with insulin surely prevents the death of the patient due to ketoacidosis and diabetic coma. But does it prevent or even delay the inevitable development of intercapillary glomerulosclerosis? Or does the treatment of polycythemia vera with radioactive phosphorus delay the progression of this myeloproliferative disorder to myelocytic leukemia?

One must remember that random variations can produce a significant false-positive rate when multiple tests (e.g., multiple blood chemistries) are done on persons who are, in fact, well. As was discussed in Chapter 1, the more tests that are ordered, the higher the probability of at least one meaningless, random positive result. One can easily see that as more screening tests are ordered, the possibility of false-positive results increases significantly. One must balance the cost of evaluating false-positive results with the benefits of diagnosing unsuspected disease. One may decrease the number of false-positive results by using a wider range for defining normal. This results in a higher number of false-negative results, however, giving false reassurance to patients who are actually ill.

With the implementation of many screening programs, there has been a concurrent examination of the true value of these programs, especially given the increased cost consciousness of the medical community. More and more authorities are questioning the value of such programs when uncovering chronic but untreatable ailments. It is generally accepted that only four conditions occurring in adult patients can be influenced by appropriate measures: hypertension, obesity, smoking, and bacteriuria. Thus, only a relatively few conditions should be sought out for treatment in the general population. In the neonatal period, phenylketonuria and congenital hypothyroidism fulfill these criteria.

If one grants that multiphasic screening procedures are worthwhile, how often should these tests be repeated? This answer is being sought at the present time. Good judgment would seem to indicate that every 1 or 2 years is a reasonable interval, but this is subject to change with the availability of new data.

Criteria for Screening Tests

Finally, which tests should be done for the purpose of screening for chronic illness? The answer to this question will vary a great deal from one laboratory to another as well as from one patient group to another. The following guidelines answer this question and outline a suggested program that may at least provide a launching pad for multiphasic screening programs tailored to fit particular needs and particular patient groups.

A number of points should be considered to define and choose a screening test.

1. The disease being tested for should occur fairly frequently in the patient population being studied. For example, the blood glucose measurement for the detection of diabetes easily satisfies this criterion.
2. The disease being tested for should eventually be fatal or result in significant disability. This criterion for the individual patient is the main point of the entire discussion—we are trying to prevent death or chronic illness. Screening for rare diseases may be justifiable if the discovery of the disease can result in a cure and the prevention of chronic and long-term disability. Testing for phenylketonuria is an example of this point.
3. A single positive test should almost always indicate that a disease is indeed present. If this is not so, follow-up and repeated testing make the entire screening program much more difficult to administer and much less agreeable to the patient.
4. The test should be simple and economical. The development of automated procedures in the clinical laboratory has been a great help. All screening procedures cannot be done this way, however, and therefore the following question must be asked with regard to certain other tests: Are they truly simple and economical?
5. Finally, the test should not be objectionable or dangerous to the patient. The bromsulphalein test was probably the best test to screen for cirrhosis. However, the occasional allergic reactions and painful extravasations of dye constituted undue risks. Protoscopy for colon cancer or the cytologic screening for cervical cancer may be objectionable to some patients. But, some of the other proposed criteria may offset these objections so that such procedures may still be considered reasonable and good screening techniques.

In the evaluation of a screening procedure, all of the above points should be considered singly and in relationship to one another, and one should be able to make a reasonable assessment of the value of including or excluding a particular test.

Table 2–1 lists a number of screening tests that have been of value in uncovering chronic diseases. One will notice that the nonspecific tests, such as erythrocyte sedimentation rate or C-reactive protein, have not been included. They are nonspecific procedures, but do indicate the presence of some significant abnormality. They may be of some use in certain cases merely to determine whether the patient has a physical illness. The screening procedures have been grouped into a number of different categories of disease so the physician may choose the procedures that are appropriate to the patient.

In addition to serving as tests to screen for chronic illness, many of these procedures also serve as helpful baseline guides for comparison with follow-up studies. (See Chapter 1 for an interpretation of significant changes either within or outside the so-called normal ranges.)

TABLE 2–1. SOME SUGGESTED SCREENING TESTS FOR CHRONIC DISEASES

Chronic Disease	Screening Procedures
Cardiovascular diseases	
Arteriosclerotic	Cholesterol, high-density lipoproteins, electrocardiogram, ? triglycerides
Hypertensive	Blood pressure
Malignancy, including leukemia	Cervical Pap smears, breast palpation and mammography, stool and urine for occult blood, proctoscopy, digital rectal examination, complete blood count
Chronic respiratory diseases	Chest x-ray, timed vital capacity, tuberculin test
Chronic renal diseases	Creatinine, urinalysis including culture (colony count)
Chronic hepatic diseases	Transaminase, bilirubin, alkaline phosphatase, iodocyanine green test*
Musculoskeletal diseases	
Gout	Uric acid
Osteomalacia, osteoporosis	Calcium, alkaline phosphatase
Endocrine diseases	
Diabetes mellitus	Two-hour postprandial or fasting blood glucose, urine glucose
Thyroid disease	Thyroxine (T_4)
Syphilis	Serologic test for syphilis (VDRL or RPR)
Acquired immune deficiency syndrome (AIDS)	HTLV-III antibody
Glaucoma	Tonometry
Hearing disorders	Audiometry
Obesity	Body weight

*Only in selected patients.

TESTING FOR SYPHILIS

The control of one disease, syphilis, has relied heavily on laboratory detection, as its clinical manifestations are evanescent and variable. These may include primary and secondary lesions, which are manifest for relatively short intervals and may mimic other diseases. If untreated the disease enters a 3- to 8-year latent phase in which no detectable manifestations are present. This is followed by a tertiary phase. The tertiary phase may include benign gummatous lesions of different tissues, cardiovascular lesions, or central nervous system lesions. The prevention of these tertiary manifestations, which occur in about one-third of untreated cases of syphilis, is the reason for the search in the completely asymptomatic patient. Although the incidence of tertiary syphilis declined markedly following the discovery of the effectiveness of penicillin therapy, one may anticipate a renewal of tertiary syphilis with the recent increase in this venereal disease.

There is no way to identify the patient with latent syphilis except by laboratory screening. Serologic testing for syphilis, therefore, has been routinely carried out for many years. Although the discovery of new cases may not be large, this screening program is deemed justifiable because tertiary syphilis results in significant disability or even death. The other criteria for screening tests are also fulfilled by the use of a serologic test for the detection of syphilis.

In general two methods of testing for syphilis are used: the complement fixation and the flocculation technique. All procedures make use of a nonspecific cardiolipin reagent, which has been modified to make the test more specific or more sensitive. However, none of these tests are truly specific; they demonstrate only the presence or absence of the reagin, a substance formed in response to exposure to, among other things, *Treponema*. A positive test is seen in all except the earliest stages of syphilis. It is also positive in other spirochetal infections such as pinta or yaws. Finally, there is a group of diseases associated with biological false-positive reactions. These include lupus erythematosus, many acute febrile diseases, leprosy, malaria, and autoimmune diseases. Negative serologic tests are seen in the absence of syphilis. But a negative test is also consistent with early primary syphilis, with some cases of treated or latent syphilis, or as a prozone phenomenon in laboratory testing for this disease.

The most widely used screening test is the venereal disease research laboratory (VDRL) procedure. If the VDRL is reactive, the titer is determined on a repeat analysis. If it is felt that the flocculation test is a biological false-positive, specialized treponemal testing can be done using the fluorescent treponemal antibody absorbed tests (FTA-ABS). These tests are usually available only in state or federal public health laboratories but should be done on those patients in whom the clinical history and serologic testing are inconsistent. If the treponemal test is reactive, syphilis is the most likely diagnosis. A nonreactive test in a patient with probable clinical evidence of syphilis should be repeated at a later time.

SUGGESTED READINGS

Ahlvin RC: Biochemical screening: A critique. N Engl J Med 283:1084, 1970.

Berwick D: Screening health fairs: A critical review of benefits, risks and costs. JAMA 254:1492, 1985.

Boucot KR, Weiss W: Is curable lung cancer detected by semiannual screening? JAMA 224:1361, 1973.

Chang YW: A guideline to serologic tests for syphilis. Diag Med 6:51, 1983.

Hodkinson HM: Biochemical Diagnosis of the Elderly. New York, Wiley, 1977.

Holland WW: Screening for disease: Taking stock. Lancet ii:1494, 1974.

Knox EG: Multiphasic screening. Lancet ii:1434, 1974.

Last J (ed): Public Health and Preventive Medicine, 12th ed. Norwalk, Conn., Appleton-Century-Crofts, 1986.

Lee TJ, Sparling PF: Syphilis: An algorithm. JAMA 242:1187, 1979.

Medical Practice Committee, American College of Physicians. Periodic health examination: A guide for designing individualized preventive health care in the asymptomatic patient. Ann Int Med 95:729, 1981.

Miller DG: Preventive medicine by risk factor analysis. JAMA 222:312, 1972.

Woo B, et al.: Screening procedures in the asymptomatic adult: Comparison of physician's recommendations, patient's desires, published guidelines, and actual practice. JAMA 254:1480, 1985.

CHEST PAIN

BASIC INFORMATION

Diagnostic Enzymology

Many enzymes are normally present in the blood, arising from the breakdown of tissues. Blood or serum concentrations of enzymes, however, are usually much lower than those within the cells. The blood clearance rates of enzymes are variable, depending on molecular size, binding proteins, and other factors. For example, lactate dehydrogenase has an estimated half-life of about 12 hours, whereas alkaline phosphatase takes 6 days for a similar clearance.

When cells are injured or destroyed, the cell membrane becomes porous and intracellular enzymes (and other intracellular substances) leak into the extracellular fluid and subsequently into the vascular compartment. One exception is the usual elevation of alkaline phosphatase in rickets. This elevation is associated with an increase in the number and activity of osteoblasts in bone. These cells are rich in alkaline phosphatase, and serum alkaline phosphatase elevations are apparently derived from production of the enzyme by the increased numbers of highly active osteoblasts.

Different enzymes are present in tissues, but each enzyme or isoenzyme may be uniquely increased in some tissues or organs. An elevation of the enzyme in the blood becomes more specific for injury to those tissues, therefore serum enzyme measurements yield diagnostic information. The serial measurement of enzyme concentrations may give information that may indicate to the physician the progression or regression of tissue injury. Thus, serum enzyme levels can be used for diagnostic purposes as well as to follow the progress of disease.

A well-known illustration of the application of diagnostic enzymology is the relation of serum creatine phosphokinase (CK) levels to acute myocardial infarction. Several hours after the actual infarction the serum CK levels begin to rise, peaking about 24 hours later and subsequently returning to normal by the third day. Figure 3–1 illustrates typical changes in the levels of several enzymes following an acute myocardial infarction. Because enzyme levels have a typical pattern of rise and fall, the clinician must correlate the estimated interval following infarction with the specific enzyme assay requested. Thus, serum lactate dehydrogenase concentrations might still be normal 36 hours after infarction, whereas by that time CK levels may be beginning to return to normal.

Although certain enzymes may originate in different tissues, an enzyme arising from one tissue can be distinguished physicochemically from one arising from another tissue, although both catalyze the same reaction. The various molecular forms of the enzyme are called isoenzymes. These isologous enzymes differ from each other in certain properties (e.g., electrophoretic mobility or optimal pH for reaction) and may arise from different tissues. However, they all catalyze the same biochemical reaction. Determination of the percentage of the various isoenzymes can be useful in the diagnosis of various

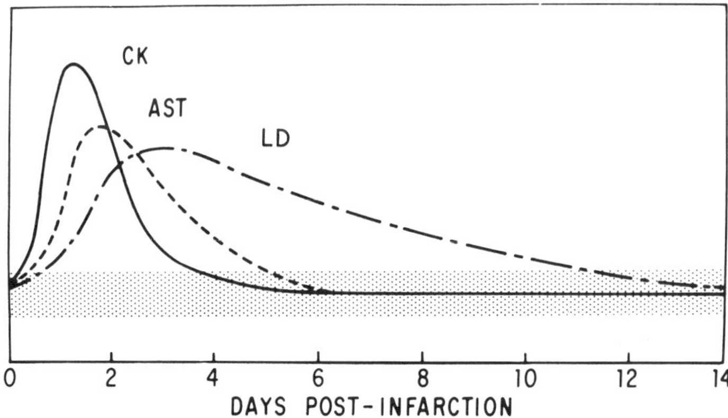

Figure 3–1. Serum enzymes in acute myocardial infarction. Shaded portion represents normal enzyme concentrations. See text for complete discussion.

diseases, e.g., in acute myocardial infarction it is useful to know the percentage of CK-MB, LD-1, and LD-2 isoenzymes.

The enzymes discussed in the following pages constitute the most widely used and clinically important in the differential diagnosis of chest pain. There is a considerable quantity of clinical experience attesting to their usefulness and correlating their concentrations with clinical disease.

Interpreting Results of Enzyme Assays

Because enzymes in serum are usually present in very low concentrations, they are not measured in absolute quantities. Rather, enzymes are measured by the rate of their catalytic activity, i.e., the quantity of substrate that is converted to product by the enzyme in a given period of time under standard conditions. The wide variety of units in which enzyme activity is expressed is due primarily to the many investigators who have studied the enzyme. Because of the variable conditions under which the enzymes are studied, it is difficult to accurately compare the units obtained from different methods. To remedy this situation, it has been recommended that enzyme activities be expressed in international units; an international unit (IU) equals 1 μmol of substrate transformed, or of product formed, per minute. It is now standard practice to express enzyme activity as IU per liter. The numerical values are identical to milliunits per milliliter, and this method will be followed. A comparison of conventional enzyme units and international units for some frequently measured enzymes is shown in Table 3–1.

Creatine Phosphokinase

The highest concentrations of the enzyme CK occur in striated muscle, although lesser amounts are present in the myocardium and brain tissue. The absence of CK in liver and erythrocytes eliminates any confusion that might arise from concurrent liver disease or hemolysis in a patient with a muscular disorder. The CK level is greatly elevated in progressive muscular dystrophy (Table 3–2), as is that of aldolase. Patients with neurogenic muscular atrophy have a negligible elevation of serum CK level. Levels of CK can also be moderately elevated immediately following strenuous muscular activity. Thus, exercise should be avoided before blood samples for CK are obtained.

TABLE 3–1. REFERENCE RANGES FOR CARDIAC ENZYMES

Enzyme	Reference Intervals (U/L)
Creatine phosphokinase (CK)	0–130
Lactate dehydrogenase (LD)	50–150
Alanine aminotransaminase (ALT)	0–35
Aspartate aminotransaminase (AST)	0–35

After several years of use it became apparent that the total CK measurement, although a sensitive test for myocardial infarction, was associated with a large number of false-positive results because of CK contamination from striated muscle activity. This lack of specificity has been considerably improved by the measurement of CK isoenzymes. The CK-MB or CK-2 isoenzyme has been shown to be both highly sensitive and highly specific for myocardial infarction. Only with some forms of muscular dystrophy and severe muscular injury is there a problem with the interpretation of the results.

The measurement of CK isoenzymes combined with the measurement of lactate dehydrogenase isoenzymes has been shown to be the most specific and sensitive test for acute myocardial injury.

Lactate Dehydrogenase

Total lactate dehydrogenase (LD) elevation is relatively nonspecific and occurs in many diseases. Elevated levels occur in certain cases of widely disseminated malignant disease (Table 3–3). Moderately elevated values follow a myocardial infarction; the test may be of value in some cases, as the elevation may persist up to 10 days after the acute episode. In liver disease, elevated values may be found in about three-quarters of cases of acute hepatitis, but normal values usually are found in obstructive jaundice, compensated cirrhosis, and chronic infections. Hemolytic anemias, because the hemolyzed erythrocytes release their LD into the plasma, are associated with elevated LD levels. Megaloblastic anemias also have elevated LD levels, presumably because of intramedullary hemolysis (within the marrow space).

Of much greater value is the measurement of individual LD isoenzymes. LD has five isoenzymes that can be separated by electrophoresis. The electrophoretically slowest fraction,

TABLE 3-2. CHARACTERISTIC CHANGES IN CREATINE PHOSPHOKINASE

Condition	CK (IU/L)
Normal male	10–200
Normal female	0–125
Increased physical activity	Up to 300
Myocardial infarction	175–1000
Intramuscular injection	Up to 700
Muscular dystrophy	Up to 3000
Neurologic injuries	Up to 800
Malignant hyperthemia	25–600
(two-thirds of cases)	

LD-5, is found in liver and skeletal muscle whereas the electrophoretically fastest fraction, LD-1, is found in the heart and erythrocytes. The isoenzyme pattern may therefore yield more specific information and greater diagnostic use to the physician.

Alanine Transaminase and Aspartate Transaminase

The enzymes alanine transaminase (ALT) and aspartate transaminase (AST), formerly known as SGPT and SGOT, are of particular value in the study of myocardial and hepatic disease. The liver is a rich source of ALT and AST. The heart and skeletal muscles also contain significant amounts of AST but contain little ALT. In acute liver cell injury, as, for example, in infectious hepatitis, changes in ALT and AST levels closely parallel each other (Table 3–4). Only AST is elevated in myocardial infarction. It is also elevated in skeletal muscle diseases, but more specific enzymes for skeletal muscle damage or necrosis are now available (see Chap. 18).

CLINICAL INVESTIGATION

Clinical Features

The causes of chest pain or discomfort with associated mild dyspnea can be divided into two major categories. The first includes myocardial infarction and other clinical disorders that may simulate myocardial infarction. The other large group of disorders associated with chest pain might be broadly termed

TABLE 3-3. CHARACTERISTIC CHANGES IN LACTATE DEHYDROGENASE

Condition	LD (IU/L)	Isoenzyme Increased
Normal	50–150	None
Malignancy	200–1000	Various
Myocardial infarct (5 days)	300–800	1
Acute hepatitis	200–500	5
Hemolytic anemia	250–800	1
Megaloblastic anemia	250–1000	1

the inflammatory chest diseases. Here, the onset of pain is usually more insidious. The pain is not quite so crushing and severe, and the evidence of infection or inflammation is more pronounced. The distinction between these two groups is by no means clear-cut; however, the tentative division made primarily on clinical grounds is useful in planning diagnostic procedures and laboratory examinations. Subsequent laboratory studies will provide confirmatory data to strengthen the clinical diagnosis. Thus, the middle-aged man who suffers the crushing substernal chest pain accompanied by mild hypotension and possible dyspnea almost surely has suffered a myocardial infarct. The mild leukocytosis, increased sedimentation rate, and elevated CK levels merely confirm the clinical diagnosis.

Unfortunately, some patients have very atypical symptoms and signs. It is in these cases that the laboratory investigation becomes important. Because of the possibility of atypical manifestations, a basic differential diagnosis of chest pain should always be borne in mind when one faces this clinical problem.

TABLE 3-4. CHARACTERISTIC CHANGES IN TRANSAMINASES

Condition	AST (IU/L)	ALT (IU/L)
Normal	0–35	0–35
Myocardial infarction	100–150	50–80
Increased physical activity	40–60	0–35
Muscular dystrophy	120	0–35
Acute hepatitis	>1000	>1000
Chronic hepatitis	40–100	40–100

Laboratory Studies

Screening Procedures

Chest X-ray. Undoubtedly the most widely used diagnostic procedure in disorders of the chest is the x-ray. With the exception of the typical episode of myocardial infarction, the roentgenogram is one of the first studies done for the patient. The indications, interpretations, and limitations of this procedure are beyond the scope of this book. On the other hand, we would be remiss in failing to indicate the prime importance of roentgenology in the study of chest diseases.

Erythrocyte Sedimentation Rate. The erythrocyte sedimentation rate (ESR), or an equivalent such as the C-reactive protein, might be considered a screening test for significant disease of any kind. The sedimentation rate is nonspecific and is elevated in most of the diseases discussed in this chapter. Conversely, a normal value rules out significant inflammatory disease and, thus, in certain cases this may provide worthwhile information.

Leukocyte Count. The white blood cell count with differential may be informative. A mildly elevated white blood cell count with granulocytosis and a mild left shift is characteristic of myocardial infarction, whereas most bacterial pneumonias lead to a significant granulocytosis (e.g., 20 to 40 x 10^9/L) with a marked left shift. Although not very common, monocytosis may indicate tuberculosis. Leukopenia or lymphocytosis, or both, point to a viral cause of the patient's chest pain.

TABLE 3–5. ENZYME LEVELS IN MYOCARDIAL INFARCTION

Enzyme	Initial Elevation (hr)	Peak Elevation (days)	Duration of Elevation (days)	Sensitivity (%)	Specificity (%)
CK, total	3–6	0.5–1.5	3–5	96	57
CK-MB isoenzyme				100	87
AST	6–12	1.5–2	4–6	92	73
LD, total	12–24	2–4	8–14	87	90
LD, isoenzymes				87	98

Definitive Procedures

Laboratory studies in chest pain that help confirm the clinical impression include chemical procedures, microbiological studies of sputum, and examination of abnormal accumulations of serous fluids such as pleural or pericardial fluid. Although examination of sputum or fluids is important, especially in ruling out certain unusual causes of chest pain (although not unusual causes of chest diseases), these tests are more appropriately included in the chapter on cough and dyspnea (see Chap. 7), and the reader is referred to those sections for further discussion. Only the more pertinent laboratory studies will be discussed.

Myocardial Infarction and Clinical Simulators of Myocardial Infarction

Electrocardiogram. Although the electrocardiogram remains an indispensable procedure in the diagnosis and follow-up of myocardial infarction, it has become evident that there are significant deficiencies in this diagnostic procedure. For example, in certain cases of infarction no changes may be demonstrable on the electrocardiogram, or prior changes may obscure evidence of fresh infarction. It is in these cases that serum enzyme determinations may be especially helpful.

Myocardial Enzymes. Three enzymes (CK, LD, and AST) have been used in the diagnosis of myocardial infarction. A comparison of these enzymes is given in Table 3–5. (see also Fig. 3–1.) It is necessary to correlate the presumed time of onset of the acute episode with the enzyme being measured. A possible infarction that occurred 1 week ago would rarely be associated with an elevated CK or AST level. On the other hand, measuring LD would be more likely to yield worthwhile information.

Recently the trend has been to use serial determinations of CK isoenzymes and LD isoenzymes in the diagnosis of acute myocardial infarction. The simultaneous use of CK and LD isoenzyme determinations combines the high degree of sensitivity offered by CK with the high degree of specificity offered by LD. Ideally three specimens are collected: one on admission, a second at 12 hours, and a third at 24 hours postadmission. In equivocal cases a fourth specimen at 48 hours can be helpful. Both total CK and LD levels are determined. If the levels are elevated, isoenzymes analyses are performed. In the classic case there is an elevated CK–MB level followed by a flipped LD pattern, i.e., the LD-1 level is greater than the LD-2 level. If enzyme and isoenzyme levels are consistently normal, a diagnosis of myocardial infarction may be excluded.

Several clinical conditions simulate myocardial infarction, and enzyme determinations are valuable in differentiating between infarction and myocardial necrosis. Elevations of cardiac enzymes (CK, LD, or AST) are rarely, if ever, seen in patients with angina pectoris or coronary insufficiency. If elevations are found, it is believed that myocardial necrosis must have occurred. If not accompanied by shock, dissecting aortic aneurysms are associated with normal serum levels of the cardiac enzyme panel. Acute or active myocarditis is manifested by increased levels of enzymes, presumably in direct proportion to the severity, extent, and duration of active disease.

In uncomplicated pulmonary embolus and infarction, an elevation of LD with normal levels of CK points toward pulmonary pathology rather than myocardial infarction. Arterial PO_2 (when breathing room air) is decreased below 80 mm Hg in practically all patients with acute pulmonary embolism. Pulmonary scans using radioactive isotopes are much more sensitive for the diagnosis of this disease.

In pneumothorax, a condition associated with sudden severe chest pain and dyspnea, cardiac enzyme levels are normal. Arterial oxygen levels are invariably decreased. The chest x-ray is diagnostic of this condition.

Patients with cardiac failure and shock for whatever reason will have moderately elevated AST and LD enzyme levels. This results from the hypoxia and cell damage within the hepatic parenchyma with resulting leak of enzymes into the circulation. The degree of enzyme elevation generally parallels

TABLE 3–6. LABORATORY DIFFERENTIATION OF TRANSUDATES FROM EXUDATES

	Transudate	Exudate
Appearance	Clear, straw colored	Turbid, cloudy, occasionally bloody
Specific gravity	<1.015	>1.015
Glucose	>60 mg/dl	<60 mg/dl
Protein	<3.0 g/dl	>3.0 g/dl
LD	<200 IU/L	>200 IU/L
Fluid/Serum LD	<0.6	>0.6
Cells	Few, mononuclear	Many, neutrophils
Cultures	Negative	May be positive

the degree of hypotension or shock associated with myocardial failure. These patients will usually have normal CK levels.

Inflammatory Chest Diseases. Although enzyme measurements on serum provide the backbone for the laboratory investigation of the myocardial infarction group, other specimens, such as pleural or pericardial fluid or sputum, are more important in the investigation of inflammatory diseases of the chest. In addition to biochemical studies, microbiological and cytologic investigations of pleural or pericardial fluid are often quite useful in determining the cause of the serous fluid accumulation.

Transudate Versus Exudate. It may also be helpful to determine whether the accumulated fluid is an exudate (resulting from inflammation) or a transudate (for example, as a result of increased venous pressure in congestive heart failure) (Table 3–6). The latter type is discussed more extensively in Chapter 6.

If the aspirated fluid is determined to be of inflammatory origin, definitive microbiological procedures are indicated. Smears of the exudate are examined for bacteria (including *Mycobacterium tuberculosis*, if indicated), and appropriate cultures are initiated, including routine aerobic and anaerobic cultures as well as cultures for tuberculosis and fungus, if indicated.

Any cloudy fluid aspirated from a serous space may be malignant. This decision is best made at the time of aspiration, as the prompt preparation of smears for Pap staining as well as cell block and membrane filter preparations yield better cytologic specimens. Romanovsky-stained smears are sometimes helpful, especially in effusions associated with a variety of lymphomas. Malignant lymphocytes and occasional Reed–Sternberg cells can be seen in these preparations. The differentiation of malignant cells from irritated mesothelial cells is at times difficult, and only an experienced cytologist should attempt such a differentiation. Clumps of variable-sized cells with large, deeply stained nuclei and possibly nucleoli are helpful in the identification of malignant cells.

Serous effusions not resulting from increased venous pressure may be caused by one of the collagen vascular diseases. The occurrence of serositis and serous effusions may be associated with systemic lupus erythematosus, rheumatoid disease, rheumatic fever, and certain hypersensitivity reactions such as serum sickness or autoimmunity. These diseases are more fully

TABLE 3-7. REFERRED PAIN IN INTRA-ABDOMINAL DISEASES*

Cholecystitis and cholelithiasis	Right sided, subscapular
Hepatitis	Right lower chest
Perisplenitis	Left back, shoulder
Subdiaphragmatic abscess	Right or left lower chest
Pancreatitis	Lumbar and dorsal back

*More complete discussions of some of these entities can be found in Chapter 8.

discussed in other chapters of this book but are mentioned here because they cause about 10 percent of cases of pericardial and pleural effusions.

The possibility that chest pain may reflect intra-abdominal disease must always be considered. The chief intra-abdominal causes of pain referred to the chest (including back and shoulders) are listed in Table 3-7.

SUGGESTED READINGS

Coodley EL: Prognostic value of enzymes in myocardial infarction. JAMA 225:597, 1973.

Galen RS: The enzyme diagnosis of myocardial infarction. Hum Path 6 (2):141, 1975.

Galen RS, Reiffel JA, Gambino SR: Diagnosis of acute myocardial infarction: Relative efficiency of serum enzyme and isoenzyme measurements. JAMA 232:145, 1975.

Hurst JW, King SB: The problem of chest "pain". JAMA 236:2100, 1976.

Hurst JW (ed): The Heart, 6th ed. New York, McGraw-Hill, 1986.

Irvin RG, Cobb FR, Roe CR: Acute myocardial infarction and MB creatine phosphokinase. Arch Intern Med 140:329, 1980.
infarction. Lab Mgmt 21:23, 1983.

Nevins MA, Saran M, Bright M: Pitfalls in interpreting serum creatine phosphokinase activity. JAMA 224:1382, 1973.

Pesce M: The CK isoenzymes: Findings and their meaning. Lab Mgmt 20:25, 1982.

Szucs MM, Brooks HL, Grossman W: Diagnostic sensitivity of laboratory findings in acute pulmonary embolism. Ann Intern Med 74:161, 1973.

Wagner G: Optimal use of serum enzyme levels in the diagnosis of acute myocardial infarction. Arch Intern Med 140:317, 1980.

Weidner N: Laboratory diagnosis of acute myocardial infarction: Usefulness of determination of lactate dehydrogenase (LDH)-1 level and ratio of LDH-1 to total LDH. Arch Pathol Lab Med 106:375, 1982.

4

HYPERTENSION

BASIC INFORMATION

Definition

There is no clear-cut difference between normal and elevated blood pressure. The usually quoted figure for the upper limit of normal, 140/90 mm Hg, is only an arbitrary figure. In fact, the arterial pressure slowly (and normally) increases with advancing age, and the interpretation of an individual patient's blood pressure should be made with this fact in mind.

Another point of considerable importance before diagnosing hypertension is the necessity of repeated measurement of the blood pressure to neutralize the psychologic factors that may considerably elevate the blood pressure. This phenomenon is well known but continually needs to be reemphasized.

General Classification

There are four major kinds of hypertension: (1) essential hypertension, i.e., without apparent cause; (2) renal vascular hypertension; (3) renal parenchymal hypertension; and (4) extrarenal hypertension.

Essential hypertension is, by far, the most common variety. Often this diagnosis is made by excluding hypertension from other causes. It most often occurs in middle-aged persons and is characterized by a relatively benign course, although at times it may be complicated by the sudden onset of malignant hypertension, which may be rapidly fatal.

Recent emphasis in the study of hypertension has been centered on the examination of the renal blood flow. Many techniques have been used to study this disorder, including intravenous pyelography (IVP), renograms using radioactive compounds excreted by the kidney, split-function renal studies, and aortography. Each method is primarily concerned with the discovery of a focal vascular stenosis in a unilateral, poorly functioning kidney. These lesions cause renal ischemia with resulting increased renin production (see next section). If focal, the lesions are often surgically correctable.

Renal parenchymal hypertension is secondary to a wide variety of diseases including glomerulonephritis and pyelonephritis. If far advanced, the disease may no longer be amendable to therapy, whereas early discovery of a treatable lesion, such as pyelonephritis, is of great benefit to the patient.

The fourth type of hypertension is the result of extrarenal causes. The adrenal gland, both cortex and medulla, is of special importance in this type of hypertension. Examples of adrenal lesions with hypertension include Cushing's disease, aldosterone-secreting adrenal adenoma, and pheochromocytoma. An uncommon cause of hypertension is polycythemia, either primary or secondary; the increased red blood cell mass directly causes hypertension in both the arterial and venous vascular tree.

The Renin–Angiotensin–Aldosterone System

The control of the blood pressure is mediated by an interplay of several substances. Some of these substances can now be measured directly, while the level of other substances may be inferred by measuring parameters known to be affected by these substances. The application of known stimulants of their

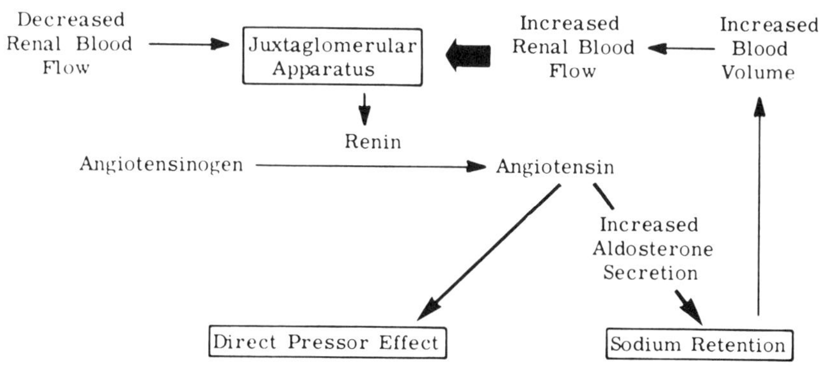

Figure 4–1. Interrelationships in the renin–aldosterone system.

secretion can further indicate the integrity of these interdependent systems. A basic understanding of the mechanisms of blood pressure control is necessary for both diagnosis and treatment of the various forms of hypertension.

The proteolytic enzyme renin is produced in the juxtaglomerular apparatus surrounding the afferent arterioles of the renal glomeruli. Increased amounts of renin are produced in response to decreased renal perfusion pressure, which is caused by decreased blood volume or total body sodium. Renin, in turn, activates angiotensin, a polypeptide that has two distinct effects on the blood pressure. One is to exert a direct pressor effect on the smooth muscle of the arterial blood vessels, thus raising the blood pressure. The second, more lasting effect, is to stimulate the production of the mineralocorticoid aldosterone; this hormone causes renal sodium retention, with subsequent increased circulating blood volume and increased arterial blood pressure. The increased renal blood pressure activates a feedback mechanism that decreases the production of renin (Fig. 4–1).

In renal vascular hypertension (renal ischemia secondary to vascular disease), renin production is increased because of the decreased amount of blood flowing through the juxtaglomerular apparatus. In extrarenal hypertension, such as primary aldosteronism, renin production is decreased because renal blood pressure and blood flow are increased and there is subsequently decreased renin production. When renin levels are being measured, the patient should be kept on a controlled salt intake. Certain manipulations of salt and water balance can be used to accentuate these changes and are discussed later in this chapter.

Catecholamine Metabolism

One of the rare but curable causes of hypertension is a tumor of the adrenal medulla called pheochromocytoma. The adrenal medulla normally produces physiologic amounts of the pressor amines epinephrine (adrenaline) and norepinephrine (noradrenaline). These compounds, collectively called catecholamines, prepare the body for stress, with an elevation in the blood pressure and an increase in the pulse rate.

Pheochromocytoma results in abnormally increased production of catecholamines with attendant paroxysmal or sustained hypertension. Catecholamines and their breakdown products are excreted in the urine, and these can be measured.

Elevated levels of one or more of these metabolites are found in patients with tumors. Surgical removal of the tumor will usually cure the patient's hypertension unless the condition has been present for many months and secondary vascular changes have occurred.

The normal scheme of catechol production and destruction is shown in Figure 4–2. The diagnosis of pheochromocytoma can be confirmed by demonstrating increases in catecholamines or their metabolites, usually metanephrines or vanillymandelic acid (VMA). These determinations are usually performed on an aliquot of a 24-hour urine specimen. Most patients will have elevated urinary VMA, metanephrines, and free catecholamines; however, in some patients one or more of these determinations may be within the reference interval. Urinary metanephrine levels have been recommended as the most accurate screening test for pheochromocytomas. It is important to remember that there are a significant number of false-positive and false-negative results with these tests. Factors that influence the levels of these metabolites include severe physical and mental stress, ethanol, incorrect specimen collection, and certain drugs (e.g., MAO inhibitors, alpha-methyldopa or L-dopa).

CLINICAL INVESTIGATION

With the variety of techniques now available for the definitive study of the hypertensive patient, it is becoming increasingly

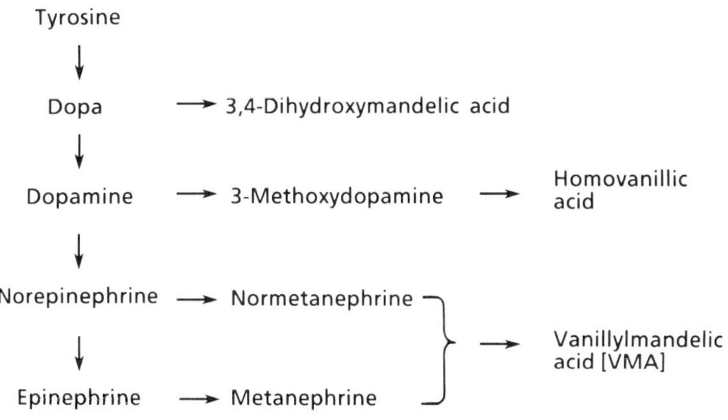

Figure 4–2. Scheme of catechol production and destruction.

important to choose procedures that will provide the essential information and to avoid unnecessary duplication as well as discomfort or even danger to the patient.

Hypertensive patients studied by laboratory techniques can be divided into two major groups on the basis of age. These are characterized by the middle-aged or elderly patient with mild or moderate hypertension and the younger patient with hypertension. More complete and vigorous investigation in the younger patient is justifiable, as there is a greater likelihood that a curable form of hypertension may be present. It is obvious that a great deal of medical judgment is required in individual cases. Thus, the discussion that follows merely provides a set of guidelines to be modified as necessary in individual instances.

Three criteria are used to select the laboratory procedures in evaluating hypertension: the ease of performance, the relative incidence of hypertension due to abnormality being sought, and the risk of injury to the patient. In younger patients hypertension caused by renovascular abnormalities or extrarenal lesions is more common; thus, the greater emphasis on screening for these abnormalities in younger patients is justified. Older patients, on the other hand, generally have essential hypertension or hypertension caused by renal parenchymal lesions, and the diagnostic program is modified accordingly.

Renal function tests offer little information in the study of the hypertensive patient, because it is only relatively late in the disease process that renal function is impaired. However, these function tests (see Chap. 11) may be of value in the long-term care of hypertensive patients in assessing the progression of the disease as well as response to therapy. These baseline studies may serve as valuable reference points.

ESSENTIAL HYPERTENSION

Clinical Features

At least 90 percent of hypertension is of the essential type. It is usually diagnosed by excluding other etiologies. This entity is seen most often in middle-aged persons. The patient is usually asymptomatic but occasionally may manifest headache, dizziness, dyspnea, or other nonspecific symptoms. The disease is

TABLE 4–1. URINALYSIS IN ESSENTIAL HYPERTENSION

Stage or Grade	Protein	Casts	Red Cells
I	0	Occasional	Occasional
II	Trace	+	Occasional
III	1–2+	+	Few
IV	3–4+	+	Many

divided into several arbitrary stages or grades from mild or benign to severe or malignant. The systolic and diastolic blood pressure increases parallel to the severity of the disease. As mortality is related to the stage of hypertension, it is helpful to delineate the stages.

Laboratory Studies

Screening Procedures

Urinalysis. Urinalysis offers a simple method to ascertain the stage of essential hypertension. Table 4–1 outlines some of the findings on urinalysis seen in essential hypertension.

Serum Creatinine and/or Blood Urea Nitrogen. These are widely available tests used to screen for renal complications of hypertension.

Creatinine Clearance. Normal kidneys have a large safety margin, i.e., many nephrons may be lost without losing excretory capacity of nitrogenous wastes. The serum creatinine will remain normal until about one-half of the nephrons are lost. The simplest and best test to quantitate renal function is the 24-hour creatinine clearance test. A gross correlation of the creatinine clearance and the stage of hypertension is found in Table 4–2 (see Chap. 11 for details of the creatinine clearance test).

TABLE 4–2. CREATININE CLEARANCE IN ESSENTIAL HYPERTENSION

Stage or Grade	Clearance (ml/min)
I	90–120
II	50–90
III	40–50
IV	15–40

Serum Potassium. A serum potassium level is useful to screen for mineralocorticoid-induced hypertension and as a baseline prior to initiating diuretic therapy.

Electrocardiogram. An electrocardiogram should be obtained to assess the patient's cardiac status and as a baseline.

HYPERTENSION CAUSED BY RENOVASCULAR DISEASE

Clinical Features

Distinctive signs and symptoms are infrequent in hypertension secondary to renovascular surgery. A bruit heard in the region of the kidney may suggest vascular stenosis. Because the renal vascular disease may be part of a generalized disease that characteristically has vascular involvement, the clinician must be aware of these associations and search for signs and symptoms of the primary vascular disease. These maladies may be as widely different as arteriosclerosis, polyarteritis, diabetes mellitus, or lupus erythematosus. All have one common denominator: partial or complete occlusion of the renal arterial or arteriolar tree.

Laboratory Studies

Screening Procedures

Renal function tests offer little help in this group of disorders. The intravenous pyelogram, the differential renal function test (Howard test), and the iodine-131 renogram may give evidence of significant differences in function between the two kidneys.

Definitive Procedures

The diagnosis of focal renal vascular insufficiency is established only by renal arteriography. As all arterial lesions are not hemodynamically significant, ancillary tests are used to assess the hemodynamic significance of the stenosis. The most widely used test involves measuring the renin activity in blood samples obtained from both renal veins and either the lower inferior vena cava or the aorta. A positive test is one in which the plasma renin activity from the involved renal vein exceeds the contralateral renal vein concentration by at least 50 percent and there is evidence of suppression of renin release from the contralateral renal vein, i.e., identical renin activity in the arterial and contralateral renal venous plasma.

HYPERTENSION CAUSED BY RENAL PARENCHYMAL DISEASE

Clinical Features

Although there are few physical findings that would direct the diagnostician to suspect renal parenchymal disease (exceptions would be costovertebral angle tenderness associated with renal infection or palpable kidneys in polycystic disease), there are a number of features in the medical history that are of help. The female patient, especially if previously pregnant, is likely to have had previous urinary tract infections. The elderly male with prostatism and urinary tract infection also is a prime candidate. Surgical manipulation, such as urethral catheterization, cystoscopy, or other procedures done on the genitourinary tract, is sometimes followed by infection. Diabetics have a significantly increased incidence of renal disease caused by either intercapillary glomerulosclerosis or more often chronic pyelonephritis.

Laboratory Studies

Screening Procedures

Urinalysis. The well-performed urinalysis, especially the microscopic examination of the sediment, is probably the most important and simplest study that can be done in the investigation of renal disease. The presence of proteinuria (albuminuria is too restrictive a term) not explained by fever, vigorous exercise, or other obvious cause should lead to more extensive investigation.

The microscopic examination of the urine sediment is invaluable if performed well and next to worthless, or even detrimental, if done poorly. Table 4–3 summarizes the usual findings in common renal parenchymal lesions.

Screening for Urinary Tract Infection. A clean-catch midstream urine specimen is required. A simple and rapid method for detecting significant bacteriuria is microscopic examination of a

TABLE 4–3. URINE MICROSCOPIC EXAMINATION IN RENAL HYPERTENSION

Lesion	White Blood Cells—HPF	Red Blood Cells—HPF	Casts—LPF
Normal	0–few	0–few	Hyaline, few
Pyelonephritis			
Acute	3–4+	0–few	White blood cell inclusion
Chronic	2–3+	0–few	Granular, white blood cell inclusion
Glomerulonephritis			
Acute	Few	3–4+	Red blood cell
Chronic	Few	1–2+	Granular
Polycystic disease*	0–few	1–4+	Hyaline, few
Diabetes mellitus*			
(Glomerulosclerosis)	Few	1–4+	Red blood cell, granular
Lupus erythematosus	0–few	0–1+	Hyaline, granular Doubly refractile lipid inclusions

HPF, high-power field; LPF, low-power field.
*Without complicating pyelonephritis.

Gram-stained smear of an uncentrifuged urine specimen. If one or more bacteria are seen per oil immersion lens field, significant infection of the urinary tract is probably present. Nitrate and leukocyte esterase tests are also useful to screen for urinary tract infection. See Chapter 11 for a more complete discussion of these tests.

Quantitative cultures of urine can be done by any of a number of acceptable methods. Bacterial counts of less than 10,000/ml are of doubtful or no significance unless the patient is receiving antimicrobial therapy. Counts greater than 100,000/ml indicate significant urinary tract infection, and the identification of the organism and the determination of its antibiotic susceptibility should be sought. Actual culture techniques are usually preferable to biochemical screening procedures for bacterial infection because, if positive, further tests can be done directly on the cultured organism. Counts between 10,000/ml and 100,000/ml must be considered in light of the clinical picture but probably represent urinary tract infection.

Definitive Procedures

If screening tests for urinary tract infection are positive, the organism should be identified and its antibiotic susceptibility determined. Anatomic abnormalities of the urinary tract should be sought because of the known association of impaired urinary flow with subsequent infection. Radiologic techniques such as intravenous and retrograde pyelography are helpful in delineating these abnormalities, which are often surgically correctable.

Percutaneous Renal Biopsy. This procedure, when carefully performed and interpreted, can provide a definitive diagnosis in equivocal renal parenchymal disease. As only a small amount of tissue can be examined, there is no substitute for sound judgment and experience in correlating the observed histologic changes with the clinical as well as laboratory findings. This is especially true in renal diseases known to be focally rather than generally distributed.

In addition to the routine hematoxylin and eosin (H&E) stains, immunofluorescent and electron microscopic examinations have become an essential part of the study of renal biopsies. Chapter 11 contains a more complete discussion of the clinical pathology of renal disease.

HYPERTENSION CAUSED BY EXTRARENAL PATHOLOY

Clinical Features

A variety of nonrenal diseases can give rise to hypertension (Table 4–4). Clinical features are those of the primary disease. The primary diagnosis most often will be easily corroborated by appropriate laboratory studies. Two adrenal lesions, pheochromocytoma and primary aldosteronism, are worthy of mention. Hypertension owing to either lesion is almost always curable by resection of the involved adrenal gland.

The pheochromocytoma, a tumor of the chromaffin tissue, produces greatly increased amounts of epinephrine or norepinephrine, or both. These substances result in either sustained or intermittent hypertension and tachycardia. In addition weight loss, headaches, nervousness, and anxiety are often present. At times, these symptoms may be triggered by emotional stress. The increased production of aldosterone by

TABLE 4–4. NONRENAL DISEASES THAT MAY LEAD TO HYPERTENSION

Hyperthyroidism
Polycythemia, primary or secondary
Diabetes
Coarctation of the aorta
Generalized arteriosclerosis
Adrenal lesions, e.g., pheochromocytoma, primary
aldosteronism, Cushing's disease

the adrenal cortex may result in increased diastolic blood pressure, but no clinical features distinguish this syndrome from other kinds of hypertension.

Laboratory Studies

Screening Procedures for Pheochromocytoma

Because of the discomfort, potential danger, and inaccuracy, the phentolamine (Regitine) test and the histamine provocative test are no longer used to screen for pheochromocytoma.

Urinary Metanephrines. Metanephrine excretion, either in a random specimen or a 24-hour specimen, will be significantly increased (greater than two times the normal value) in about 95 percent of patients with pheochromocytoma (Table 4–5). As

TABLE 4–5. URINARY CATECHOL EXCRETION

Catechol	Present Reference Interval	Present Unit	Conversion Factor	SI Reference Interval	SI Unit Symbol
Epinephrine (fluorimetric)	<10	μg/24 hr	5.458	<55	nmol/day
Homovanillate (as homovanillic acid)	<8	mg/24 hr	5.489	<45	μmol/day
Metanephrines (as normetanephrine)	0–2.0	mg/24 hr	5.458	0–11.0	μmol/day
Norepinephrine (fluorimetric)	<100	μg/24 hr	5.911	<590	nmol/day
Vanillylmandelic acid (VMA)	<6.8	mg/24 hr	5.046	<35	μmol/day

was discussed earlier, it must be kept in mind that there are a significant number of false-positive and false-negative determinations secondary to stress and/or various drugs.

Definitive Procedures for Pheochromocytoma

Other biochemical tests that can screen for pheochromocytoma include urinary VMA, urinary catecholamines, and plasma catecholamines. The sensitivity of these tests is only slightly less (about 90 to 95 percent) than the urinary metanephrine excretion (about 95 percent). The VMA test has one definitive advantage in that it is a technically more simple procedure and may be more readily available in smaller laboratories. Table 4–5 lists the reference or normal values for the urinary catechols.

Once the diagnosis of pheochromocytoma is strongly suspected from the results of biochemical testing certain radiographic procedures are useful to localize the tumor. These procedures include IVP, CT scanning and selective adrenal arteriography.

Screening Procedures for Primary Aldosteronism

Serum Potassium. Spontaneous hypokalemia (<3.8 mmol/L), with or without alkalosis, is an indication for further definitive studies. Hypokalemia may be accentuated by sodium loading. Ingestion of greater than 200 mmol of sodium per day for 4 days results in no significant changes of potassium levels in normal or hypertensive patients without aldosteronism. Patients with primary or secondary hyperaldosteronism have a reduction of serum potassium levels to less than 3.5 mmol/L when on a high sodium intake.

Definitive Procedures for Primary Aldosteronism

Urinary Potassium. A urinary potassium at over 30 mg/day in the presence of hypokalemia is presumptive evidence for primary hyperaldosteronism.

Plasma Renin Activity (PRA). As the sodium loading procedures are positive in both primary and secondary aldosteronism, measurement of aldosterone excretion will add little to differentiate these two conditions. By taking advantage of the known interrelationships between renin, angiotensin, and aldosterone, the measurement of PRA is helpful. Plasma renin activity is low in patients with primary aldosteronism, its production being suppressed. Renin activity is usually within the normal range in essential hypertension. Conversely, increased renin levels are found in malignant hypertension and renovascular hypertension. Two stimuli for renin production, sodium deprivation and upright posture, are used to corroborate suppressed renin activity. If the specimens are carefully collected under the proper clinical conditions and measured in a reputable laboratory, this determination will distinguish primary aldosteronism from secondary forms as well as from essential hypertension.

Aldosterone Suppression Test. The patient is taken off diuretics and placed on a diet containing 200 mmol of sodium and 80 mmol of potassium daily for 3 days. A 24-hour urine is collected and sodium, potassium, creatinine, and aldosterone levels are measured. Serum potassium and creatinine levels as well as the blood pH are also measured.

If the 24-hour sodium excretion exceeds 100 mmol and the creatinine excretion exceeds 15 mg/kg in 24 hours (a complete collection), a persistent hypokalemia and/or the excretion of more than 40 mmol of potassium are strongly suggestive of primary aldosteraldosteronism. Systemic alkalosis supports this diagnosis. The aldosterone excretion should normally be less than 20 µg/day unless the patient has aldosteronism with an increased aldosterone excretion.

Fluorocortisone Suppression Test. With a normal sodium intake (around 120 mmol/day), 200 ng of the synthetic mineralocorticoid fluorocortisone is given two times a day for 3 days. Plasma or urinary aldosterone is measured just before and on the third day of fluorocortisone administration. Failure to significantly decrease aldosterone excretion is evidence for an adrenal adenoma with increased aldosterone secretion.

SUGGESTED READINGS

Atuk N: Pheochromocytoma: Diagnosis, localization, and treatment. Hosp Pract 18(4):187, 1983.

Burke MD: Hypertension—Exploring the great unknown. Diag Med 1:34, 1978.

Burke MD: Hypertension: Test strategies for laboratory diagnosis. Postgrad Med 67(6):77, 1980.

Gernst J, Kuchel O, Hamet P, Contin M: (eds): Hypertension. McGraw Hill, New York, 1983.

Kaplan NM: Adrenal causes of hypertension. Arch Intern Med 133:1001, 1974.

Kaplan NM: Renin profiles—the unfulfilled promises. JAMA 238:611, 1977.

Maronde RF: The hypertensive patient: An algorithm for diagnostic workup. JAMA 233:997, 1975.

Melby JC, Finnerty FA: Extensive hypertensive work-up: Pro and con. JAMA 231:399, 1975.

Noth RH: Interpretation of plasma renin activity. Arch Intern Med 138:528, 1978.

Sacks TG, Abramson JH: Screening tests for bacteriuria. JAMA 201:1, 1967.

The Joint National Committee on Detection, Evaluation, and Treatment of High Blood Pressure. The 1980 Report of the Joint National Committee on Detection, Evaluation, and Treatment of High Blood Pressure. Arch Intern Med 140:1280, 1980.

Weinberger M, et al.: Primary aldosteronism: Diagnosis, localization, and treatment. Ann Intern Med 90:386, 1979.

HYPOTENSION AND SHOCK

BASIC INFORMATION

Pathologic Physiology of Shock

The practitioner approaching a patient in shock must bear in mind the various causes of shock, because rational therapy must be correlated with etiology. A great deal of investigation into the pathogenesis and treatment of shock has been done in recent years. These studies indicate that prompt and specific therapy will greatly improve the outcome.

Three different kinds of shock are seen clinically: hypovolemic shock, cardiogenic shock, and septic shock. A fourth variety, neurogenic shock, is associated with dilatation of the peripheral capillary bed, which results in the loss of an effective circulating blood volume. An infrequently seen variety, hypoxic shock, resulting from the inadequate oxygenation of arterial blood secondary to respiratory difficulties, is seldom recognized as a distinct entity and will not be discussed.

Any condition that results in a significant loss of fluid from the intravascular space, either as whole blood or plasma, will result in hypovolemic shock (Table 5–1). These losses may be external, such as through wounds or burns, or internal, into extravascular spaces or body cavities. The primary manifestations include hypotension with decreased blood volume, compensatory high peripheral resistance because of arterial constriction and decreased cardiac output. In this case, therapy is primarily directed toward replacement of the intravascular volume with fluids (crystalloids), colloids, or blood, as well as a direct attack upon any localized area of bleeding or fluid loss.

Cardiogenic shock is secondary to the primary failure of the heart to pump adequate amounts of blood. This may have several causes, of which myocardial infarction is probably the most common. Cardiac arrhythmias, cardiac tamponade secondary to intrapericardial hemorrhage or pericarditis, or pulmonary emboli may likewise result in cardiogenic shock.

Septic shock is secondary to the toxicity of infection that may be produced by the bacteria themselves (endotoxin) or bacterial products (exotoxin). In either case there is peripheral pooling of blood in capacitance (primary venous) vessels, causing a decrease in the effective circulating blood volume but without actual blood loss.

The body responds to shock by attempting to redistribute the flow of blood, i.e., a relatively larger fraction of the cardiac output is diverted to vital structures such as the heart and the brain, and perfusion to the rest of the body is diminished and inadequate. If shock is prolonged, there is a deepening cellular hypoxia. It will be recalled that glucose requires oxygen for efficient metabolism via the Krebs cycle, i.e., aerobic metabolism. If cellular hypoxia is produced, as in shock, cell metabolism shifts to the relatively inefficient anaerobic energy metabolism. This results in the shunting of pyruvate into the production of increasing amounts of lactic acid, and metabolic acidosis occurs. There is concurrent decreased storage of energy as adenosine triphosphate (ATP). Because of the lack of energy production, the sodium–potassium differential across the cell membrane is not maintained and intracellular potassium is released into the extracellular space. If no therapy is given or if it is ineffective, further impairment of energy production occurs and finally the cells are irreversibly damaged. It is evident that with the impairment of the microcirculation most organ and tissue functions will be compromised and eventually lost. Renal failure resulting from acute tubular necrosis (ATN) is the most common early consequence of shock and the onset of renal failure following an episode of shock is

TABLE 5–1. ACUTE BLOOD LOSS AND REPLACEMENT REQUIREMENTS

Blood Loss		Clinical	Transfusion
(%)	*(ml)*	Symptoms	Requirement
10–15	500–750	Simple faint	Not necessary
15–25	750–1250	Incipient shock	Desirable
25–35	1250–1750	Moderate shock	Necessary
35 +	>1750	Profound shock	Urgent

an ominous sign. Liver failure, adrenal failure, and other evidences of functional decompensation of various organ systems are also found.

In many cases of severe shock, there is increased platelet aggregation and resulting disseminated intravascular coagulation. Most coagulation factors are consumed in this process, and widespread capillary hemorrhage ensues. This complication may be seen in all types of shock. A more complete discussion of this entity can be found in Chapter 15.

The development of techniques for the placement and use of catheters in the vena cava (central venous catheters) and pulmonary artery (Swan–Ganz catheters) have been invaluable in the study as well as the therapy of shock. The pressures noted in the vena cava reflect the status of volume replacement and the ability of the right heart to pump blood. The Swan–Ganz catheter is used to obtain the cardiac output and pulmonary wedge pressure; the wedge pressure more accurately reflects the status of the left heart function. Using the information obtained from these catheters, one can accurately assess volume status and myocardial function, and thus help determine the need for additional volume replacement, removal, or cardiac support drugs.

CLINICAL INVESTIGATION

Clinical Features

In clinical shock it is now known that hypotension is a comparatively late manifestation, having been postponed and prevented by normal body defense mechanisms such as arteriolar pressor reactions and adrenal cortical discharge. The hypotension is accompanied by tachycardia. Respiration may be increased in both depth and rapidity. If shock has persisted for a significant period of time, urine output is decreased, and any urine that is produced has a very high specific gravity. The patient with hypovolemic shock frequently has a history and clinical evidence of blood loss such as that following injury or burns. Prompt and specific therapy must be initiated before the completion of extensive diagnostic studies. Patients with cardiogenic shock may exhibit the clinical manifestations of myocardial infarction with chest pain or have evidence of pulmonary emboli; thus, the diagnosis will be evident following the clinical history and physical examination.

Laboratory Studies

Screening Procedures

Urinalysis. The urinalysis may reveal both a decreased minute volume of urine as well as an increased specific gravity and/or osmolarity. If the shock is secondary to an incompatible transfusion reaction, free hemoglobin and sometimes distinctive hemoglobin (not red blood cell) casts will be found in the urine.

Hematocrit. This measurement as well as the hemoglobin and red blood cell count will be lowered when shock is due to blood loss, as, for example, in a bleeding peptic ulcer or bleeding secondary to trauma. The hematocrit is probably the most convenient test for monitoring acute blood loss in critical care areas such as emergency rooms, operating rooms, recovery rooms, and intensive care facilities. Blood loss from the intravascular space is compensated by the mobilization of extracellular fluid into the vascular compartment or by plasma or other intravenous fluid replacement. These changes result in dilution of the red blood cell mass (hemodilution) and a decreased hematocrit. It must be remembered that in acute blood loss situations, before mobilization of extracellular fluid or intravenous fluid replacement, the hematocrit may still be in the normal range. It is only after restoration of the intravascular volume that the hematocrit will reflect the true extent of blood loss.

Blood pH. The measurement of blood pH provides a simple yet accurate estimation of the severity of the shock syndrome with its concomitant metabolic acidosis, as well as a gauge of the response to therapy. The normal pH is 7.41 ± 0.03. A pH below 7.20 indicates severe acidosis.

Blood Gases (P_{CO_2} and P_{O_2}). In shock, oxygen levels fall and carbon dioxide levels increase. The deviations from normal parallel the severity of the shock.

Definitive Procedures

Most of the test findings discussed previously are abnormal in shock resulting from any cause. Only the hemoglobin and/or hematocrit levels, if markedly decreased, will point to a particular variety of shock, e.g., hypovolemic. The reader is referred to more specific and definitive procedures of various organ dysfunctions in other portions of this book to expand the laboratory evaluation.

Myocardial Enzymes. If cardiogenic shock from myocardial infarction is a consideration, serum cardiac enzymes may be of help in diagnosis. The more specific, CK, is preferred because the other enzymes (ALT, AST, and LD) may be elevated in shock for any number of reasons. The latter enzymes may arise from a poorly oxygenated liver in hypovolemic or septic shock, and any great value in differential diagnosis is lost. (See Chapter 3 for a more complete discussion.)

Blood Volume. The measurement of the blood volume is usually not of great help in the diagnosis and management of many cases of hypovolemic shock. However, in complicated cases, for example, following prolonged use of cardiopulmonary bypass procedures in open heart surgery, this measurement may be useful. In most cases measurement of the plasma volume with use of radioiodinated human serum albumin, if available, is preferred because of the simplicity and speed.

Blood Cultures. The drawing of blood for one or more cultures before the initiation of antibiotic therapy, although not of immediate benefit to the patient, may later provide valuable information. The identification of the responsible organism and the determination of its antibiotic susceptibility may, in fact, be lifesaving.

Coagulation Studies. Disseminated intravascular coagulation results in consumption of most of the clotting factors, including platelets, Factor VIII, prothrombin complex, and fibrinogen. Decreased levels of these and other coagulation factors point to intravascular coagulation. See Chapter 15 for a more complete discussion of this coagulation problem.

Lactic Acid. Elevated levels of lactic acid are the result of the shift of cellular energy production from the aerobic to the anaerobic pathway. Studies have shown that arterial blood lactate levels are a good indicator of prognosis in patients with acute myocardial infarction and myocardial failure.

SUGGESTED READINGS

Bane A: Recent developments in the study and treatment of shock. Surg Gynecol Obstet 127:849, 1968.

Bane A, Chandry J, Wurth M, Sayeed M: Cellular alterations with shock and ischemia. Angiology 25:31, 1974.

Boyan CP: Hypovolemic shock. Anesth Analg 46:746, 1967.

Byrne JJ: Current concepts: Shock. N Engl J Med 275:543, 1966.

Doty DB, Weil MH: Comparison of microcirculatory and central hematocrit as measure of circulatory shock. Surg Gynecol Obstet 124:1263, 1967.

Hardaway RM: The role of intravascular clotting in the etiology of shock. Ann Surg 155:325, 1962.

Parker M, Parrillo J: Septic shock. JAMA 250:3324, 1983.

Pinsky M: Cause-specific management of shock. Postgrad Med 73:127, 1983.

Shoemaker W: Pathophysiology and therapy of shock syndromes. In Shoemaker W, et al. (eds): Textbook of Critical Care. Philadelphia, Saunders, 1984.

Swan H, Ganz W: Measurement of right atrial and pulmonary arterial pressures and cardiac output: Clinical applications of hemodynamic monitoring. Adv Inter Med 27:453, 1982.

Wilson RF, Chiscano AD, Quadrios E: Some observations on 58 patients with cardiac shock. Anesth Analg 46:764, 1967.

6

EDEMA AND ASCITES

BASIC INFORMATION

Etiology of Edema

The maintenance of the normal passage of metabolites from the circulating plasma into the tissue spaces as well as the return of waste products of metabolism into the plasma compartment is a function of two interacting mechanisms. These mechanisms are the osmotic gradient between the vascular and tissue spaces (a function primarily of the plasma proteins) and the intracapillary vascular pressure. These relationships are most easily appreciated by inspecting a simplified diagram of the vascular system (Fig. 6–1).

The accumulation of increased amounts of fluid in the interstitial space is called edema. Special terms are used when edema is found in certain areas (e.g., ascites, if the fluid accumulates in the abdominal cavity) or if it is caused by certain disorders (e.g., lymphedema, if it is caused by blockage of the lymphatic channels). Alterations in any of the factors found in Figure 6–1 may result in localized or generalized edema.

If there is a significant decrease in the plasma protein concentration, especially albumin, edema results. Chronic liver disease with decreased albumin production or chronic renal disease with associated increased protein losses are good clinical examples of this process. Gram for gram, albumin exerts four times as much osmotic pressure as do the globulins; this is because albumin is a protein of much lower molecular weight than globulin.

Plasma protein concentration can also be effectively decreased by plasma dilution. The retention of fluid due to the

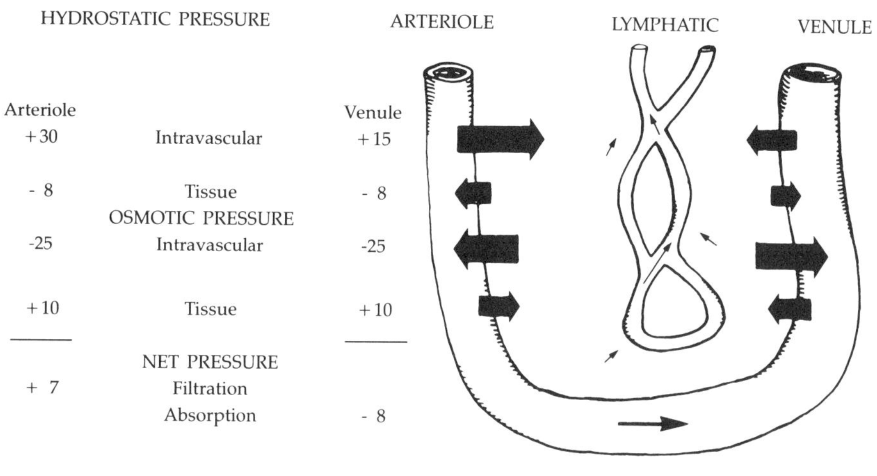

Figure 6–1. Factors affecting interstitial fluid flow. The size of the arrows is proportional to the pressures. The direction of flow is also indicated.

action of estrogens, aldosterone, or other hormones is an example of this type of edema production.

On the other hand, if venous or lymphatic intravascular pressure is increased, there is an effective decrease in the fluid reabsorption pressure, and fluid therefore accumulates in the interstitial tissues. A common example of this process is found in heart failure, with increased venous pressure and resultant peripheral and/or pulmonary edema. As venous pressure is greater in the more dependent tissues, edema is first noted in the feet (pedal edema) or lung bases (pulmonary edema).

Increased arteriolar or capillary pressure also results in edema. This is a major mechanism of edema and tissue swelling in the inflammatory process and also in local or generalized edema caused by application of heat to the body. In these cases the capillaries are dilated, and there is at least a partial transmission of the higher arteriolar pressure into the capillary bed. Arterial hypertension, on the other hand, does not result in edema because the arterioles are actually constricted and only the proximal portion of the arterial tree is subject to increased pressures.

There are a wide variety of causes of edema in a patient. Many of these are evident from the history and physical examination of the patient. At other times laboratory investigations may be helpful in determining the cause.

Secondary Aldosteronism

Almost all the clinical conditions discussed have an associated elevation of adrenal aldosterone production. The exact mode of production is not completely understood, although it is believed that the following sequence may occur; the juxtaglomerular cells of the kidney secrete increased amounts of renin into the blood, which leads to increased production of angiotensin; angiotensin, in turn, stimulates the zona glomerulosa layer of the adrenal cortex to increase the production of aldosterone. The primary action of aldosterone is directed on the renal tubular cells to retain sodium. This results in increased amounts of extracellular sodium and water. A corollary action of aldosterone is to increase the renal excretion of potassium and magnesium.

It should be stated that in some types of renal disease the loss of sodium and water may directly stimulate aldosterone production. In cirrhosis and cardiac failure, however, the exact stimulus for increased aldosterone production is not yet known because the extracellular fluid space is already expanded, a condition that one would think should decrease the production of aldosterone. The common denominator of all edematous states is increased aldosterone production with its associated effects.

In contrast to hypertensive states caused by possible primary aldosteronism, there appears to be no reason for measuring aldosterone levels in edematous states because secondary aldosteronism is almost invariably present. Also, in secondary aldosteronism there is usually no evidence of hypokalemic alkalosis, an almost universal finding in the primary variety. (See Chapter 4 for a discussion of primary aldosteronism.)

CLINICAL INVESTIGATION

The clinical history and physical examination of the edematous patient often point directly to the cause of edema, and only a minimal number of laboratory tests are necessary to confirm the clinical diagnosis. In some cases, such as in patients with prominent ascites, the diagnosis may be equivocal, the laboratory procedures also tend to be borderline or nondiagnostic. Sometimes the edema secondary to disease in one organ may interfere with the normal function of other important organs whose malfunction may also cause edema. A good example of this would be a patient with cardiac failure who consequently develops both hepatic and renal congestion that in turn leads to impaired hepatic and renal function and further edema. In this case both the clinical and, more importantly for this discussion, the laboratory findings would indicate impaired function of multiple organs.

The three most important causes of edema are cardiac failure, cirrhosis, and renal disease. These three causes should always be the primary consideration, and only after they have been satisfactorily ruled out, other less common causes may be considered. As one philosopher put it, "When you hear hoofbeats, think of horses, not zebras." More unusual causes of edema are particularly associated with ascites and include conditions such as intra-abdominal infection (e.g., acute peritonitis or tuberculous peritonitis), intra-abdominal neoplasia (e.g., ovarian or gastrointestinal), or parasitic infestation (e.g., schistosomiasis or echinococcosis). Diagnostic paracentesis, including appropriate bacteriologic and cytologic studies, will yield a positive diagnosis in cases of intra-abdominal infection or neoplasia. Portal vein obstruction (Budd–Chiari syndrome) requires sophisticated x-ray examination or exploratory laparotomy for a definitive diagnosis.

Localized edema is most often a result of lymphatic obstruction. This may be caused by various chronic inflammatory, parasitic, or neoplastic processes. Some congenital forms are also known. Diagnostic biopsy may be helpful but may also worsen the edematous condition by further compromising the lymphatic flow. Many chronic inflammatory reactions can lead to lymphatic destruction and edema secondary to the lymphatic blockage. Microbiological cultures may not be particularly helpful in these chronic cases.

The parasitic infection most commonly associated with localized edema is filariasis, particularly that caused by *Wuchereria bancrofti*. This is an important disease in the tropics, and patients who have traveled to those countries may be suspected of harboring this parasite. The blood smear, preferably taken at night, is examined for the diagnostic microfilaria.

Neoplastic lymphatic blockage, as well as blockage of lymphatics secondary to treatment for neoplasia by radical surgery or irradiation, or both, is a well-known cause of localized edema, especially of the extremities.

The congenital variety of localized (lower extremities) edema is called Milroy's disease and apparently results from a defective lymphatic network.

Focal edema often accompanies deep vein thromboses in the lower extremity. This disease is discussed in Chapter 15.

Laboratory Studies

Screening Procedures

Complete Blood Count. The complete blood count may show significant changes depending on the primary cause of edema. Often a moderate anemia is associated with cirrhosis and chronic renal disease but is usually not associated with cardiac failure. The anemia of cirrhosis is often macrocytic. Chronic renal disease is associated with hypochromic microcytic anemia and the red blood cells may show burring on the films. The association of mild neutropenia and thrombocytopenia with cirrhosis may also be helpful. Finding peppered platelets (increasingly prominent platelets) in the blood smear points to renal disease.

Urinalysis. A grossly abnormal urinalysis frequently points to the kidneys as the primary cause of edema. The urinalysis findings may be only minimally abnormal in cases of renal congestion caused by primary cardiac failure. Chapter 11 discusses the urinalysis in renal disease in more detail.

Serum Proteins. Hepatic parenchymal disease is associated with significant decreases in the serum albumin concentration. Cardiac or renal disease affects serum proteins to a lesser degree.

Definitive Procedures

Results of the following laboratory procedures will be helpful in differentiating edema caused by hepatic disease, especially cirrhosis, cardiac failure, and renal failure. As indicated, cardiac edema is usually accompanied by few, and essentially nondiagnostic, laboratory abnormalities. The silent myocardial infarction is the exceptional case. The patient's age, clinical evidence of cardiac disease (such as atrial fibrillation or cardiac enlargement), and the absence of evidence of hepatic or renal failure may point to the diagnosis. A therapeutic trial of digitalis may provide the best evidence for the diagnosis.

Urea Nitrogen and Creatinine. If grossly elevated, these analyses indicate that renal function is impaired. Mild elevations of these substances may be noted in cardiac failure with concurrent renal congestion. If the urea nitrogen level is decreased, hepatic failure is a likely cause, as urea synthesis is a normal function of the liver. (Chapter 11 contains additional comments on these substances and their relation to renal function.)

Bilirubin. The total bilirubin concentration may be grossly elevated in edema resulting from hepatic disease but only mildly elevated (1 to 5 mg/dl) in cardiac edema, and usually normal in renal failure.

Transaminase. The transaminase levels (AST and ALT) may be of considerable diagnostic help. The levels of both enzymes may be moderately elevated (e.g., 50 to 300 IU/L) in cirrhosis. In cardiac failure with hepatic congestion there may be similar elevations. If, however, only the AST is elevated (e.g., 50 to 150 IU/L) the patient may have suffered a silent myocardial infarction that has led to myocardial failure and edema. In this case other enzymes, e.g., CK, or an electrocardiogram may help diagnose the cause of the edema (see Chap. 3).

Alkaline Phosphatase. Another enzyme assay that may be of considerable help is the alkaline phosphatase assay. If elevated it usually points to hepatic edema, and if normal, cardiac or renal failure is a more probable cause.

SUGGESTED READINGS

Brenner B, Stein J: (eds): Sodium and Water Homeostasis. New York, Churchill Livingstone, 1978.

Guyton A: Edema. In Guyton A (ed): Textbook of Medical Physiology, 6th ed. Philadelphia, Saunders, 1981.

Levy M, Seely JF: Pathophysiology of edema formation. In Brenner BM, Rector FC (eds): The Kidney, 2nd ed. Philadelphia, Saunders, 1981.

7
COUGH AND DYSPNEA

BASIC INFORMATION

General Comments

Diseases of the respiratory system can be divided into infectious and noninfectious types. Although this seems quite straightforward, the clinical cases are frequently more involved. For example, a patient with cancer of the lung (a noninfectious disease) often presents with pneumonia superimposed on the poorly aerated lung distal to the tumor.

This chapter discusses the diseases of the respiratory system that are manifested primarily by cough or dyspnea, or both. Although pain may sometimes be associated with several of these entities, this symptom is usually relatively minor (see Chap. 3). A division between diseases associated with cough and those associated with dyspnea may be helpful in correlating the clinical laboratory manifestations of chest disease. But frequently both cough and dyspnea occur in a patient, and the clinician must be alert to this possibility.

The various laboratory procedures discussed in this chapter add specific and useful information that is directly applicable to the care of the patient. For example, the determination of the antibiotic susceptibility of the organism causing the patient's acute pneumonia is important in the patient's treatment. Cooperation among the clinician, radiologist, and clinical pathologist will result in maximal patient benefit. Each physician can contribute important information that will aid in both diagnosis and treatment.

Blood Gases

The primary function of the lungs is the exchange of gases; oxygen moves from the inspired air to the capillary blood, and carbon dioxide moves from the capillary blood into the alveolar air. Both oxygen and carbon dioxide move between air and blood by simple diffusion, from areas of higher to areas of lower partial pressures (Table 7–1).

The exchange of gases is accomplished in the alveoli, 300 million tiny air pockets whose walls are lined with delicate capillaries. Air flows into these alveoli by the process known as ventilation. The interface between the alveolar air and the pulmonary capillaries is normally thin and delicate, allowing for rapid diffusion of gases. If, for any reason (infection, edema, or fibrosis), this surface is thickened, gaseous diffusion will be impaired. The patient will become hypoxic (low oxygen concentration) and hypercarbic (high carbon dioxide concentration).

There are other reasons for hypoxemia. For example, hypoventilation will lead to hypoxemia. Likewise, the shunting of blood from the right to the left heart with some blood bypassing the pulmonary circulation will lead to hypoxemia.

Another cause of hypoxemia, ventilation–perfusion inequality, is felt to be the most common but also the most difficult to understand. In this condition significant mismatches of ventilation and blood exist in various regions of the lung. A final cause of hypoxemia is decreased cardiac output. However, it is seldom the sole cause of hypoxemia.

Although the differentiation of these conditions can best be done in the pulmonary function laboratory, initial informa-

TABLE 7–1. OXYGEN, CARBON DIOXIDE, AND pH VALUES IN AIR AND BLOOD

	Room Air	Alveolar Air	Mixed Venous Blood (Pulmonary Artery)	Pulmonary Capillary	Systemic Artery
P_{CO_2}	0 mm Hg	41 mm Hg	45 mm Hg	41 mm Hg	41 mm Hg
P_{O_2}	150 mm Hg	103 mm Hg	40 mm Hg	98 mm Hg	93 mm Hg
pH	—	—	7.38	7.40	7.40
Oxygen saturation	—	—	70%	98%	96%

tion that may help to sort out these conditions is available from the clinical laboratory. Recognition of hypoventilation is based on two blood gas determinations: an elevated $PaCO_2$ in a normal alveolar–arterial oxygen gradient (PAO_2–PaO_2). Alveolar oxygen tension is calculated as follows:

$$PAO_2 = (\text{Barometric pressure} - 47)\ FIO_2 - 1.2\ (PaCO_2)$$

where FIO_2 is the fraction of inspired oxygen. The normal alveolar–arterial oxygen gradient (PAO_2–PaO_2) is 3 to 10 mm Hg; by age 65 the gradient has increased to 25 mm Hg.

Ventilation–perfusion inequalities are identified by noting that, although the alveolar–arterial oxygen gradient widens, the PaO_2 is corrected with supplemental oxygen. In a patient with a shunt (i.e., blood bypasses ventilated areas of the lung), on the other hand, the decreased PaO_2 is not corrected when given supplemental oxygen.

In diffusion impairment, oxygen has difficulty diffusing through the alveolar–capillary membrane. The dysfunction is usually identified by calculating the CO_2 diffusing capacity.

It can be seen that the evaluation of pulmonary function is at times quite straightforward and at other times quite confusing, especially if several different processes are occurring simultaneously. Nevertheless, the arterial blood gases do give an accurate picture of the patient's condition even though it may be difficult or even impossible to pinpoint the cause.

CLINICAL INVESTIGATION

Clinical Features

Cough is usually caused by irritation and inflammation of the respiratory mucous membranes; if infection is present, the cough may be associated with variable amounts of sputum produced by the accompanying inflammatory reaction. Thus, cough and sputum production are regarded as manifestations of pulmonary infection.

Dyspnea, on the other hand, is often caused by a decreased or impaired oxygenation of arterial blood as it flows through the pulmonary vasculature. Implicit in this situation is some impairment of gaseous exchange between the alveolus and the pulmonary capillary bed.

Infections of the respiratory tract are of two types: upper respiratory tract infections and lower respiratory tract infections of the lungs and bronchial tree.

The signs and symptoms of upper respiratory tract infections (common cold) are well known and need only be mentioned: coryza, sneezing, headache, sore throat, nasal drainage, pharyngitis, fever, and possibly cervical lymphadenopathy with a purulent tonsillar exudate.

The majority of diagnosed upper respiratory infections are due to the common cold (caused by innumerable cold viruses) or streptococcal pharyngitis. Allergic disease (caused by a wide variety of allergens in susceptible individuals) may mimic an upper respiratory tract infection. Many other diseases (e.g., measles, infectious mononucleosis, whooping cough) may initially present as a common cold only to evolve into the more generalized disease.

Cough, sputum production, fever, and other systemic manifestations indicate significant involvement of the lower respiratory tract, most commonly caused by bacterial infection. This infection may be either primary or secondary to other problems such as pulmonary neoplasia or emboli.

Laboratory Studies

Upper Respiratory Infections

Clinical laboratory studies are usually not necessary in most cases of upper respiratory tract infections clinically presenting as a common cold. If there is a question of the differentiation of common cold symptoms from possible streptococcal pharyngitis or early manifestations of infectious mononucleosis, several laboratory studies may be helpful. The identification of streptococcal infections is especially important because of the potential complications of this disease.

Methods for Identifying Infections

Throat Culture. Throat cultures done on blood agar plates identify infections caused by group A streptococci. Special media for the isolation of *Mycoplasma pneumoniae* or other agents associated with acute pharyngitis are not yet generally available but will undoubtedly become more commonly used in the future.

Anti-Streptolysin O Titer. A rising ASO titer serves to identify a streptococcal infection positively, but only after the infection has subsided. (See Chapter 20 for a complete discussion of the serologic tests that are helpful in diagnosing a streptococcal infection.)

White Blood Cell Count. Only minimal changes are noted in the total or differential white blood cell count in the uncomplicated common cold. With secondary bronchitis or other complicating infections, a mild elevation of the white blood cell count with a left shift in the differential count may be present.

In allergic reactions, a mild to moderate eosinophilia may be found, although it may be masked by the neutrophilia of any complicating infection. At times, smears of nasal mucus stained with Wright's stain may reveal a large proportion of eosinophilic granulocytes, pointing to allergy as the cause of the patient's problem.

Careful examination of well-prepared peripheral blood smears may reveal the abnormal lymphocytes seen in certain diseases initially manifested by upper respiratory tract involvement. These include the variant (atypical) lymphocytes of infectious mononucleosis and the giant lymphocytes of whooping cough. The characteristic white blood cell count changes in infectious mononucleosis are a relative (>50 percent) or absolute (>4.5 × 10^9/L) lymphocytosis. In addition, variant (atypical) or reactive lymphocytes (>10 percent) are found on the differential blood smear.

Infectious Mononucleosis Tests. The standard heterophil antibody test (Paul–Bunnell) has been almost completely replaced by the more convenient slide or spot tests. These tests, the precision of which is much improved, have been found to be entirely satisfactory for detecting heterophil antibodies.

Epstein-Barr Virus (EBV) Antibody Titers. About 95 percent of infectious mononucleosis cases are caused by EBV, with cytomegalovirus (CMV) accounting for the remainder. This test is not ordinarily available, but EBV antibody titers may be useful in the study of the occasional atypical case.

Productive Cough

Methods for Identifying Infections with Productive Cough

Chest X-ray. X-rays of the chest by routine and specialized techniques (e.g., bronchograms in bronchiectasis) are the primary method for differentiating the wide variety of infectious and noninfectious causes of cough and dyspnea.

Leukocyte Count. There is usually an elevation of the total white blood cell count with a neutrophilia and left shift in most lower

TABLE 7–2. ETIOLOGY OF PURULENT PNEUMONIA

Etiologic Agent	Gross Characteristics
Staphylococcus	Grossly purulent, yellow, thick
Pneumococcus	Grossly purulent, may be tinged with blood
Escherichia coli	Purulent, foul smelling
Proteus	Foul smelling
Klebsiella–Aerobacter	Stringy or mucoid, purulent
Pseudomonas	Greenish
Myobacterium tuberculosis	Caseous
Pneumocystis carinii	No unusual features

respiratory tract infections. These changes may be less prominent in infants and the elderly. They are also less marked when the infection is confined to the bronchial tree (e.g., bronchitis, bronchiectasis) or when it is caused by viruses. With bacterial infection of the pulmonary parenchyma, neutrophilia is usually prominent.

Sputum Examination. One major difficulty in the laboratory examination of respiratory infections is the collection of a specimen of actual sputum. All too often, for a variety of reasons, merely saliva is sent to the laboratory for examination. Obviously, this is unsatisfactory. Good and poor sputa should be rated on the basis of the numbers of leukocytes and epithelial cells found upon microscopic examination of a Gram- or methylene blue-stained smear. Generally, specimens containing mucus, few (less than 25) squamous epithelial cells, and many (at least 10) leukocytes per low power field are adequate sputum specimens. Gross and microscopic examination of sputum may be helpful in determining the cause of pulmonary infection. Tables 7–2 and 7–3 characterize the sputa of certain infections. If the microscopic examination is positive, an imme-

TABLE 7–3. MICROSCOPIC EXAMINATION OF SPUTUM

Etiologic Agent	Microscopic Examination
Staphylococcus	Gram-positive cocci in small clumps
Streptococcus pneumoniae	Gram-positive cocci in pairs
Streptococcus	Gram-positive cocci in chains
Coliforms var.	Gram-negative bacilli
Candida	Gram-positive budding yeast and hyphae

diate (albeit tentative) diagnosis can be made and appropriate antibiotic therapy begun.

Often, the gross and microscopic examination of the sputum specimens may be inconclusive, and it is then necessary to examine the cultures. Sputum specimens are ordinarily plated on several media to culture most of the common bacterial pathogens. These media usually include blood agar (for gram-positive bacteria and fungi), enteric agar (e.g., eosin methylene blue for gram-negative organisms), and chocolate agar (for *Haemophilus influenzae*). If unusual organisms are suspected, the appropriate culture techniques should be specifically requested of the laboratory. Examples of such organisms include *Mycobacterium tuberculosis*, all varieties of fungi, and the pleuropneumonia-like organisms (PPLO).

Recently, the addition of a colony count to the sputum culture procedure has been advocated. In this procedure a semiquantitative estimation of the numbers of bacteria present is made. The rationale is entirely similar to that of urine colony count (qv). One obvious difficulty is obtaining true sputum, undiluted with saliva. Another is obtaining a fairly homogeneous mixture of sputum. This technique requires further evaluation before it can be advocated for routine use.

Antibiotic Susceptibility Testing. There are several methods of antibiotic sensitivity testing. The mixed flora of the sputum culture may be plated and sensitivity discs applied immediately. The advantage of this technique is speed. The results are usually available within less than 18 hours. This method, however, is not recommended by most authorities. If, on the other

TABLE 7–4. ROUTINE SPUTUM ANTIBIOTIC SUSCEPTIBILITY TESTING

	Organisms			
	Enterics (coliforms)	*Pseudomonas*	*Staphylococci*	*Streptococci*
Antibiotics Routinely Tested	Amikacin	Amikacin	Cephalothin	Ampicillin
	Ampicillin	Carbenicillin	Clindamycin	Penicillin
	Cefazolin	Cefotaxime	Erythromycin	Vancomycin
	Chloramphenicol	Ceftazidine	Methicillin	
	Gentamicin	Gentamicin	Penicillin	
	Tetracycline	Tobramycin	Tetracycline	
	Tobramycin		Vancomycin	

hand, the individual organisms are first identified and then antibiotic susceptibilities are determined, an additional day or more is required before the clinician obtains the information desired. Close liaison with the diagnostic microbiology laboratory results in a mutually advantageous system of identification combined with a maximum of clinical usefulness.

Table 7–4 lists antibiotics that are useful against respiratory infections. The list will, of course, be modified to include newer antibiotics or to compensate for unusual varieties of respiratory infections in certain clinical settings.

If staphylococci are cultured, methicillin and vancomycin may be included. If *Pseudomonas* are cultured, carbenicillin should be included in the antibiotic susceptibility testing.

Suspected Pulmonary Embolism and Infarction

Pulmonary embolization and infarction may occur in a wide variety of conditions (thrombophlebitis, pelvic thrombosis, fat embolism) and give rise to nonspecific signs and symptoms such as dyspnea, cough, blood-tinged sputum, chest pain, and hypotension. In addition, secondary pneumonia may become evident. Laboratory tests in pulmonary embolism are not helpful. Pulmonary angiography or radioisotope scanning techniques are required for definitive diagnosis.

Dyspnea

The complete laboratory study of the dyspneic patient is usually done in a specialized pulmonary function laboratory.

Spirometry (Forced Expiration Studies).

A useful yet simple test of pulmonary function is the analysis of the single forced expiration. Obstructive diseases (e.g., bronchial asthma) can be easily distinguished from restrictive pulmonary problems (e.g., pulmonary fibrosis). Mixed patterns may also be seen. A pulmonary physiology text should be consulted for a complete discussion of pulmonary function tests.

Blood Gases.

Blood gas analyses are now commonly performed in the laboratory. These studies (blood carbon dioxide and oxygen concentrations), combined with blood pH measurements, are adequate in the initial evaluation of the dyspneic patient (Table 7–5). See Chapter 12 for a more complete discussion of blood gases.

None of these measurements can absolutely differentiate between the many causes of dyspnea such as asthma, pulmonary edema, and pulmonary fibrosis. It is here that the sophis-

TABLE 7–5. ARTERIAL BLOOD GAS PATTERNS IN SPECIFIC DISEASES

Disease	P_{O_2}	P_{CO_2}	pH
Normal	90–100 mm Hg	35–45 mm Hg	7.38–7.44
Chronic obstructive pulmonary disease (COPD)			
Type A (emphysematous, "pink puffer")	↓	N	N
Type B (bronchial, "blue bloater")	↓ ↓	↑	N or ↓
Asthma			
Between attacks	N	N	N
Moderate attack	↓	↓ or N	↑ or N
Severe attack	↓ ↓	↑	↓
Adult respiratory distress syndrome (ARDS)			
Early	↓	N or ↓	N or ↑
Advanced	↓ ↓	↑	↓
Pulmonary edema			
Early	↓	N or ↓	N or ↑
Advanced	↓ ↓	↑	↓
Pulmonary embolism	↓	↓ or N	↑ or N
Pulmonary fibrosis	N or ↓	N or ↓	N
Cystic fibrosis			
Early	↓	N or ↓	N or ↑
Late	↓ ↓	↑	N or ↓

N, normal; ↓, decreased; ↑, increased.

ticated pulmonary function studies offer information that, in conjunction with the history and physical examination, is helpful in sorting out these conditions.

Red Blood Cell Measurements. Lowered blood oxygen levels stimulate erythropoiesis; therefore, all red blood cell parameters, such as the hemoglobin, hematocrit, and red blood cell count, may be increased in chronic hypoxemia.

Cystic Fibrosis

Clinical Features. Cystic fibrosis is the most common lethal autosomal recessive inherited disorder in whites, with an estimated gene frequency of 1 in 2000 live births. The prognosis for these patients is poor, with a median survival age of 21 years. Cystic fibrosis is characterized by viscous secretions ob-

TABLE 7-6. SWEAT ELECTROLYTE CONCENTRATIONS (mmol/L) IN CYSTIC FIBROSIS PATIENTS AND NORMAL CONTROLS

	Sodium		Chloride		Potassium	
	Mean	*Range*	*Mean*	*Range*	*Mean*	*Range*
Normal controls	28	16–46	28	8–43	10	6–17
Cystic fibrosis patients	111	75–145	115	79–148	23	14–30

structing the exocrine glands. The organs most affected are the lungs, pancreas, small intestine, sweat glands, liver, and reproductive system. The organ dysfunctions can lead to chronic pulmonary disease (e.g., recurrent bronchopneumonia), pancreatic insufficiency, abnormal sweat electrolytes, biliary cirrhosis, and decreased fertility. The metabolic defect is unknown. There is no cure for cystic fibrosis, nor is there a suitable screening technique currently available.

Diagnosis of cystic fibrosis is based on a positive sweat test (discussed in the next section) and one or more of the following: chronic pulmonary disease, pancreatic insufficiency, or a family history of cystic fibrosis.

Laboratory Studies

Sweat Test. Sweat testing is fraught with problems. In 1975 it was estimated that 10 to 13 percent of all sweat tests performed were in error. The errors were attributed to unreliable methods, evaporation and contamination of the sample, and poorly trained laboratory personnel. The Gibson Cook quantitative pilocarpine iontophoresis test is the standard assay currently used at cystic fibrosis centers and is the method recommended by the Cystic Fibrosis Foundation. Generally the test should be run in duplicate or repeated before a diagnosis is made. This method uses pilocarpine to stimulate sweat production. Patients with cystic fibrosis have elevated sweat sodium, chloride, and potassium concentrations (Table 7–6). Sweat potassium is not diagnostically valuable. Sweat chloride concentration provides the greatest discrimination in the diagnosis of cystic fibrosis. In the pediatric population sweat chloride concentrations above 60 mmol/L are considered positive for cystic fibrosis. Sweat chloride concentrations between 40 and 60 mmol/L are considered borderline and require further investigation. As a person matures, sweat electrolytes normally increase in concentration, therefore, up to 80 mmol/L of chloride may be normal for an adult. Sodium values in normal patients and patients with cystic fibrosis can overlap, therefore sweat sodium levels are less reliable than chloride levels. However, a sweat sodium value above 70 mmol/L is considered abnormal.

Neonatal Screening Tests. Serum trypsin is an enzyme that is produced in the pancreas. Serum immunoreactive trypsin is elevated early in the course of cystic fibrosis because of mechanical obstruction of the pancreatic ducts by mucus, but eventually decreases below normal levels as the pancreatic cells are destroyed. This leads to an overlap with healthy persons in the transition stage between elevated values and decreased values, therefore only unequivocally high or low values are significant. Also, 10 to 20 percent of infants with cystic fibrosis will not have pancreatic involvement and therefore will be missed. Currently there is controversy concerning mass screening for cystic fibrosis. Some of the critical issues include the validity and reliability of the serum immunoreactive trypsin assay, the benefits of screening, the technical and counseling follow-up services available, and the advantages of early diagnosis on prognosis.

Focal Pulmonary Lesions

Pulmonary cancer may have a wide variety of clinical manifestations; at times there may be a complete absence of any signs or symptoms, and the lesion will be discovered by chest x-ray. Therefore, the clinician must be especially alert to this possibility and always include it in the differential diagnosis.

The disease may be present initially as an acute pneumonitis, which may persist with a nonproductive cough. Secondary infection frequently occurs, and sputum production or hemoptysis may be evident. As the disease progresses, persistent chest pain, weight loss, and other evidence of advancing disease are noted.

Chest X-ray and Related Studies. At any stage a chest x-ray may be done, and a focal or coin lesion may be found. In later stages focal pneumonia, lobar collapse, or hilar masses signal more advanced disease.

Several other procedures may be appropriate in the study of suspected pulmonary carcinoma. For example, a variety of roentgenologic techniques (such as tomograms or CT scans) are used in the study of suspected pulmonary carcinoma as well as bronchoscopy and percutaneous needle biopsy.

Pulmonary Cytology. The laboratory investigation centers around pulmonary cytologic examination. Sputum (appropriately collected, promptly fixed and prepared, and expertly examined) yields diagnostic information in a large number of cases, particularly centrally located tumors. A series of sputum examinations rather than a single specimen significantly improves the diagnostic yield.

If pleural fluid accumulates, this material should be aspirated and examined using the Papanicolaou technique or a Cytospin preparation. Here, as with sputum, the differentiation of a malignant cell from irritated bronchial epithelial or mesothelial cells is difficult and only a person experienced in such studies should make the final diagnosis.

Bronchial aspiration or biopsy done during fiber–optic bronchoscopy may be necessary before a positive diagnosis of pulmonary neoplasia can be made.

SUGGESTED READINGS

Boener D: The value of the sputum Gram stain in community acquired pneumonia. JAMA 247:642, 1982.

Cugell DW, Buckingham WB, Webster JR Jr, Kettel LJ: The limitations of laboratory methods in the diagnosis of pulmonary embolism. Med Clin N Am 51:175, 1967.

Davidson M, et al.: Bacteriologic diagnosis of acute pneumonia: Comparison of sputum, transtracheal aspirates, and lung aspirates. JAMA 235:158, 1976.

DesJardins T: Clinical Manifestations of Respiratory Disease. Chicago, Year Book Medical, 1984.

Gerding D: Etiologic diagnosis of acute pneumonia in adults. Postgrad Med 69:136, 1981.

Hammond K, Johnson B: The sweat test for cystic fibrosis: Improving its reliability. Lab Med 12:56, 1981.

Komaroff AL: A management strategy for sore throat. JAMA 239:1429, 1978.

LeGrys V: The Laboratory Diagnosis of Selected Inborn Errors of Metabolism. New York, Praeger, 1984, pp 65–76.

Murray PR, Washington JA: Microscopic and bacteriologic analysis of exporated sputum. Mayo Clin Proc 50:339, 1975.

Polachek AA, Zoneraich S, Zoneraich O, Sass M: Pulmonary infarction and serum lactic dehydrogenase. JAMA 204:811, 1968.

Rosenow E, et al.: Pulmonary embolism. Mayo Clin Proc 56:161, 1981.

Saccomanno G: Sputum cytology: Collection, fixation, and concentration of sputum, bronchial aspirates and bronchial brushings. Lab Med 10:523, 1979.

Sivak E: Blood-gas measurements in respiratory failure. Diag Med Oct:3l, 1983.

Tecson F, Louria D: Infectious pneumonias: A review. J Fam Pract 4:201, 1977.

Tuller MA: Acid-base Homestasis and its Disorders. Flushing, NY, Medical Examination, 1971.

THE ACUTE SURGICAL ABDOMEN

BASIC INFORMATION

Gastric Analysis

Gastric juice is the product of several different gastric mucosal cells, the secretion of which are governed by several interrelated stimuli but chiefly by the vagal (or neurogenic) and the intrinsic hormonal mechanisms, i.e., gastrin. The most easily measured product of the secretory cells is hydrochloric acid. It is also the most useful clinical measurement and closely parallels gastrin pepsin production; therefore, the measurement of pepsin or pepsinogen in gastric juice, plasma, or urine is rarely indicated.

Hydrochloric acid was formerly measured as free acid and total acid. Both measurements were arbitrary and nonphysiologic, because free acid is an acid content below pH 3.5 and total acid includes titration not to neutrality but to pH 8, as phenolphthalein is used as the acid-base indicator. The quantitation of total acid production per unit time has, on the other hand, been shown to be a clinically valuable measurement under basal conditions as well as after histamine stimulation. Therefore, multiple samples are now analyzed to acquire these data.

A variety of agents have been used to produce maximal acid output (MAO) by the stomach. Histamine was the first standard stimulant to be used. However, it required simultaneous administration of an antihistaminic agent to inhibit untoward systemic side effects. The drug betazole produces maximal histaminelike stimulation without prior antihistamine preparation, but maximal stimulation is somewhat delayed. Pentagastrin is currently the preferred stimulus for maximal acid secretion. It contains the C-terminal tetrapeptide of gastrin linked to a substituted alanine and acts as a physiologic gastric acid secretagogue.

Test for Gastric Secretion

The patient is instructed to take no food or fluid after the evening meal of the day preceding the test. The following morning a gastric tube is passed, and all the gastric contents are withdrawn. The tube is left in place. Fluoroscopic control may be indicated, as blind placement frequently fails to position the tube in the gastric antrum. If hydrochloric acid is found in the initial specimen, as shown by using a drop of Töpfer's reagent (it changes to red below pH 3.5), the procedure can be discontinued if one is searching only for the presence of achlorhydria.

All the contents obtained, at 15-minute intervals, over a 1-hour period are withdrawn and placed in separate, properly labeled containers. Following the completion of the basal collections, pentagastrin is given (6 μg/kg of body weight). Four additional 15-minute specimens are collected, and each is placed into a clean, labeled container. Specimens of gastric juice are then submitted for analysis. The following determinations are usually performed on each sample of the fractional collection:

- Volume in milliliters
- pH, by using pH meter or narrow-range pH paper
- Acid concentration, expressed as millimols per liter, determined by titration to pH 7.0 with the use of phenol red as an indicator. The millimols per liter units are numerically equal to the formerly used degrees or clinical units. Table 8–1 helps in interpreting the laboratory data.

Tubeless Gastric Analysis

If one is interested in merely checking for the presence or absence of acid production, as for example, in pernicious anemia, the tubeless gastric analysis may be satisfactory. No gastric tube is inserted, and only two samples of urine are required, the analysis of which is considerably simpler than the multiple titrations necessary in the tube test.

Urine voided prior to the test is discarded. The patient takes two tablets of sodium benzoate with one glass of water. One hour later the patient urinates, and all the urine is placed in a container labeled control urine.

TABLE 8–1. GASTRIC ACID SECRETION*

Condition	Basal	Maximal
Normal	0–5	1–20
Gastric ulcer	0–5	1–20
Duodenal ulcer	>5	20–60
Achlorhydria	0	0
Zollinger-Ellison syndrome	>20	35–60

*Millimols of HCl per hour.

Granules of resin-coated azure A are placed into one-fourth glass of water and stirred well. The granules will not dissolve. The patient drinks this suspension. If any granules remain in the glass, the patient should drink them with a little more water. The granules should not be chewed.

Two hours after swallowing the granules, the patient again urinates and all of the urine is placed into another container marked test urine.

If hydrochloric acid is present in the stomach, the resin coating the dye is dissolved, and the azure A is absorbed and subsequently excreted in the urine. Normally greater than 0.6 mg is excreted within 2 hours. If no dye is found in the urine, achlorhydria is assumed to be present, if the test was done properly. It is usually wise to do this test with pentagastrin stimulation, as in the tube gastric analysis; a number of patients, especially in the older age group, may exhibit achlorhydria that will respond to histamine stimulation and therefore is not truly achlorhydria.

The patient may continue to pass blue or green urine for a few days, but this has no significance; it occurs because of colonic bacterial digestion of the resin granules.

Leukocyte Counts in Infection and Inflammation

The leukocyte count is an important laboratory indicator of infection. Included in this count is the total white blood cell count with a white cell differential count. In bacterial infections the total white count is characteristically elevated owing to a neutrophilic granulocytosis with a left shift of the neutrophils to more immature forms, i.e., bands or metamyelocytes.

There are several types of leukocytosis, the terms of which are sometimes used incorrectly. The most common abnormality of the white blood cell count is a relative as well as absolute granulocytosis. This reaction is characteristic of pyogenic infections including abscesses and massive tissue necrosis. The counts generally are between $15 \times 10^9/L$ and $30 \times 10^9/L$, with greater than 80 percent granulocytes. A left shift is usually evident; sometimes this change may be the only indicator of a problem. Finally, the presence of toxic granulation in the neutrophils and the formation of Doehle bodies is characteristic of more severe infections.

Other types of white blood cell changes are also found with different types of infection and may give valuable clues to the cause of the patient's complaints. Some characteristic white blood cell changes, as well as frequent causes, are catalogued in Tables 20–1 and 20–2.

Patients vary in their hematologic reactivity to infection or inflammation. For example, infection usually causes a greater degree of neutrophilic leukocytosis in children than in adults. Conversely, elderly patients may respond minimally or not at all to infection. Weakened and debilitated patients often fail to respond to infection with a leukocytosis.

In one study about 40 percent of infected patients had white blood cell counts of less than $11 \times 19^9/L$. Generally, however, the degree of neutrophilia parallels the amount of inflamed tissue because the factors promoting leukocytosis are thought to be derived from necrotic cells. Therefore, an abscess or localized inflammatory process may result in a more significant leukocytosis than a generalized process such as septicemia.

Bone marrow formation of granulocytes is divided between two compartments, namely, the production and the storage compartments. The production or dividing compartment is composed of myeloblasts, promyeloblasts, and myelocytes, whereas the storage compartment contains metamyelocytes and band and segmented neutrophils, which are available for release to the peripheral tissues if necessary. With an increased demand for granulocytes in the periphery, the storage pool of segmented neutrophils is depleted and the number and proportion of bands released from the marrow steadily increases. In severe, overwhelming infections, however, the marrow pool may be totally exhausted.

The response to inflammation with the rapid passage from the maturing or storage neutrophil pool to the peripheral circulation can be reflected in the differential white count. By applying specific and strict criteria for the differentiation of band and segmented neutrophils the laboratory can provide significant information to the clinician regarding infectious (and inflammatory) processes in patients. These criteria are given in Chapter 14.

CLINICAL INVESTIGATION

Basic Evaluation

The sudden occurence of severe abdominal pain is commonly called a surgical abdomen because most of the conditions and diseases causing severe and sudden abdominal pain are probable indications for surgical exploration and therapy. In contrast, the so-called medical diseases of the abdomen are characterized by chronicity; severe pain is infrequent, except in acute porphyria or lead colic, for example.

What approach does the astute physician or surgeon take in treating the patient with an acute abdomen? What are the major diagnostic features that help the physician come to a diagnosis? How can the laboratory help? The answers to some of questions are found in this chapter. The major criteria for diagnosis are based primarily on the physical examination. This examination is predicated on a history of the present illness, although a past medical history suggestive of chronic abdominal disease should not be ignored. In fact, the past history often provides significant clues to the present diagnosis.

After the history is taken, the next question to be answered is: What is the objective clinical or laboratory evidence of inflammation? On physical examination these signs include fever, tachycardia, deep abdominal tenderness, muscle guarding, and rebound tenderness. These signs may be absent in the early stages, therefore periodic reexaminations for these signs are important.

The laboratory examinations that may be of help in the initial evaluation include a white blood cell count with differential and possibly a sedimentation rate. These tests are nonspecific indicators of inflammatory reactions whenever they may occur.

If it is evident that there is an inflammatory reaction within the abdomen, the next step is to find evidence of localization within a particular organ system as well as the location within the abdomen. Again, the history of the present illness coupled with the physical examination are the best means of answering this question. Questions directed toward previous symptoms of peptic ulcer (e.g., epigastric discomfort relieved by food or antacids), biliary tract disease (e.g., dyspepsia, intolerance to fatty foods, or previous jaundice), and abnormalities of intestinal function or the urinary tract may again provide worthwhile clues.

When a tentative diagnosis or differential diagnosis is made, roentgenographic or laboratory procedures are used to provide valuable positive or negative evidence to corroborate the diagnosis or to eliminate other conditions that may simulate the disease. Because of the rapid progression of many of these diseases and the benefits of prompt surgical intervention, there is a need for the rapid performance and reporting of these ancillary studies. Fortunately, the number and complexity of helpful laboratory procedures are not great and thus pose no particular problem to the laboratory. Unfortunately, acute disease cannot be scheduled to occur during regular working hours. Around-the-clock laboratory coverage must be provided.

In the discussions that follow it is presumed that a tentative diagnosis has been made on clinical grounds and the attending physician is in a position to acquire confirmatory laboratory evidence. Only the most common x-ray examinations are mentioned and then only briefly. The reader is referred to other texts for more detailed discussion of such studies.

ACUTE APPENDICITIS AND DIVERTICULITIS

Clinical Features

Both diseases are characterized by mild to severe abdominal pain, which is accompanied by fever, nausea, vomiting, and, at times, constipation. The term left-sided appendicitis is often applied to diverticulitis, as the clinical features of both diseases are similar except for the right-sided localization of appendicitis versus left-sided localization with diverticulitis. Diverticulitis is by definition an inflammation within a diverticulum of the colon (which became more pronounced only with advancing years). This disease usually occurs in middle or older aged patients. Appendicitis, on the other hand, is more common in younger patients.

Laboratory Studies

Screening Procedures

Leukocyte Count. The elevation of the white blood cell count with a granulocytosis and left shift is almost always found in patients with acute appendicitis or diverticulitis. There are, of course, exceptions to this generalization, the most common occurring in patients who have been treated with antibiotics. In these cases both clinical and laboratory evidence of disease is partially suppressed. Elderly patients may fail to show significant leukocytosis even with bowel rupture and peritonitis.

Urinalysis. A urinalysis is useful in excluding genitourinary conditions that may mimic acute appendicitis or diverticulitis.

Definitive Procedures

There are no laboratory tests specific for acute inflammatory disease of the appendix or large bowel diverticula.

ACUTE CHOLECYSTITIS

Clinical Features

Although the stereotypic fair, fat, and 40-year-old woman has a higher probability of suffering from gallbladder disease, it should be remembered that this disorder can occur in any age group, including children, and should therefore be considered in any patient with acute abdominal disease.

These patients may give a history of recurrent episodes of right upper quadrant pain after heavy, fatty meals. The pain characteristically radiates into the region of the right scapula. Nausea and vomiting may accompany the pain. Abdominal muscular rigidity in the right upper quadrant is found on physical examination.

Jaundice may occur if the common bile duct is obstructed by a stone or edema of the wall of the bile duct. Usually the jaundice is mild and can be missed if not carefully sought (see also Chap. 9).

Laboratory Studies

Screening Procedures

Leukocyte Count. The nonspecific granulocytosis with left shift merely indicates the presence of an inflammatory reaction, site unspecified. A normal white blood cell count would militate against any acute reaction. But again, remember that elderly patients may not respond with a significant elevation of the white blood cell count. In these cases, however, a left shift almost invariably occurs, and therefore, a differential white blood cell count is indicated even in the absence of leukocytosis.

Transaminases. In acute cholecystitis slightly less than one-half of patients have mild elevations (40 to 80 IU/L) in serum transaminases, i.e., ALT, formerly SGPT, and AST, formerly SGOT. Elevations can also occur in other diseases such as myocardial infarction, hepatic congestion, hepatitis, or pancreatitis.

Alkaline Phosphatase. Alkaline phosphatase levels do not usually rise until the biliary tract obstruction is moderately advanced and therefore, is not of prime importance in the laboratory investigation of acute cholecystitis.

Bilirubin. The bilirubin level may be increased in slightly less than one-half of patients with acute cholecystitis.

Hemoglobin and Red Blood Cell Morphology. It is well known that hemolytic anemias are associated with an increased incidence of biliary calculi. These pigmented stones tend to be small and multiple and, therefore, are more prone to result in biliary colic than the larger cholesterol stones. Thus, the finding of anemia as well as evidence of abnormal erythrocytes associated with hemolytic disease (e.g., microspherocytes) may be a valuable clue.

Definitive Procedures

There are no laboratory tests specific for acute cholecystitis.

PEPTIC ULCER DISEASE

Clinical Features

The symptoms of peptic ulcer disease are well known. The epigastric pain may be dull or severe depending on the localization and extent of ulceration. It is aggravated by fasting and relieved by foods or antacids. Nausea and vomiting may occur. On physical examination there may be localized tenderness corresponding to the site of ulceration, but otherwise the physical examination may be quite unrewarding.

Because the disease is usually chronic, there may be progression to any of several well-known complications. The signs and symptoms of each are characteristic. These complications include gastrointestinal bleeding, penetration of the ulcer into surrounding structures such as the pancreas, perforation into the peritoneal space, and cicatrization with gastric obstruction. Although each of these complications has a characteristic clinical picture, it may be considerably modified in chronic disease.

Laboratory Studies

Screening Procedures

There are no laboratory examinations that serve as screening procedures for peptic ulcer disease. If any of the complications noted above occur, however, several laboratory procedures might be of some help.

Hemoglobin. The measurement of the hemoglobin or the hematocrit in the peptic ulcer patient who is bleeding will help monitor the extent and duration of hemorrhage. This may also be assessed clinically by noting the amount of bloody vomitus or melena. Stool examination for occult blood may be of some aid in the anemic patient with a mild or equivocal clinical history for peptic ulcer (see also Chap. 13).

Amylase. The ulcer may penetrate into the pancreas, the surrounding tissue, or may perforate. In these cases there may be an elevation of the serum amylase levels. These elevations are usually moderate (200 to 720 IU/L) and are related to the duration of perforation. An elevated amylase level does not necessarily indicate penetration into the pancreas itself but may denote focal peritonitis in the lesser omental sac and the peripancreatic tissues.

Definitive Procedures

Radiography and Endoscopy. The demonstration of an ulcer with a barium swallow or upper GI endoscopy are the definitive procedures for the diagnosis of peptic ulcer disease.

Gastric Analysis. Gastric analysis may be helpful although not diagnostic in peptic ulcer disease. A maximal acid output (MAO) greater than 40 mmol in 1 hour in a patient with dyspepsia is strongly suggestive of duodenal ulcer. The presence of hydrochloric acid in all samples of basal cell secretion indicates active duodenal ulcer, although, again, the finding cannot be considered diagnostic (Table 8–1).

The presence of large volumes of highly acidic gastric juice collected without pentagastrin stimulation is characteristic of Zollinger-Ellison syndrome, a major feature of which is severe peptic ulcer disease. A gastrin-secreting tumor of the pancreas causes this problem. The measurement of serum gastrin levels helps greatly in the diagnosis of this disorder.

ACUTE PANCREATITIS

Clinical Features

In an alcoholic patient, excruciating upper abdominal pain that radiates into the dorsolumbar region and is accompanied by nausea and vomiting is characteristic of acute hemorrhagic pancreatitis. The patient usually exhibits abdominal distention and decreased peristalsis as well as fever and tachycardia. The acute episode may progress to prostration, peripheral vascular collapse, and death. Often the patient continues to have recurrent acute episodes of the disease, which finally result in deficiencies of both exocrine and endocrine pancreatic function.

Because the disease may be adversely affected by surgical exploration, it is important to make a positive diagnosis. This disease mimics many other causes of acute abdominal symptoms that are aided by surgical treatment. The differentiation is greatly aided by fast and accurate serum amylase and lipase determinations.

Laboratory Studies

Screening Procedures

Leukocyte Count. Laboratory studies, such as the white blood cell count and the differential count, as well as the sedimentation rate will be nonspecific in the patient suffering from acute pancreatitis.

Serum Amylase. As soon as the diagnosis is suspected, the measurement of the serum amylase is mandatory. Serum amylase levels greater than 1000 IU/L are practically diagnostic of acute pancreatitis if opiate administration has been ruled out. In acute pancreatitis the serum amylase begins rising within about 8 hours, reaches a peak in 24 to 48 hours, and in uncomplicated cases, returns to normal in 3 to 5 days. Failure of the amylase to return to normal by 5 days or so should raise the possibility of some complication of pancreatitis, e.g., pseudocyst or pancreatic abscess.

Alpha-amylase is an enzyme that hydrolyzes polysaccharides such as glycogen and starch. It is found in large concentrations in the pancreas and the salivary gland. In addition to pancreatitis, other diseases can cause elevations of amylase. With the onset of mumps, serum amylase is usually elevated, but by the end of the second week the serum levels return to normal. Morphine and codeine, by closing the sphincter of Oddi, increase the intraductal pressure in the pancreas, and therefore can cause significant elevations of serum amylase. These increases in amylase are usually maximal 5 hours after administration of the drug and return to normal within 24 hours.

In any acute inflammation in the region of the pancreas, even if the pancreas is not primarily involved, increased levels of amylase may be noted, e.g., in lesions such as a peptic ulcer penetrating into the pancreas. Mild elevations of amylase levels can also be associated with biliary tract disease, alcoholism, mesenteric thrombosis, generalized peritonitis, renal insufficiency, and hepatitis.

Urine Amylase. Because the serum levels may return to normal within a few days, it is helpful to measure urinary amylase levels in patients seen several days after the onset of symptoms of pancreatitis. The amylase levels may remain elevated up to 7 to 10 days following the acute episode.

Serum Lipase. Other serum enzyme determinations, such as lipase, increase the accuracy of the laboratory diagnosis of acute pancreatitis. When both serum amylase and lipase are used in a suspected case of acute pancreatitis, the sensitivity has been reported as high as 90 to 97 percent. This test is probably indicated when the clinical diagnosis is strongly suspected but the amylase studies are only mildly abnormal.

Amylase Clearance. The ratio of amylase clearance to creatinine clearance has been proposed as an aid in the differentiation of acute pancreatitis from several clinically similar disorders. A random urine sample rather than a 24-hour collection is required. The calculation is as follows:

$$\frac{\text{Urine amylase}}{\text{Serum amylase}} \times \frac{\text{Serum creatinine}}{\text{Urine creatinine}} \times 100 = \frac{\text{Amylase}}{\text{clearance ratio}}$$

This ratio is normally less than 4 percent. In acute pancreatitis it is usually greater than 4 percent, and often in the range of 7 to 15 percent. In about one-third of patients with acute pancreatitis, however, the ratio is normal, and elevated ratios may be found in diagnoses other than acute pancreatitis. Table 8–2 lists the diagnostic efficiency of the various laboratory tests in acute pancreatitis.

Calcium. On occasion severe pancreatitis is associated with symptomatic hypocalcemia. The etiology is not well understood. To prepare for this complication, the measurement of a serum calcium level during the acute episode is helpful as a baseline measurement. If the serum calcium level falls below 8 mg/dl within the first 48 hours, the disease is considered severe.

TABLE 8–2. DIAGNOSTIC EFFICIENCY OF VARIOUS LABORATORY TESTS IN ACUTE PANCREATITIS

Test	Sensitivity (%)	Specificity (%)
Serum amylase	70–98	70–76
Urine amylase	80–98	80–90
Serum lipase	75–100	70–86
Amylase/creatinine clearance ratio	93–100	80–97
Amylase isoenzymes	100	92

From Van Lente F: Diagnosing acute pancreatitis the enzymatic way. Diag Med 5:53, 1982.

GYNECOLOGIC CAUSES OF ACUTE ABDOMINAL DISEASE

Clinical Features

Women in the childbearing years may present with an acute abdomen, and in these cases the clinician must take into consideration two additional disorders. First, there is the possibility of a pregnancy in which the fertilized egg is implanted in a location other than the uterus (ectopic pregnancy). The most common site is the fallopian tube. The abnormal progression of the pregnancy is easily understood, as is the almost certain possibility of hemorrhage into the fallopian tube and into the lower abdomen. The clinical features of lower abdominal pain and tenderness, possibly with vaginal bleeding or a palpable mass in an adnexal area of the uterus, accompanied by anemia, tachycardia, and possibly shock should alert the clinician to this condition. Investigation into the menstrual history as well as the examination for secondary signs of pregnancy may clinch the diagnosis.

The second consideration is pelvic inflammatory disease (PID), which is widely seen and usually diagnosed almost solely on clinical grounds. The initial episode is usually a gonococcal salpingitis. At this time, a positive diagnosis is sometimes possible (discussed in the next section). Later episodes are complicated by the development of adhesions and blockage and dilation of the fallopian tubes. Secondary invasion by several bacteria as well as gonococci leads to an indolent infection with pelvic exacerbations. Severe lower abdominal pain and tenderness, leukorrhea, and palpable masses in the adnexal areas indicate such complications.

An occasional female patient in this age group will have an acute, although short-lived, episode of lower abdominal pain that may mimic the early stages of either of the above entities. The cause is a small amount of bleeding that arises at the site of ovulation. The menstrual history will be most helpful. This condition, called mittelschmerz (German for middle pain), is self-limited.

Laboratory Studies

Screening Procedures

Pregnancy Test. The pregnancy test is a valuable aid in the assessment of patients with a possible ectopic pregnancy. The most sensitive hemagglutination inhibition tube tests may miss up to 50 percent of ectopic pregnancies. Therefore, the most sensitive pregnancy tests must be used, e.g., radioimmunoassay procedures. See Chapter 21 for a more complete discussion of these tests.

Complete Blood Count. The nonspecific tests for inflammation (leukocyte count, differential count) as well as the hemoglobin or hematocrit level will reflect the inflammatory and hemorrhagic components of this complication of pregnancy. PID is usually accompanied by significant leukocytosis and a left shift of the granulocytes.

Definitive Procedures

Bacterial Cultures. A culture of any cervical discharge in patients with suspected PID may reveal the presence of gonococcus, staphylococcus, streptococcus, or other etiologic bacteria including anaerobes. The percentage of definitive cultures is, however, quite low. As the problem must be handled quickly, the results of such cultures arrive too late to be of help in the initial management of these patients.

ACUTE URINARY TRACT INFLAMMATION INCLUDING URINARY CALCULI

Clinical Features

There are several important conditions occurring in the urinary tract that may mimic the acute surgical abdomen. These conditions include acute pyelonephritis, renal or ureteral calculi, and acute cystitis.

The patient with acute pyelonephritis usually presents with high fever, chills, lumbar pain, and urinary frequency and urgency. In addition, nausea, vomiting, and diarrhea may be present. This type of infection can mimic acute appendicitis, diverticulitis, or pancreatitis. The disease is more common in women or following urinary tract manipulations. Costovertebral angle tenderness and a tender palpable kidney help to make the diagnosis.

Acute cystitis presents a similar picture. The pain, however, is usually suprapubic rather than lumbar. Also, gastrointestinal manifestations are less prominent.

The passage of a renal calculus down the ureter is usually accompanied by severe colicky flank pain, which localizes to the periumbilical area as the stone progresses down the ureter. Urinary frequency and urgency as well as dysuria may be present.

Laboratory Studies

Screening Procedures

Urinalysis. The gross and microscopic examination of the urine provides a reliable and easy method for the investigation of acute disorders within the urinary tract.

In acute pyelonephritis many polymorphonuclear leukocytes as well as white blood cell casts are found in the urinary sediment. Significant numbers of bacteria are usually found in the Gram-stained sediment (more than five bacteria per oil immersion field). In acute cystitis the urinary findings are similar, although true white blood cell casts are not seen. See Chapter 11 for a more complete discussion of the urinalysis in renal disease.

The urine from patients passing a calculus will contain considerable numbers of erythrocytes because of the trauma to the ureter caused by the passing stone. White blood cells are variable depending on the duration and the course of the disease.

Definitive Procedures

Urine Colony Count. The measurement of the concentration of bacteria in the urine, or colony count, done on a freshly voided urine specimen is of great help in the evaluation of urinary tract infections. More than 100,000 organisms per cubic milliliter (or colony-forming units (CFUs)) is indicative of significant infection. Smaller numbers of bacteria ($<$50,000 per cubic milliliter) usually indicate contamination of the specimen during the collection rather than infection. If the specimen is collected using a catheter, greater than 10,000 CFUs indicates a significant infection. The exception to these criteria is in patients receiving antimicrobial treatment in which smaller numbers of bacteria may be found even in active, albeit treated, infections.

If significant numbers of organisms are found, identification and antimicrobial sensitivity testing should be done. The disc method of sensitivity testing is usually satisfactory, but minimal inhibitory concentration (MIC) determinations for antibiotic susceptibility studies are being done more frequently, especially in complicated cases.

Stone Analysis. In patients with renal calculi, it is important to retain for qualitative chemical analysis any calculi passed or surgically removed. All urine that is voided should be strained and any stones or suspicious material submitted to the laboratory for analysis. Although the majority of calculi are composed of a variety of calcium crystalloids that arise from nonspecific causes, an occasional patient will form calculi because of specific metabolic abnormalities, such as gout and cystinuria. If the diagnosis is previously known, there is no particular advantage in repeating the analysis. The laboratory personnel will appreciate analyzing all stones, however, to improve and maintain their techniques of stone analysis.

Tests in Patients with Renal Calculi. If the kidney stone is not analyzed, several analyses of urine or serum are indicated to check for metabolic causes of stone formation. These include: serum calcium in hyperparathyroidism; serum uric acid in gout; urine microscopy for cystine crystals or urine chromatography or electrophoresis to determine excessive cystine or other amino acid excretion in cystinuria.

In acute urinary tract disorders these definitive procedures are of little help for an immediate diagnosis. Because they are important in the future management of these patients, however, they probably should be measured at the time of the acute illness to acquire the maximal amount of diagnostic information.

PORPHYRIA

Clinical Features

The porphyrias are a group of diseases characterized by defects in heme biosynthesis resulting in an abnormal porphyrin metabolism and overproduction of heme precursors. Clinically, they may be characterized by a wide variety of acute symptoms, which mimic many of the acute disorders previously discussed in this chapter. The patient may present with symptoms of severe periumbilical abdominal pain, which may radiate into the back, thighs, or chest. There is accompanying nausea, vomiting, and constipation. The resemblance to acute appendicitis, pancreatitis, or peptic ulcer is at times striking. Recurrent episodes are a feature of the disorder, and pregnancy, infection, and use of barbiturates and certain other drugs may precipitate an acute episode.

The clinical features that help distinguish this disorder are the presence of neurologic disturbances such as foot drop, wrist drop, and hypesthesia. The abdominal examination is inconsistent with the clinical signs, as only minimal tenderness is found in a soft, mildly distended abdomen.

Although this disorder is uncommon, it should be included in the differential diagnosis of the acute abdomen, otherwise these patients may be operated on needlessly.

Laboratory Studies

Screening Procedures

Urinary Porphobilinogen. The Hoesch test for porphobilinogen is an excellent screening procedure for acute intermittent porphyria, although it may be negative in the other, even less common porphyrias. This test is usually positive even during remissions of the disease. False-negative results are rare in acute intermittent porphyria. False-positive results can be reduced to a miminum by the knowledge that the red color produced with the Ehrlich's aldehyde reagent is insoluble in chloroform or butanol.

Porphyrins. All porphyrins have a characteristic absorption spectrum related to the conjugated bond system of the tetrapyrrole ring. They all exhibit an absorption band near 400 nm, the Soret band. When irradiated with light of this wavelength, all free porphyrins exhibit an intense red fluorescence. This is the basis of screening tests for porphyrins in blood, urine, and feces. The general procedure involves extraction of the porphyrins into an organic solvent system followed by extraction into hydrochloric acid.

Definitive Procedures

Quantitation of Individual Porphyrins. The quantitation of the porphyrins or related compounds in urine may be desirable to establish more firmly the diagnosis of porphyria. The differentiation of the various forms of porphyria is made on clinical,

TABLE 8–3. PROPHYRIN STUDIES IN THE PORPHYRIAS

	Porphyrin				
Porphyria	δ-*Aminolevulinic Acid*	*Porphobilinogen*	*Uroporphyrin*	*Coproporhyrin*	*Erythrocyte Protoporphyrin*
Erythropoietic	N	N	↑	↑	↑
Hepatic					
Acute intermittent porphyria	↑	↑	↑	N	N
Hereditary coproporphyria	↑	↑	N	↑	N
Variegate porphyria	↑	↑	N or ↑	N or ↑	N
Porphyria cutanea tarda	N	N	↑	N or ↑	N
Protoporphyria	N	N	N	N or ↑	↑
Present reference interval (quality/24 hr)	1–7 mg	0–2 mg	5–20 μg	45–180 μg	15–50 μg/dL
SI reference interval (quantity/day)	8–53 μmol	0–8.8 μmol	6–24 nmol	68–276 nmol	0.28–0.90 μmol/L

genetic, and laboratory grounds. The laboratory diagnosis is shown in Table 8–3, which summarizes these differences.

OTHER UNCOMMON CAUSES OF ACUTE ABDOMEN

Clinical Features

Vascular Accidents

With increased numbers of geriatric patients, the syndrome of an acute abdominal crisis secondary to a vascular accident and accompanying bowel infarction is seen more frequently. The clinical features include those associated with bowel obstruction. Frequently the apparent good clinical condition of the elderly patient belies the severity of the episode.

Trauma and Other Mechanical Disturbances

Trauma to the abdomen may cause a variety of injuries to organs as well as blood vessels. Likewise, the various mechanical disturbances, such as volvulus, intussusception, or strangulated hernia, should always be included in the differential diagnosis of the acute abdomen.

Laboratory Studies

Blood counts and chemical determinations show only the nonspecific changes associated with acute inflammation or bowel obstruction. Therefore, they are not of great help in the differential diagnosis of these disorders.

If there is significant internal hemorrhage, the hemoglobin and hematocrit will reflect these changes.

SUGGESTED READINGS

Batsakis JG, Briere RG: Interpretive Enzymology. Springfield, Charles C. Thomas, 1967.

Eckfeldt J, et al.: Serum tests for pancreatitis in patients with abdominal pain. Arch Pathol Lab Med 109:316, 1985.

Goldberg A, Moore M (eds): The Porphyrias. Clinic Haematol. 9:2, 1980.

Lifton LJ, et al.: Pancreatitis and lipase. JAMA 229:47, 1974.

Mathy KA, Koepke JA: The clinical usefulness of segmented vs stab neutrophil criteria for differential leukocyte counts. Am J Clin Pathol 61:947, 1974.

Moossa A: Diagnostic tests and procedures in acute pancreatitis. N Engl J Med 311:639, 1984.

Salt W, Schenker S: Amylase—Its clinical significance: A review of the literature. Medicine 55:269, 1976.

Sell A, Isenberg J: Duodenal ulcer diseases. In Sleisenger W, Fortrans J (eds): Gastrointestinal Disease, 3rd ed. Philadelphia, Saunders, 1983, pp 625–674.

Sparberg M, Kirsner JB: Current episodes of gastric analysis. Am J Diag Dis 9:567, 1964.

Van Lente F: Diagnosing acute pancreatitis the enzymatic way. Diag Medicine 5:53, 1982.

With T: Diagnostic tools for porphyria. Lab Med 11:446, 1980.

9
JAUNDICE

BASIC INFORMATION

Bilirubin Metabolism

Bilirubin comes from the hemoglobin of disintegrating red blood cells that have been broken down in the reticuloendothelial cells. After its formation, bilirubin is tightly bound to plasma albumin, forming a lipid-soluble conjugate. This moiety is measured as the unconjugated (indirect) bilirubin in the clinical laboratory. Bilirubin is transported by the blood (bound to albumin) to the liver. Transport of bilirubin into the hepatocyte involves dissociation of bilirubin from albumin. In the liver the hepatocyte bilirubin is conjugated with glucuronide, forming a water-soluble conjugate, which is excreted into the biliary passages. Excreted bilirubin, regurgitated or forced back into the bloodstream in cases of biliary obstruction, results in an elevated serum bilirubin of the conjugated (direct) type. Conjugated bilirubin, or bile, entering the gastrointestinal tract by way of the common bile duct is acted on by anaerobic bacteria to form several substances, collectively known as urobilinogens. These substances are excreted in the feces as such or as the oxidation product urobilin. A portion of the pigments, however, is reabsorbed and carried back to the liver by way of the portal circulation. In the liver a portion of the urobilinogen is reconverted to bilirubin. Also a small amount escapes into the general circulation and is excreted by the kidney. Small amounts of urobilinogen are normally found in the urine, and these traces are rapidly oxidized into urobilin when voided specimens are allowed to stand (Fig. 9–1).

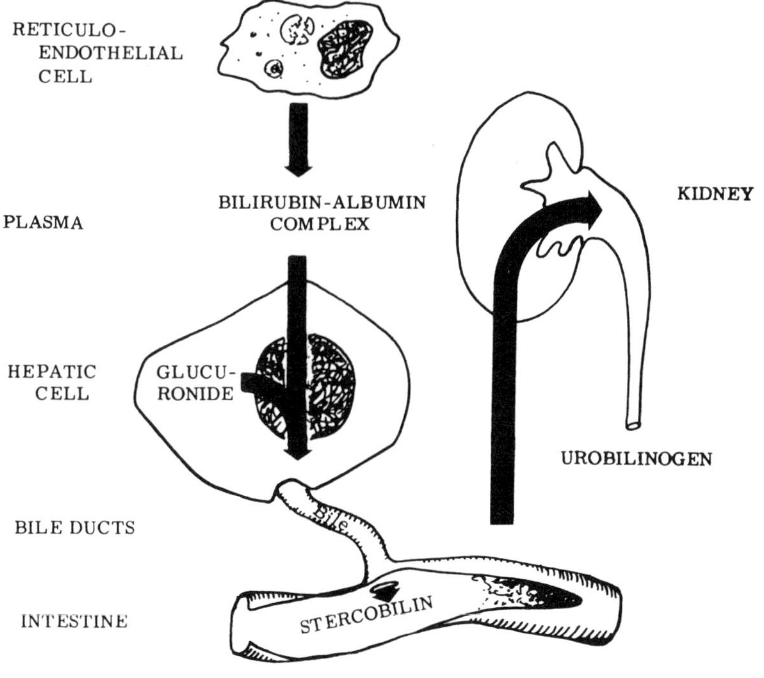

Figure 9–1. Normal bilirubin pathways. In this and the following figures the arrows indicate major pathways of hemoglobin catabolism. See the text for a more complete discussion.

Classification of Jaundice

Although classifications of jaundice are numerous, most include only three major categories. These three types (prehepatic, hepatic, and posthepatic) are named for the anatomic site at which there is a derangement of normal bilirubin metabolism. Sometimes more than one site may be the focus of disease, and a more complex clinical and laboratory pattern emerges. An example would be the patient with spherocytic anemia and complicating biliary calculi.

Prehepatic Jaundice—Hemolytic Jaundice

In uncomplicated prehepatic jaundice there is no intrinsic disease in the liver or biliary tract. It is only an increased amount of bilirubin presented to the liver for excretion. As indicated in Figure 9–2, the normal pathways of bilirubin metabolism are crowded with excessive quantities of bilirubin or related com-

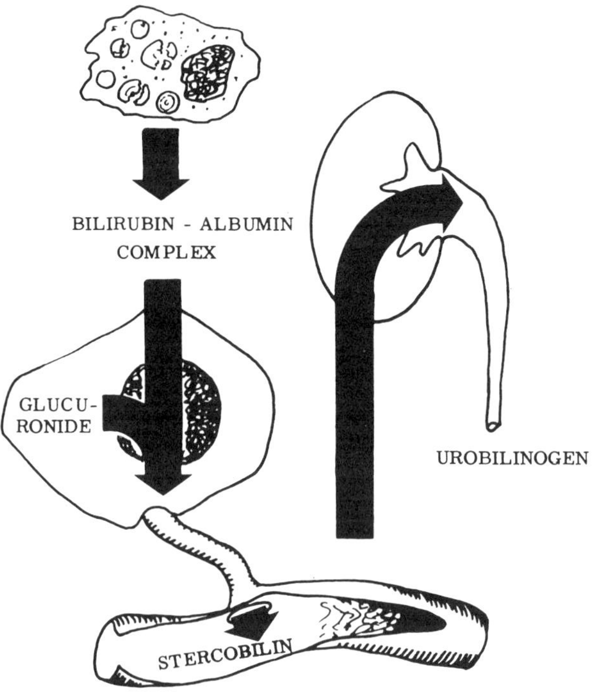

Figure 9–2. Hemolytic jaundice. Although the normal pathways remain intact, the concentration of hemoglobin breakdown products is markedly increased in all compartments.

pounds. Because there is no blockage of the biliary tract, no excess bilirubin glucuronide is forced back into the bloodstream, and no significant increase in serum conjugated bilirubin is found. On the other hand, increased amounts of urobilinogen (more correctly but less commonly called stercobilinogen) are found in the intestinal tract, which are absorbed and subsequently excreted by the kidneys.

Hepatic Jaundice—Hepatoceliular Jaundice

This type of jaundice is secondary to intrinsic hepatic parenchymal injury or disease. The hepatic cellular dysfunction may result from infections with hepatitis virus or bacteria, anoxia, certain drugs, neoplasia, and injury from a wide variety of toxic substances including alcohol, phosphorus, or benzene. Inefficient or even almost total lack of bilirubin transfer by the hepatic cells results in both a piling up of unconjugated bilirubin and an increased amount of conjugated bilirubin in the

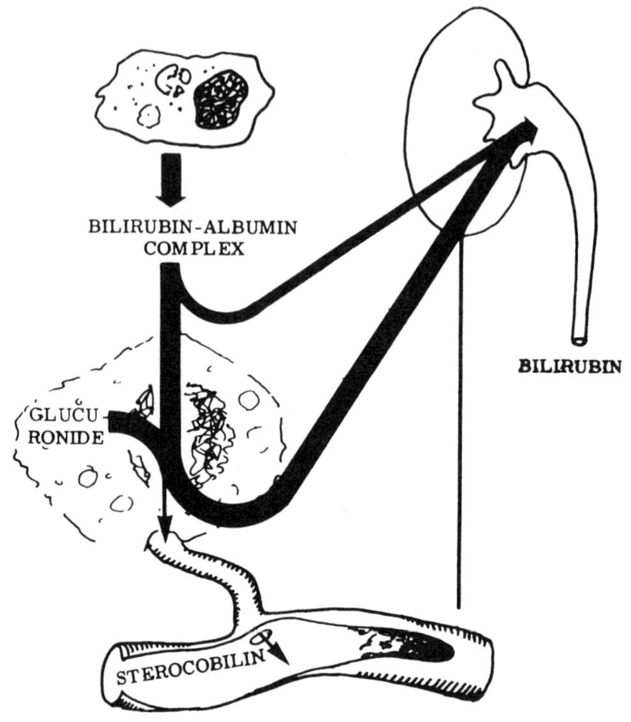

Figure 9–3. Hepatic jaundice. A variety of hemoglobin catabolic products accumulate in various compartments.

circulation. The latter effect is most likely from blockage of biliary canaliculi within the hepatic parenchyma because of cellular and intracellular swelling and inflammation (Fig. 9–3).

Clinically, an enlarged and tender liver with or without splenomegaly may be found. Loss of appetite, nausea, and vomiting are frequent accompanying symptoms. It is hoped that a history of chemical or drug exposure will be elicited in cases of toxic hepatitis. Blood contaminated with various viruses (e.g., hepatis B virus) can cause hepatitis.

Posthepatic Jaundice—Obstructive Jaundice

Partial or complete blockage of the biliary tract by calculi, tumor, inflammatory reactions, fibrosis, or extrinsic pressure results in a regurgitation or backup of conjugated bilirubin into the lymphatic and vascular spaces (Fig. 9–4). Secondary intrinsic hepatic injury may become evident after prolonged blockage, resulting in biliary cirrhosis.

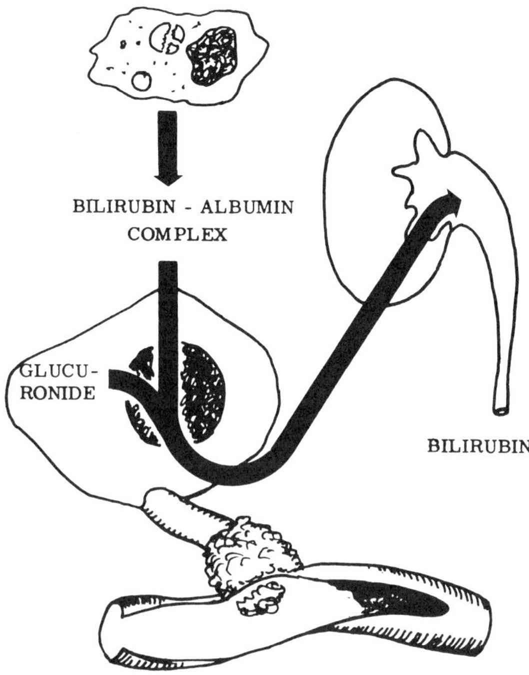

Figure 9–4. Obstructive jaundice. The normal excretion of bilirubin is blocked (in this case by a tumor) and the conjugated bilirubin spills into the circulatory compartment, with considerable amounts being excreted in the urine.

Colicky abdominal pain in the right upper quadrant with radiation into the right shoulder and accompanied by intermittent or increasing jaundice is the classic picture of biliary calculi. Obstruction of the biliary tract by tumor, on the other hand, tends to be painless, with increasing and unremitting jaundice.

In addition to the extrahepatic obstruction, intrahepatic obstruction secondary to neoplasia, drugs (e.g., chlorpromazine jaundice), or intrahepatic calculi also occurs. Biochemical tests are usually not able to differentiate the site of obstruction.

CLINICAL INVESTIGATION

Clinical Features

The most effective method in the differential diagnosis of jaundice and hepatic disease is a detailed clinical history, thoughtfully analyzed with the known mechanisms of each disease and supplemented by a careful and complete physical examination. Frequently, supplementary information from liver function tests is necessary. Such tests have great value if their use is understood and certain general principles are kept in mind. First, there is no abnormal liver function test (LFT) that is pathognomonic of a specific lesion. Far advanced and even fatal liver disease may exist without markedly abnormal hepatic function. When the results of the tests are at variance with the clinical impression, both sets of data should be carefully reviewed. In general, if a laboratory test is not compatible with the clinical data, the latter should be relied upon. Such discrepancies may only be settled with a liver biopsy.

Correlation of the results of hepatic function tests with the histologic changes in the liver may be limited. Extrahepatic biliary obstruction seldom exists for long without the production of intrahepatic parenchymal damage. Conversely, inflammatory swelling with breakdown and increased permeability of biliary ducts gives rise to intrahepatic obstructive phenomena or other changes simulating obstruction in many cases of hepatocellular disease.

Faced with a confusing clinical picture and a great number of possible laboratory tests, how can the clinician most effectively use the laboratory to arrive at a diagnosis?

Laboratory Studies

Screening Tests

Fortunately, several procedures are available that can direct further laboratory testing. These tests check primarily for prehepatic, hepatic, or posthepatic causes of jaundice. The recommended panel includes the following: bilirubin, total, conjugated and unconjugated, transaminases (AST and ALT), alkaline phosphatase (with gamma-glutamyl transpeptidase, if elevated), and urine bilirubin (bile).

Bilirubin. The serum bilirubin measurement gives an accurate indication of the total amount of bile pigment in the blood as well as an estimate of the excretory function of the liver. If this is almost all of the unconjugated (indirect) type, it is probable that the jaundice results from excessive hemolysis. Hyperbilirubinemia caused by hemolysis rarely exceeds 5 mg/dl. The conjugated (direct) bilirubin is elevated in parenchymal disease of the liver or biliary obstruction. In these cases levels of 20 mg/dl or greater are not uncommon. Neither the absolute amounts nor the ratio of unconjugated to conjugated bilirubin is always valid in differentiating biliary obstruction from hepatic parenchymal disease. Levels of the conjugated portion which constitute between 20 and 40 percent of the total bilirubin are more characteristic of hepatic jaundice, whereas levels in excess of 50 percent are more characteristic of posthepatic obstruction.

Bilirubin levels determined at frequent intervals and plotted will yield diagnostic information when the trend is observed.

- In complete biliary obstruction there is a rapid rise with high plateau levels (30 to 40 mg/dl).
- Obstruction caused by a calculus shows a rapid rise but a gradual fall after the stone is passed. If partial obstruction persists or if it is complicated by biliary cirrhosis, a low plateau may be seen.
- In severe acute hepatitis, after peaking over several days or up to 2 weeks, there is a rapid fall of the bilirubin levels if recovery occurs.
- Chronic hepatitis shows low fluctuating curves. Each small rise indicates additional liver damage or increased blood destruction with liver insufficiency.

Transaminases. The measurement of serum transaminases, AST or ALT, is especially valuable in the assessment of hepatic cell injury. These enzyme levels show significant elevations even before jaundice is noted. In all cases of acute hepatitis, toxic or viral, there are significant (10 to 25 times normal) elevations of these enzymes. Almost all patients with chronic hepatitis, active cirrhosis, as well as posthepatic obstruction show only mild to moderate elevations of these enzymes. ALT is more specific for hepatic necrosis than AST, although elevated AST levels persist longer than ALT levels.

As with serial bilirubin determinations, serial transaminase measurements yield information about the course and prognosis in chronic liver disease. In chronic hepatitis with intermittent acute episodes, low-grade elevations with interspersed peaks of marked elevation will be seen. In chronic hepatitis or cirrhosis without significant hepatic cellular damage, no interspersed peaks will be seen. In acute, subsequently fatal hepatitis there is a terminal drop in transaminase levels caused by complete necrosis and lysis of essentially all liver tissue; there is no more transaminase to be released into the circulation.

Alkaline Phosphatase (ALP). The serum ALP is often elevated in obstructive diseases of the hepatobiliary system. Obstructive jaundice tends to produce marked and early elevation, whereas hepatocellular disease produces only a slight if any elevation. This determination does not, however, unequivocally separate hepatic from obstructive jaundice. Abnormal elevation of the serum ALP is seen in more than half of the patients with metastatic tumors in the liver and may be the only abnormal liver function test in such instances. Many other diseases, such as metabolic bone disease, affect the serum ALP level and, as is the case with any other test, the procedure is also subject to technical difficulties.

The measurement of ALP isoenzymes is sometimes helpful in determining the cause of elevated ALP. Bone has a different phosphatase than liver.

Gamma-Glutamyl Transpeptidase (GTT). The enzyme GTT is useful in distinguishing osseous from extraosseous elevations of ALP. It parallels the rise in ALP in liver disease whereas it remains normal in bone disorders associated with elevated phosphatase concentrations.

Urine Bilirubin. The determination of conjugated bilirubin in urine (formerly misnamed bile) is a simple yet effective method to detect patients with hepatic disease who may not exhibit clinical jaundice. It is also a valuable procedure to differentiate hepatic from prehepatic jaundice. Only conjugated bilirubin is excreted in the urine, and therefore, this determination serves to differentiate prehepatic (i.e., hemolytic) jaundice from the hepatic or posthepatic forms. In hemolytic jaundice, bilirubin is not found in the urine unless coexisting hepatic disease is also present.

Table 9–1 summarizes the general patterns of laboratory findings in the three major types of jaundice.

Supplementary Liver Function Tests

The clinical evaluation coupled with information gained from the screening laboratory tests described previously should suggest a definitive, or at least a presumptive, diagnosis in the jaundiced patient. Sometimes, however, this information may be equivocal or even misleading, and supplementary information may be necessary before a diagnosis can be made. In the following sections, a number of these more definitive determinations are discussed. They are grouped according to a presumed or tentative diagnosis, but one must remember that at

TABLE 9–1. SCREENING TESTS IN JAUNDICE

Test	Prehepatic	Hepatic	Posthepatic
Bilirubin, conjugated	0	+ +	+ + to + + +
Bilirubin, unconjugated	+	0	0
Transaminases	0 to +	+ + + +	0 to +
Alkaline phosphatase	0	+	+ + +
Urine bilirubin (bile)	0	+ +	+ to + +

times overlapping occurs between these categories. A discussion on laboratory tests in chronic liver disease and cirrhosis is also included.

Presumptive Prehepatic Jaundice

Urine Urobilinogen. Excessive destruction of red blood cells leads to increased bilirubin formation and, correspondingly, to the excretion of large amounts of conjugated bilirubin into the intestine. There, the conjugated bilirubin is acted on by anaerobes, and increased amounts of urobilinogen (stercobilinogen) are formed and excreted in the stools. Excessive amounts are also absorbed and carried to the liver. If the liver is normal it can usually handle this excess and there is only a mild increase in urobilinogen levels in the urine. Hence, in mild prehepatic jaundice there are high stool values and close to normal urine levels. If hemolysis is very brisk, however, urine urobilinogen levels will be quite elevated.

In hepatitis with edema and inflammation of the liver there is blockage of the bile canaliculi. Low stool and urine values of urobilinogen are noted in these cases.

In partial biliary obstruction (posthepatic jaundice) without liver damage, conjugated bilirubin is formed as usual, but little gets into the intestine, therefore, both stool and urine urobilinogen levels are low. The stool levels can easily be confirmed by noting the characteristic light or clay-colored stools associated with biliary obstruction.

The reader is referred to the discussions on the various types of hemolytic anemias in Chapter 13 for additional studies indicated in prehepatic jaundice.

Presumptive Hepatic Jaundice

Serum Enzymes. In addition to the transaminase levels, other serum enzyme levels are abnormally increased in liver disease.

TABLE 9–2. FEATURES OF THE VARIOUS FORMS OF VIRAL HEPATITIS

Feature	Type A Hepatitis	Type B Hepatitis	Non-A, Non-B Hepatitis
Agent	Hepatitis A virus 27 nm RNA virus	Hepatitis B virus 42 nm DNA virus	Unknown
Antigens	HA Ag	HBsAg, HBcAg, HBeAg	Unknown
Antibodies	Anti-HAV	Anti-HBs, Anti-HBc, Anti-HBe	Unknown
Transmission	Fecal–oral	Parenteral	Parenteral
Mortality	0.1%	1–3%	1–2%
Chronicity	None	5–10%	6–60%
Incubation period	15–45 days	40–180 days	15–150 days

For instance, lactate dehydrogenase (LD) parallels elevations of transaminase. But over the years the transaminases have proved to be both sensitive and specific for hepatic cell injury.

Prothrombin Time. Prothrombin production is decreased in both posthepatic (obstructive) jaundice and hepatic parenchymal disease. The hypoprothrombinemia associated with parenchymal liver disease is caused by defective hepatic synthesis of clotting factors whereas in posthepatic jaundice it is caused by intestinal malabsorption of vitamin K because of a lack of bile salts.

Viral Hepatitis. There are at least three types of viral hepatitis: type A (infectious) hepatitis, type B (serum) hepatitis, and non-A, non-B hepatitis. The viruses of type A and type B hepatitis have been identified and are well characterized. Sensitive and specific assays for the viral antigens and antibodies associated with these diseases are now available. The virus of non-A, non-B hepatitis has yet to be identified, and there are no reliable assays to identify antigens or antibodies of this disease.

Once acute hepatitis has been diagnosed on the basis of clinical history and biochemical laboratory tests (i.e., markedly elevated serum transaminases, mildly elevated ALP, and elevated conjugated and unconjugated serum bilirubin), specific serologic assays should be performed to determine whether the disease is type A, type B, or non-A, non-B hepatitis. The diagnosis of non-A, non-B hepatitis is a diagnosis of exclusion and should only be made after the many other causes of acute hepatitis are ruled out. Some of the contrasting features of the three forms of viral hepatitis are summarized in Table 9–2.

The clinical, biochemical, and serologic course of a typical case of type A hepatitis is summarized in Figure 9–5. The IgM-specific antibodies appear early in illness and the detection of these antibodies in a single serum specimen supports the diagnosis of a recent primary infection. The presence of IgG-specific antibodies alone indicates a more remote postinfection and immunity to reinfection. At present it is not practical to test for the hepatitis A antigen.

The clinical biochemical and serologic course of a typical case of type B hepatitis is summarized in Figure 9–6. The diagnosis of type B hepatitis is made by the detection of hepatitis B surface antigen (HBsAg) in the blood. The HBsAg disappears with recovery. The finding of HBsAg, which persists for 6 months, is indicative of a chronic infection. The anti-HBs is

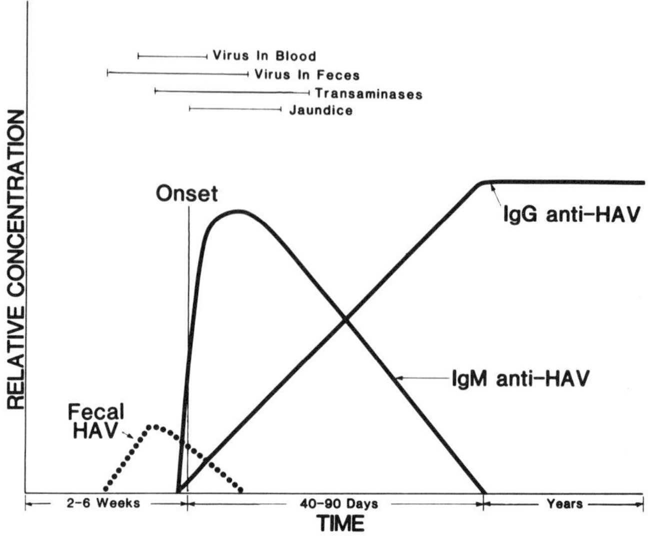

Figure 9-5. Clinical and laboratory findings in type A viral hepatitis. *(From Testmeir GE, Bayer WL: Those "other agents" in the differential diagnosis of posttransfusion hepatitis. In Keating LJ, Silvergleid AJ (eds): Hepatitis. Washington, DC, American Association of Blood Banks, 1981, p. 69.)*

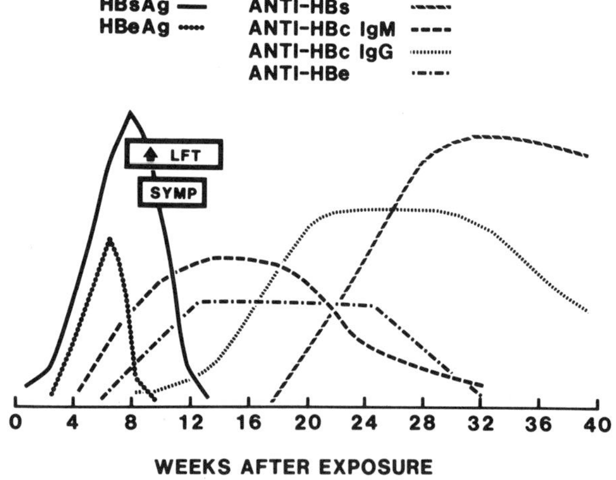

Figure 9-6. Serologic markers in acute hepatitis B infection. These findings illustrate a typical case, in which the disease resolved and immunity developed. *(From Polesky H, Hanson M: Hepatitis B—serologic markers. In Keating LJ, Silvergleid AJ (eds): Hepatitis. Washington, DC, American Association of Blood Banks, 1981, p. 20.)*

found in the serum of patients who have recovered from type B hepatitis. Its presence indicates recovery and immunity to reinfection. There may be a window period between the time that HBsAg disappears and anti-HBs appears. During this window period anticore antibody (anti-HBc) may be the only serologic marker present in the serum.

Percutaneous Liver Biopsy. If the tests of parenchymal function fail to indicate the nature of the damage to the hepatic parenchyma, a biopsy study must be done to find the exact nature of the hepatic injury. It is necessary to remember, however, that focal lesions may be missed in a needle biopsy specimen.

Presumptive Posthepatic Jaundice ·

X-Ray Studies. Additional examinations in the presumed posthepatic jaundice are essentially confined to specialized x-ray techniques such as cholecystography, ultrasonography, radionucleotide cholescintigraphy, and upper gastrointestinal studies with special reference to gastric and pancreatic pathologic changes that may be affecting the biliary tract.

Percutaneous Liver Biopsy. It should be noted that obstructive jaundice may be caused either by intrahepatic or extrahepatic disease and that the previously mentioned tests may not locate the site of obstruction. In such circumstances, liver biopsy or surgical exploration, or both, may be necessary for a positive diagnosis.

Presumptive Chronic Liver Disease and Cirrhosis

Dye Clearance Studies. These studies are very sensitive tests of hepatic function. In recent years, however, there has been a decreasing use of these procedures because of their adverse reactions and because the information they provide can be obtained by other testing. These tests depend on three factors, i.e., the hepatic blood flow, the integrity of the reticuloendothelial system, and the function of the hepatic parenchymal cells. An abnormality in any of these areas may affect the result of the test. Because allergic reactions to bromsulphalein (BSP) do occur, this dye is now used only rarely. Iodocyanine green (CardioGreen) has been proposed as a substitute. It has a biologic half-time of 2.5 to 3.0 minutes, and less than 1

TABLE 9–3. SERUM PROTEIN CHANGES IN HEPATIC DISEASE

Disease	Albumin	Globulins			
		α_1	α_2	β	γ
Cirrhosis, nutritional	↓	N˙	N	↑	↑↑
Cirrhosis, biliary	↓	N	↑	↑↑↑	↑
Acute hepatitis	N or ↓	N	N	↑	↑
Liver cancer, primary or metastatic	↓	↑	↑↑	N	N
Obstructive jaundice	N or ↓	N	↑	↑↑	N

N, normal; ↓, decreased; ↑, increased.

percent of the dye should be recovered from the blood at 20 minutes. In general, if reticuloendothelial disease, hepatic congestion resulting from heart failure, and extrahepatic biliary obstruction are absent, reduction of dye clearance indicates hepatic parenchymal disease.

Serum Proteins Including Electrophoresis. Hepatic disease is often accompanied by alterations of various serum protein fractions. Serum electrophoresis is the best method for evaluating these changes, although the fractionation of proteins into albumin and globulins can reveal significant changes in the comparative quantities of these substances. Table 9–3 categorizes the characteristic changes of serum proteins in liver disease. In general the gamma-globulin fraction is increased in almost all types of hepatic disease, whereas the albumin fraction is decreased. This is as expected, because albumin is synthesized in the liver, whereas γ-globulins are synthesized in the reticuloendothelial cells.

Antimitochondrial Antibody. This antibody level is elevated in most patients with primary biliary cirrhosis, whereas it is almost invariably negative in secondary biliary cirrhosis.

Alpha-Fetoprotein. Hepatoma is a complication of cirrhosis. Alpha-fetoprotein is a major serum protein of the fetus that declines to undetectable levels after the first year of life. Interestingly, patients with primary hepatocellular carcinoma (hepatoma) have markedly increased levels, and its presence, in high concentrations, is considered diagnostic of hepatoma. More sensitive methods indicate that the protein may be mildly elevated in several nonneoplastic hepatic diseases. Moderately elevated levels may also be seen in a small proportion of other neoplasms, germ cell tumors, as well as pancreatic, lung, and gastrointestinal tract tumors.

SUGGESTED READINGS

Bloomer JR, Waldmann TA, McIntire KR, Klatskin E: α-Fetoprotein in non-neoplastic hepatic disorders. JAMA 233:38, 1975.

Boucher I: Diagnosis of jaundice. Br Med J 283: 1282, 1981.

Elibol T, Winkelman EI, King JW, Brown CH: Lack of diagnostic significance of serum alkaline phosphatase values in differentiating hepatocellular and obstructive jaundice. Cleve Clin Q 35:159, 1968.

Ellis G, et al.: Serum enzyme tests in diseases of the liver and biliary tree. Am J Clin Path 70:248, 1978.

Mushawan I, et al.: Interpretation of various serologic profiles of hepatitis B virus infection. Am J Clin Path 76:773, 1981.

Nordyke RA: Surgical vs. nonsurgical jaundice. JAMA 194:949, 1965.

Ostrow JD: Jaundice in older children and adults. JAMA 234:522, 1975.

Schiff E: Evaluating jaundice: Obstructive or not? Patient Care 14:70, 1980.

Snydman D, et al.: Use of IgM-hepatitis A antibody testing. JAMA 245:827, 1981.

Thaler MM: Jaundice in the newborn: Algorithmic diagnosis of conjugated and unconjugated hyperbilirubinemia. JAMA 237:58, 1977.

10

INDIGESTION AND DIARRHEA

BASIC INFORMATION

The Normal Process of Digestion

The breakdown of foodstuffs into smaller molecules that can be absorbed from the intestinal tract is the process of digestion. This process is aided by enzymes secreted by several glands in the upper gastrointestinal tract, notably the salivary glands, the stomach, and the exocrine pancreas. The salivary glands are relatively unimportant in digestion; they secrete ptyalin (salivary amylase), a starch-splitting enzyme, which is inactivated in the acidic environment of the stomach.

Gastric juice contains two major secretions that are important in digestion. First, gastric pepsin is secreted by the gastric chief cells in an inactive form, pepsinogen. It is activated by the hydrochloric acid secretion of the parietal cells. Pepsin breaks down proteins into large proteose and peptone subunits.

The pancreas produces several important enzymes including chymotrypsin and trypsin (both of which break down proteins, proteoses, and peptones); amylase, which digests starch; and lipase, which breaks down neutral fats into glycerol and fatty acids. Relatively less important pancreatic enzymes are carboxypeptidase, ribonuclease, and deoxyribonuclease.

Although the major function of the small intestine is that of absorption rather than digestion, several enzymes are secreted in this portion of the bowel. Aminopeptidase and dipeptidase further break down the protein subunits. The production of several enzymes that catalyze the division of disaccharides, such as sucrase, maltase, and lactase, is another digestive function of the small bowel.

Mechanisms of Absorption: Intestinal Transport

In contrast with the digestive processes outlined previously, absorption is primarily a function of the small bowel. It should be mentioned, however, that one other organ system, the liver and the biliary tract, is at least indirectly responsible for absorption. The secretion of bile is necessary for the absorption of fat as well as fat-soluble substances such as certain vitamins (carotene and vitamins A, D, and K).

The digestive process breaks down foodstuffs into basic molecules that can be absorbed across the intestinal mucosa. Monosaccharides, for instance, are phosphorylated and transported across the mucosa. Other sugars, such as pentoses, are absorbed without phosphorylation, but the rate of absorption is slower.

Fats are primarily absorbed by a pinocytic process in the small bowel. The small globules of neutral fat and the breakdown products are carried across the mucosal cell and subsequently enter the submucosal space and the intestinal lymphatic and venous channels as chylomicrons (Fig. 10–1).

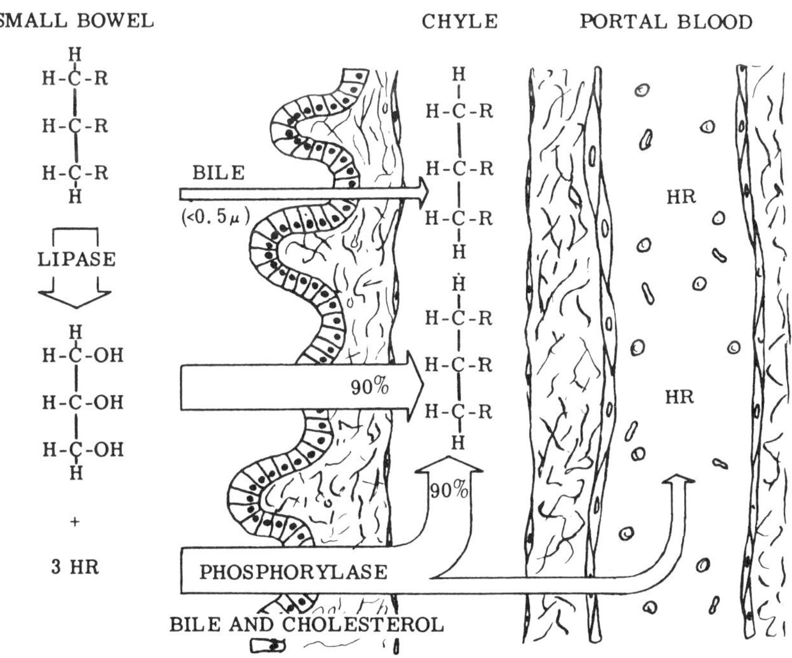

Figure 10–1. Fat absorption schema. R denotes any of a variety of fatty acid molecules that can be found in the neutral fat molecule.

Proteins are probably completely broken down into amino acids before these substances are absorbed by active transport across the mucosa. Interestingly, the L-isomers participate in an active transport mechanism, whereas the D-isomers are absorbed only by diffusion. Absorption of larger protein fragments also occurs and may be responsible for some forms of the sensitization phenomenon. In fact, newborn infants can absorb intact gamma-globulins and apparently acquire immunity in this manner.

CLINICAL INVESTIGATION

Clinical Features

Diarrhea, either chronic or acute, is a nonspecific symptom that may be caused by a wide variety of conditions. By definition it is the intermittent or continual occurrence of frequent and loose stools. With food poisoning, diarrhea, nausea, and vomiting are regularly seen as a reaction to the bacterial toxins. Diarrhea may be secondary to deficient or excessive secretion of gastrointestinal fluids or to defects in intestinal absorption or motility. It may also be secondary to intrinsic intestinal diseases, including infection and injury. Finally, it may be a manifestation of systemic disease. It is evident, therefore, that the clinical picture may be quite variable. Symptoms range from mild food intolerance to severe crampy abdominal pain. Abdominal discomfort or pain is more common with disorders accompanied by hypermotility. Such discomfort may follow eating and, if specific defects of secretion or absorption exist, the symptoms may be precipitated by the ingestion of certain foods. An excellent example of such a defect is disaccharide intolerance in persons with a deficiency of specific intestinal disaccharidases.

Chronic intermittent diarrhea caused by deficient digestion and absorption of certain disaccharides has been described recently both as a congenital and an acquired disorder. In these disorders disaccharides are not hydrolyzed in the mucosal cells of the small bowel. The unabsorbed carbohydrate is fermented by bacteria, leading to excretion of greatly increased amounts of the disaccharide as well as short chain organic acids in the feces. Clinical syndromes arising from congenital intestinal disaccharidase deficits include lactase, invertase, isomaltase, and combined invertase–isomaltase deficiencies. The various disorders in which acquired disaccharidase deficiencies are found include sprue and celiac disease, cystic fibrosis, ulcerative colitis, regional enteritis, peptic ulcer, and as a sequela of segmental small bowel resection.

Many diseases of the small bowel result in impairment of digestion and absorption of fat with a resultant abnormal increase in the content of fat in the stool, termed steatorrhea. In contrast with diarrhea, steatorrhea always indicates the existence of an organic abnormality of the small bowel itself or organs directly related to digestion, i.e., the pancreas, the hepatobiliary tract and, at times, the stomach. When fat is not absorbed properly, there is often an associated malabsorption of other metabolites including protein, vitamins, and minerals.

Chronic diarrhea or steatorrhea of significant duration and degree usually results in malnutrition, although this is not invariably the case. Deficiencies of protein, iron, prothrombin, and calcium may become manifest as the disease continues.

Laboratory Studies

Screening Procedures in Acute Indigestion or Diarrhea

Gross Examination of Stools. Other than increased amounts of fluid, the stools in acute disease may be quite unremarkable. The rice water stools of shigellosis or the foul-smelling watery stools of salmonellosis are seen only rarely.

Blood streaking may be present in bacterial infection, but gross blood is rare. Gross or microscopic evidence of pus may be present. In amebic colitis there may be accompanying blood and mucus with the passage of watery stools. In ulcerative colitis there may be similar stools, whereas in regional enteritis, diarrhea is not as severe and gross blood is usually absent.

Chemical examination for blood usually offers no significant additional information in acute conditions, although sometimes pH and some chemical determinations are requested by pediatricians.

Examination for Fecal Leukocytes. A small fleck of mucus or liquid stool mixed with an equal volume of methylene blue stain is examined for the presence of fecal leukocytes. Table 10–1 lists the possible diagnoses.

Stool Culture for Enteric Pathogens. Bacterial culture of the stool for pathogenic organisms should be done if symptoms persist beyond a reasonable time. Plating media should routinely include media specially designed to grow *Salmonella, Shigella*, and *Campylobacter*. *Yersinia* and *Vibrio* cultures should be requested in appropriate cases. In infants the culture of *Escherichia coli* may represent the offending pathogenic organism. Serologic identification of pathogenic *E. coli* can be done in this age group, but only for epidemiologic study of nursery outbreaks of disease.

Patients receiving broad-spectrum antibiotic therapy may experience an overgrowth of pathogenic fungi, especially *Candida*. A Gram stain of the stool may be diagnostic. *Clostridium difficile* causes most cases of pseudomembranous colitis. This organism may be cultured on selective media but it is usually diagnosed by detection of cytotoxin in the stool.

Examination of Stools for Parasitic Organisms. Most parasitic nematodes pass ova in the stool, which are easily found when appropriate concentration and flotation techniques are employed. In addition, the rhabditiform larvae of strongyloides can be found by using this technique.

In the case of *Entamoeba histolytica* infestation, positive diagnosis is best established by prompt examination of fresh, warm stool on a warmed microscope stage before the organisms become immotile. The prompt transportation to the laboratory of a freshly purged or even proctoscopically obtained specimen is often rewarded by a positive diagnosis. In stools that have been allowed to remain at room temperature or the examination of which has been otherwise delayed, it is impossible to see trophozoites of *E. histolytica*. Special stains (iron-hemotoxylin) should be done to document the infection.

TABLE 10–1. FECAL LEUKOCYTES IN VARIOUS ENTERITIDES

Leukocytes Present	Leukocytes Absent
Shigella	Staphylococcal toxin
Salmonella	*E. coli* toxin
Escherichia coli, invasive strains	*C. perfingens* toxin
	Vibrio cholerae toxin
Yersinia	*Giardia lamblia*
Ulcerative colitis	*Entamoeba histolytica* (usually)
Clostridium difficile	*Dientamoeba fragilis*
Campyolobacter	Viruses

Definitive Procedures in Acute Indigestion or Diarrhea

Blood Culture in Salmonellosis. Blood culture (early) and serologic studies (late) positively establish a diagnosis of typhoid fever. Bacteremia may not be present in other varieties of salmonellosis (paratyphoid fever).

Viral Studies. Prominent gastrointestinal symptoms may be secondary to many viral infections, including rotovirus, adenovirus, ECHO virus, or Coxsackie virus. Serologic confirmation requires evidence of a significant rise in serum antibody titers from the acute to the convalescent serum specimen.

Culture of stool specimens for viruses is not readily available at present and, if done, usually is only of epidemiologic importance.

Testing for Intestinal Disaccharidase Deficiency. The patient is prepared as for a glucose tolerance test. In addition, he or she should be free of diarrhea for 2 or more days before the test is done. The disaccharide (e.g., lactose, sucrose, or isomaltose), as a 10 percent aqueous solution, is given orally. The usual dose is 50 g, although some investigators advocate larger doses of up to 100 g. Higher doses will, of course, be associated with more severe symptoms in enzyme-deficient patients.

Blood for glucose, i.e., reducing substances, is collected at fasting or zero time, $\frac{1}{2}$, 1, $1\frac{1}{2}$, and 2 hours. Stools are collected for 12 hours following the ingestion of the test disaccharide dose and are examined for pH and sugar using Clinitest tablets.

Normally the blood sugar elevation parallels that of a one-dose oral glucose tolerance test. In the various disaccharidase deficiency states, the blood sugar curve is flat, with a less than 25 mg/dl increase in blood sugar concentration. Typically a large excess of the disaccharide in the stool can also be detected. The stool pH, measured with nitrazine paper, falls to pH 4 to 5 (normal >7) within 6 to 18 hours. Inadequacy of digestion and absorption is also indicated by development of the symptoms of intestinal discomfort and diarrhea after the disaccharide is ingested.

If the disaccharide tolerance is abnormal, a control test may be performed by determining the response to the two constituent monosaccharides. Testing on blood and stool is identical to that outlined above.

Screening Procedures in Chronic Diarrhea and Malabsorption

Gross Examination of the Stool. In a nontropical sprue, the defect in absorption results in stools that are characteristically bulky, foul smelling, and greasy because of the presence of large amounts of neutral fats and fatty acids.

In pancreatic insufficiency, in addition to increased amounts of fat, undigested protein and carbohydrate may be indicated by the presence of meat fibers and starch granules on microscopic examination.

The stools of regional enteritis and ulcerative colitis usually have increased mucus and pus. In addition, feces from patients with ulcerative colitis may be grossly bloody.

Fat Absorption (Screening). Although this test lacks quantitative accuracy, it is useful because of its rapidity and simplicity. The fasting patient is given a drink containing 50 ml of corn oil that has been homogenized with 240 ml of skimmed milk. A blood specimen is drawn into heparin before and again at 4 and 6 hours after the corn oil drink is given. If fat is absorbed, the optical density of either or both postingestion samples normally should rise more than 0.10 OD unit above the fasting level.

Qualitative Fecal Fat Determination. The microscopic examination of the stool for increased fat content is a simple but very worthwhile procedure in the evaluation of the patient with possible steatorrhea. To ensure validity, the diet should contain adequate amounts of fat, i.e., at least 60 g/day.

Fat in the feces can be stained with Sudan III dye. Normally neutral fat stains as bright orange droplets but fatty acids do not stain. By using heat and hydrolysis, however, fatty acids and neutral fats can be converted to stainable fatty acids. The preparation can then be stained and examined again and the number of droplets will increase from the first examination. Large amounts of stained neutral fat globules are suggestive of pancreatic insufficiency. Large amounts of saponified fat are seen in patients with absorptive defects.

Glucose Tolerance Test. A glucose tolerance test may provide useful information in the study of patients with gastrointestinal disorders associated with malabsorption as well as hypermotility. Because the blood levels of glucose at any one time are dependent on many factors, including gastric emptying, intestinal motility, rate of glucose metabolism in the liver and other tissues, and rate of clearance by the kidney, the results should be interpreted with some caution.

In malabsorption caused by intrinsic small bowel disease, a flat glucose tolerance curve is frequently found. Keep in mind, however, that about 20 percent of healthy persons also have a flat glucose tolerance curve. On the other hand, the majority of patients with pancreatic insufficiency will have a diabetic glucose tolerance curve due to associated islet destruction. The details of conducting and interpreting glucose tolerance studies can be found in Chapter 17, which includes a discussion on the diagnosis of diabetes.

Because of the difficulties in interpreting this test, it has been largely replaced by the xylose absorption test (discussion follows).

Serum Carotene. Because carotene and vitamin A are fat-soluble, their absorption is impaired in the diseases in question. Low serum levels of carotene (>100 mg/dl) are highly suggestive of fat malabsorption. However, one can see low serum levels in patients with a poor diet, severe liver disease, or high fever.

Blood Levels of Other Nutrients. There are certain constituents found in the peripheral blood that may reflect poor intestinal absorption or poor nutrition. These indicator substances include total protein, albumin, calcium, hemoglobin or iron, vitamin B_{12}, folate, ferritin, and prothrombin. The frequency and extent of abnormality more or less parallel the extent and severity of the primary disease.

Definitive Procedures in Chronic Diarrhea and Malabsorption

The following sections are confined to clinical laboratory aids in the evaluation of chronic gastrointestinal disorders. It should be remembered, however, that definitive diagnosis of many of these disorders may be best made with specialized x-ray studies, sigmoidoscopic examination, or biopsy confirmation.

Culture of Small Bowel Contents. A sample of small bowel secretions is obtained using a double lumen tube. The tube is placed under fluoroscopic control. Exactly 1 ml of material is diluted with 9 ml of fresh thioglycolate broth, and a quantitative culture is done.

Greater than 10^6 organisms per milliliter of intestinal contents indicates a significant bacterial overgrowth. Gram-negative coliforms and *Bacteroides* species are especially significant.

Bacterial overgrowth is seen in a diverse group of intestinal diseases. These include surgical blind loops, jejunal diverticula, diabetic enteropathy, gastrojejunocolic fistula, bowel strictures, scleroderma, and tropical sprue.

Endocrine Disorders and Chronic Diarrhea. The association of chronic diarrhea with hyperthyroidism and hypoadrenalism is now generally appreciated, and laboratory efforts to evaluate the function of these endocrine glands should not be overlooked (see Chap. 17 on endocrine disorders).

A relatively rare but extremely interesting endocrine disorder, the Zollinger-Ellison syndrome, may have associated diarrhea. This syndrome was first described as severe peptic ulcer disease in association with hypersecretion of gastric hydrochloric acid apparently caused by a single adenoma or by multiple adenomas of the pancreas. More recently other endocrine gland adenomas have also been found to be associated with this disorder. The primary laboratory tests used to diagnose this disorder are the plasma gastrin levels and the measurement of gastric hydrochloric acid secretion; 10 to 20 times the normal amount may be found. This increase is due to a continual hypersecretion of gastric juice.

The details of conducting and interpreting gastric analysis studies can be found in Chapter 8, which discusses the acute surgical abdomen.

Xylose Absorption Test. This test is a measure of the intestinal absorption attributable to diffusion. The absorption of the pentose D-xylose does not require phosphorylation in the bowel mucosa. The amount absorbed is a function of the absorptive surface of the small bowel. Thus, normal values are found in exocrine pancreatic insufficiency and a variety of other digestive disturbances and help in differentiating these entities from primary absorptive defects of the small bowel. Of the D-xylose absorbed, a large portion is subsequently excreted unaltered in the urine and can be measured.

The fasting patient is given 25 g of D-xylose as a 5 percent solution. No food is taken during the test, but 200 ml of water are given hourly. The bladder is emptied at the beginning of the test, and all urine passed during the 5 hours after ingestion of D-xylose is collected and pooled into a single container. The total amount of D-xylose excreted is then measured. A blood specimen is obtained at 2 hours to determine the serum D-xylose level.

The mean urinary excretion is about 6.5 g in healthy persons. Less than 5 g is excreted in patients with sprue or other primary malabsorptive disorders of the small bowel. The test may be falsely abnormal in poorly hydrated patients or in patients with poor renal function, ascites, edema, bacterial overgrowth of the bowel, or rapid gastric emptying and intestinal transport. In patients with poor renal function (e.g., the elderly), delayed gastric emptying, or liver disease with ascites, the 2-hour serum xylose level may be helpful diagnostically. Normal values are above 25 mg/100 ml and values below 20 mg/100 ml are strongly suggestive of malabsorption.

Fat Absorption Studies Using Radiolabeled Fats. The use of neutral fat and split fatty acids labeled with radioactive iodine may be useful in the evaluation of steatorrhea. However, the hoped for advantage, i.e., the avoidance of collecting and measuring fat in the stool, has not been realized. Stool collections are still necessary to avoid errors of interpretation of blood levels of radioactivity.

This test is conducted in two stages. In the first part, labeled neutral fat (glycerol triolein) is given orally with a test meal. If pancreatic lipase is present the neutral fat will be split into glycerol and three oleic acid fragments. The oleic acid portions will subsequently be absorbed if the small intestinal mucosa is normal. If the neutral fat is not absorbed and increased amounts are recovered from the stool, either the pancreas or the small intestine may be at fault. In the follow-up procedure radioactively labeled oleic acid is given; it does not require pancreatic lipase for absorption. If it is absorbed the small intestine is presumed to be normal, and the trioleate malabsorption is caused by pancreatic insufficiency. If, on the other hand, there is poor absorption of both glycerol trioleate and oleic acid, disease of the small intestine is the cause of the malabsorption (Fig. 10–1).

Peak blood levels of radioactivity usually occur at about the third hour and normally are above 5 percent of the ingested radioactivity. Recovery of less than 7 percent of the ingested radioactivity on 3- or 4-day fecal collection is considered normal.

Quantitative Fecal Fat Determination. The measurement of fecal fat on a 72-hour (3-day) stool collection is the single best

TABLE 10–2. DUODENAL DRAINAGE IN SECRETIN TEST

Disorder	Volume (ml/kg)	Bicarbonate (meg/L)
Normal	2.1–4.3	90–125
Cystic fibrosis	Low	Low
Chronic pancreatitis	Normal	Low
Carcinoma of pancreas		
Head	Low	Normal
Tail	Normal	Normal

test for the evaluation of steatorrhea. Close supervision of fat intake (about 100 g/day) as well as complete collection of stool are essential. Normally less than 7 g of fat per day are present in the stool.

Secretin Test. Secretin, which stimulates exocrine pancreatic secretion, is administered to the patient suspected of having chronic exocrine pancreatic insufficiency. Pure synthetic L-secretin (1 unit/kg) is injected intravenously over a 1-minute period. Duodenal contents are collected (four 20-minute samples) and measured. They are also analyzed for bicarbonate and amylase content. The placement of the double lumen tube is critical.

A positive test is indicated by a less than normal volume or amounts of amylase and bicarbonate in the duodenal drainage (Table 10–2). Elevation of serum amylase or lipase levels, or both, above normal can also constitute a positive test.

Carcinoid Syndrome

This syndrome is a rare cause of abdominal symptoms. It includes pain, diarrhea, nausea, and vomiting and may be accompanied by dyspnea and weight loss. These patients may also exhibit episodic flushing and cyanosis, tachycardia, hypotension, and hepatomegaly. This unusual set of clinical manifestations may be associated with a carcinoid tumor. The tumor is most common in the small bowel but may arise in any portion of the gastrointestinal tract. Patients with metastatic disease are more likely to have clinical manifestations. In addition, certain bronchial adenomas have similar histologic characteristics. Patients with these adenomas may have a similar clinical picture.

The signs and symptoms result from increased amounts of metabolites of serotonin being released into the circulation.

The principal degradation product, 5-hydroxyindoleacetic acid (5-HIAA), is excreted in the urine and is easily measured. Normally less than 5 mg of 5-HIAA are excreted per day, but this may be increased 5 to 100 times in the carcinoid syndrome.

SUGGESTED READINGS

Bliss C: Fat absorption and malabsorption. Arch Intern Med 141:1213, 1981.

Chey WY, Shay H, Nielsen OF, Lorber SH: Evaluation of tests of pancreatic function in chronic pancreatic disease. JAMA 201:374, 1967.

Dreiling D, et al.: Pancreatic secretory testing in 1974. Gut 16:653, 1975.

Fordtran JS, Soergel KH, Ingelfinger FJ: Intestinal absorption of D-xylose in man. N Eng J Med 267:274, 1962.

Greenberger N: Gastrointestinal Disorders: A Pathophysiologic Approach, 2nd ed. Chicago, Year Book Med., Pub., 1981.

Hershfield NB, Lind JF, Hildes JA: Clinical correlations with pancreatic function tests. Can Med Assoc J 98:185, 1968.

Kalser MH: Laboratory aids in diagnosis of steatorrhea. JAMA 188:37, 1964.

Kern F Jr, Struthers JE Jr: Intestinal lactase deficiency and lactose intolerance in adults. JAMA 195:927, 1966.

Krawitt E, Becken W: Limitations of the usefulness of the D-xylose absorption test. Am J Clin Pathol 63:261, 1975.

Rogers A: Answers to questions on diarrhea. Hosp Med 14:267, 1983.

Satterwhite TK, DuPont HL: The patient with acute diarrhea. JAMA 236:2662, 1976.

11
RENAL DISEASE

COMMENTS ON THE ROUTINE URINALYSIS

Because the routine urinalysis is an integral part of any medical examination, the presence of any abnormality in the basic urinalysis findings (rather than the patient's symptoms of disease) serves as our starting point for further laboratory investigation. Especially important is evidence of increased glucose or protein excretion or abnormal constituents in the microscopic examination of the urinary sediment. If abnormalities are found, a more definitive examination is required to delineate the cause. Additional testing may be required to quantitate the extent of intrinsic renal disease or to assess the evolution of such disease. Although the finding of glucose in the urine is discussed more fully in the sections on diabetes mellitus in Chapter 17, the remaining abnormalities are discussed in this chapter.

BASIC INFORMATION

Renal Structure and Function

Homeostasis of the extracellular fluid environment, or milieu, is regulated by two organs: (1) the lungs, which primarily regulate levels of oxygen and carbon dioxide and (2) the kidneys, which control the nongaseous chemical environment. This regulation by the kidney is in addition to its other main function, i.e., the removal of metabolic waste products.

The nephron is the basic functional unit of the kidney, and its various portions perform specific tasks in the overall regulation of the extracellular fluid composition. For example, the

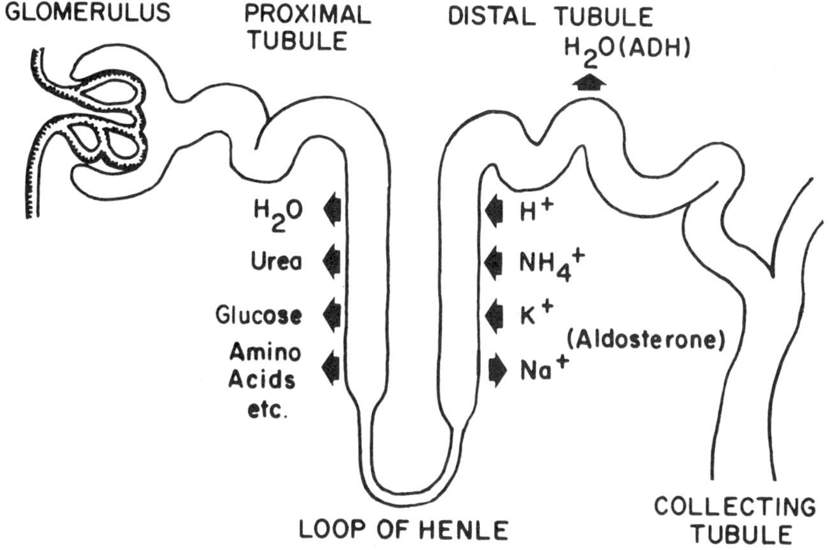

Figure 11–1. The nephron. Some of the important tubular reabsorption and exchange functions are indicated.

glomeruli act primarily as filters of the plasma, nonselectively removing large quantities of water and low molecular weight compounds as well as inorganic ions from the plasma. High molecular weight substances (such as plasma proteins) are not filtered except when the glomeruli are damaged by disease. In these cases proteins and even blood cells may gain access to the forming urine.

The renal tubules act on the dilute urine of the glomerular filtrate in three specific ways. The tubular cells selectively reabsorb certain substances, e.g., glucose, water, or electrolytes, the conservation of which is necessary to the overall body economy. In addition, certain substances such as creatinine, uric acid, and potassium are secreted into the tubular lumina. Finally, the body's acid-base balance is maintained by the exchange of secreted hydrogen ions for filtered sodium ions as well as the production of ammonia and its exchange for sodium ions. These tubular actions profoundly change the composition of the original glomerular filtrate, all having the primary purpose of maintaining the normal composition of the plasma and hence the extracellular and intracellular fluid compartments (Fig. 11–1).

A wide variety of inborn errors of tubular function are known; the usual mechanism being the failure to reabsorb various substances such as amino acids, phosphate ion, or carbohydrates from the glomerular filtrate.

It is quite apparent that either focal or generalized diseases can selectively destroy renal tissue. Because there are an estimated two million nephrons and there is a comparatively large reserve capacity, renal function will not be compromised until the disease process is fairly far advanced. It is the responsibility of the physician to discover any evidence of renal dysfunction or disease as early as possible and to treat it adequately and completely to prevent the progression of such disease.

The basic urinalysis, including a well-performed microscopic examination, provides an excellent laboratory test to screen for abnormalities of the kidneys or the urinary tract. It is unfortunate that this simple procedure is so often delegated to those least prepared to perform the examination properly, thus shortchanging the patient. The availability of excellent simple and reliable test reagents and procedures has done much to standardize the procedure. The microscopic examination, however, still requires adequate training and experience.

The following sections provide a logical approach to the laboratory investigations of the kidney and the urinary tract from the starting point of the basic urinalysis.

CLINICAL INVESTIGATION

Laboratory Studies

Basic Urinalysis

The basic or routine urinalysis includes the following procedures: pH, specific gravity, tests for reducing substances (primarily glucose), and protein, and a microscopic examination of the urine sediment. Abnormalities in any of these tests may point to certain disorders of the urinary tract or may indicate that additional studies are necessary. In the following sections some of the major abnormalities found on urinalysis are discussed.

The urine sample should be collected in a clean and dry container. A voided specimen is adequate for chemical and microscopic analysis. The specimen should be examined within 1 hour of voiding because red blood cells, white blood cells, and casts decompose in urine allowed to stand at room temperature. Also various chemical measurements may change over time, e.g., glucose may be consumed by cells and bacteria, pH may change due to bacterial growth, and bilirubin may decrease with exposure to light.

pH. Normal kidneys are capable of producing urine that can vary from a pH of 4.5 to about 8.0. Freshly voided urine from patients on a normal diet has a pH of about 6.0. Excessively acid urine may be excreted by patients on high protein diets or by patients with systemic acidosis. Alkaline urine occurs in patients consuming diets high in vegetables, citrus fruits, and milk or in patients with renal tubular acidosis or systemic alkalosis. In urinary tract infections the urine tends to be alkaline. Urine standing at room temperature may become alkaline due to bacterial overgrowth.

Specific Gravity. The normal specific gravity of urine ranges from 1.010 to 1.035. The specific gravity is one parameter of renal tubular function, i.e., it is a measure of the kidney's ability to concentrate urine. Low specific gravities are seen in diabetes insipidus, a disease caused by the absence of, or impairment to, the normal functioning of antidiuretic hormone. Low specific gravities may also occur in patients with glomerulonephritis, pyelonephritis, and various other renal anomalies due to extensive renal tubular damage. High specific gravities may be seen in diabetes mellitus, adrenal insufficiency, hepatic disease, and congestive heart failure.

Glycosuria. This is discussed in the section on diabetes mellitus (Chap. 17).

Proteinuria. Normally there is only a very small amount of protein in the urine, i.e., less than 150 mg/24 hours. Detection of an abnormal amount of protein in the urine is evidence of increased glomerular basement permeability. Because the albumin molecule is smaller than that of globulin, it passes more easily through a damaged glomerulus. Thus, the commonly used term albuminuria is often correct. Other plasma proteins have also been found in urine and certain patterns of proteinuria are emerging that may prove to be diagnostically helpful in the future (discussion follows).

Microscopic Examination of the Urine Sediment. Although a microscopic urinalysis in the asymptomatic patient is associated with a low yield of abnormalities, the urine sediment from the symptomatic patient can provide valuable information to differentiate the various intrinsic renal abnormalities associated with proteinuria. It must be examined within a rea-

TABLE 11–1. CHARACTERISTIC URINE MICROSCOPIC FINDINGS IN RENAL DISEASE

Lesion	Protein	Bacteria	White Blood Cells (per hpf)	Red Blood Cells (per hpf)	Casts (per lpf)
Normal	0–tr	0	0–few	0–few	Hyaline, 0 or few
Pyelonephritis					
Acute	0–2+	+	3–4+	0–few	White blood cell inclusion
Chronic	2–4+	±	2–3+	0–few	Granular, white blood cell inclusion
Glomerulonephritis					
Acute	2–4+	0	Few	3–4+	Red blood cell
Chronic	2–3+	0	Few	1–2+	Granular
Nephrotic syndrome	4+	0	Few	0–few	Fatty, oval fat bodies
Orthostatic proteinuria	0–3+	0	0–few	0–few	Hyaline, few

hpf, high power field; lpf, low power field.

sonable time after the urine is voided, however, preferably within 1 hour.

Table 11-1 summarizes the characteristic findings in these renal lesions. The various types and stages of nephritis present a complicated picture that may finally be resolved only by renal biopsy. The characteristic urine microscopic findings are often overlapping and equivocal. Only in the nephrotic syndrome are there characteristic blood findings that may be of significant help for definitive diagnosis. These findings include the depletion of serum proteins and the characteristic serum protein electrophoretic patterns (low albumin and gamma-globulin with elevated alpha- and beta-globulins) plus markedly elevated cholesterol levels.

Percutaneous Renal Biopsy

This is the final definitive procedure in the evaluation of intrinsic renal disease. When carefully performed and expertly interpreted, this procedure can usually provide a definitive diagnosis in otherwise equivocal renal parenchymal lesions. As only a small amount of tissue is available for examination, there is no substitute for sound judgment and experience in correlating the observed histologic changes with the clinical and laboratory findings. This is especially true in renal diseases known to be focal rather than general.

Proteinuria

If proteinuria is found on urinalysis and repeated examination indicates that it is not related to fever, exercise, possible emotional tension, or contamination by vaginal secretions or feces, the cause must be sought.

There are many causes of proteinuria including postural (or orthostatic) proteinuria, congestive heart failure, febrile illnesses, myeloma, renal glomerular diseases (e.g., diabetes mellitus, collagen vascular diseases), renal tubular diseases, (e.g., Fanconi's syndrome), renal interstitial diseases (e.g., pyelonephritis), and bladder tumors.

Although not common, postural proteinuria may be ruled out by collecting urine after the patient has been recumbent. If no protein is excreted during this time, orthostatic proteinuria is the likely cause. In glomerular diseases proteinuria may vary from 1 g/24 hours to more than 40 g/24 hours. The largest single component of glomerular proteinuria is albumin, which constitutes 70 percent or more by weight of the total protein excreted. In contrast, the maximal urinary excretion of protein in renal tubular disease is usually less than 1 g/24 hours. Tubular proteinuria is characterized by excessive excretion of proteins of low molecular weight (less than 50,000 daltons) with albumin constituting only a minor fraction of the total protein present. Because a positive result for proteinuria is significant, it should be confirmed by a second, different method. The laboratory tests for proteinuria are discussed in the next sections.

Laboratory Measurement of Urine Proteins

Dipstick Method. The principle of the dipstick method involves a color reaction between bromphenol blue and albumin. The sensitivity of the test is such that 20 to 30 mg/dl of albumin is detected. Dipsticks are insensitive to globulins and Bence Jones protein. A trace to 1+ dipstick reading roughly corresponds with 0.5 to 1.5 g protein/24 hours. A 2+ reading corresponds with a protein excretion between 1.5 and 7.5 g/24 hours. The dipstick test may give false-positive results with alkaline urine.

Sulfosalicylic Acid Test. A positive dipstick screen should be confirmed with sulfosalicyclic acid. Sulfosalicylic acid is one of several reagents used to precipitate protein from urine but is considered the method of choice. These tests can be interpreted qualitatively or quantitatively. Sulfosalicylic acid detects most proteins including albumin, globulins, Tamm-Horsfall protein, and Bence Jones proteins. False-positive results may occur in some patients receiving penicillin as well as after the use of some radiographic contrast media.

Protein Electrophoresis. This procedure is useful to distinguish between glomerular and tubular proteinuria. In tubular proteinuria, the albumin fraction is relatively small, i.e., 10 to 20 percent of the total protein present, whereas in glomerular proteinuria albumin makes up 70 percent or so of the total protein excreted.

Immunoelectrophoresis. This is the method of choice for characterizing monoclonal light chains (i.e., Bence Jones proteins) in multiple myeloma.

Hematuria

Hematuria is defined as the presence of abnormal numbers of intact red blood cells in the urine sediment. Hemoglobinuria, on the other hand, indicates the presence of free hemoglobin in the urine. It usually accompanies hematuria caused by the lysis of the red blood cells in the urine. In hemolytic reactions occurring within the plasma compartment, only free hemoglobin will be present in the urine. Hematuria may be discovered by the microscopic examination, red blood cells being evident. Free hemoglobin specifically reacts with orthotolidine (dipstick procedure); it also gives positive reactions for protein as expected. Finally, one must not forget that red urine can also be due to myoglobinuria following skeletal muscle damage and screening tests for hemoglobin or protein are positive.

Probably the most common cause of hematuria is mixing of the urine with menstrual blood. This cause can be eliminated by proper collection techniques or by avoiding doing urinalyses when the patient is menstruating.

Urinary blood may originate from any part of the urinary tract: the upper tract (kidneys), the middle tract (ureters, bladder, prostate, and related structures), and the lower tract (primarily the urethra). Blood present throughout urination usually originates in the upper or middle tract, whereas blood present only during initial or final portions of urination comes from the lower urinary tract.

The causes of hematuria include infection, neoplasia, trauma, calculi, systemic diseases such as vascular or bleeding disorders, and a group of miscellaneous disorders. The history and physical examination of the patient with hematuria may quickly uncover the cause; however, if not, a systematic search for the cause is mandatory.

Glomerulonephritis is the most common cause of hematuria in children, whereas urinary tract infection is the most frequent cause in adults. After infection, tumors and trauma are frequent causes of hematuria in men, whereas women seem more often to harbor renal calculi. Infection as a cause can easily be eliminated or implicated by the search for increased numbers of white blood cells or white cell casts. If these are present in abnormal numbers, a urine culture is indicated. An occasional patient with long-standing calculi surrounded by an inflammatory reaction may show increased numbers of white blood cells, although the cultures may be sterile.

In the case of hematuria with few additional urine abnormalities, the possibility of tumor or calculus should be strongly considered. Intravenous or retrograde pyelography and cystoscopy are probably the examinations best suited to check for these possibilities.

Diagnosis of Urinary Tract Infection

A fresh clean-catch midstream specimen or a catheterized specimen is essential for the following tests.

Screening Procedures

Nitrite and Leukocyte Esterase Tests. A positive nitrite test indicates that bacteria, which reduce urinary nitrate to nitrite, are present in significant numbers. Esterase activity has been demonstrated in the primary granules of neutrophils. Esterase activity is not present in urine in the absence of inflammation. These two tests are now available on dipsticks. When both tests are positive, a urinary tract infection is strongly indicated. When both tests are negative, the probability of significant bacteriuria is about 5 percent.

Microscopic Examination of the Urine Sediment. One or more bacteria per oil immersion lens field in a Gram-stained uncentrifuged urine specimen suggests significant bacteriuria, i.e., greater than 100,000 CFUs/ml. In the centrifuged urine specimen, however, more than four or five bacteria per oil immersion field indicate probable infection.

As discussed previously, the urinary sediment in urinary tract infections usually contain significant numbers of white blood cells. If white cell casts are seen, pyelonephritis should be suspected. White blood cell clumps are found in acute cystitis.

Definitive Procedures

Microbiology Cultures. If screening tests for urinary tract infection are positive, the organism should be identified by any of a number of acceptable culture methods. The concentration of the bacteria should be determined. Bacterial counts of less than 100,000 CFUs/ml are of doubtful or no significance unless definite clinical manifestations are present or if the patient is receiving antimicrobial therapy. Counts greater than 100,000 CFUs/ml indicate a significant urinary tract infection. Antibiotic susceptibility testing should also be determined to aid in therapy. Efforts should also be made to determine if there are any structural abnormalities of the urinary tract because of their known association with impaired urine flow and consequent infection. Radiologic techniques such as intravenous and retrograde pyelography and renal arteriography help to delineate these abnormalities, which are often correctable by surgical intervention.

Repeated sterile cultures in the setting of persistent increased numbers of leukocytes in the urine should suggest tuberculosis or lupus nephritis.

Antibody-Coated Bacteria. One of the problems encountered in urinary tract infection is finding the exact location of the infection. Pyelonephritis and prostatitis require more intensive therapy than cystitis. It has been found that bacteria in urine from kidney and prostate infections become coated with antibody by the time they reach the bladder. Thus a simple direct immunofluorescence procedure may be used to visualize bacteria that are coated with antibody, thus localizing the infection.

Laboratory Evaluation of Renal Failure

Screening Procedures

Urea Nitrogen. In humans, urea is an end product of protein metabolism. When the kidney is not able to clear urea sufficiently, urea accumulates in the blood. Serum urea is not a sensitive indicator of renal disease, as 50 to 70 percent of nephrons must be destroyed before serum urea levels reach the upper limits of the normal range.

Creatinine. Creatinine is derived from muscle metabolism. Serum creatinine levels also rise in renal disease. Like urea levels, creatinine levels do not exceed the upper limit of the normal range until about 50 percent of the nephrons are destroyed. However, serum creatinine levels fluctuate less with diet or the state of hydration than serum urea levels do and therefore this measurement is preferred over urea nitrogen as a screening test for renal disease.

Creatinine Clearance. Glomerular function is most conveniently measured with the creatinine clearance test. The creatinine clearance is a renal function test based on the rate of excretion by the kidneys of metabolically produced creatinine. It is one of the more sensitive tests of renal failure. The amount of creatinine produced by endogenous protein metabolism is constant and proportional to the body surface area. The amount present in the urine is dependent on a combination of glomerular filtration and tubular secretion of this material. The test is carried out as indicated below.

The bladder is emptied at the beginning of the test period, and all urine passed in the following 24 hours is collected into a single container. The specimen is refrigerated because creatinine is unstable at room temperature. No preservatives should be added to the collection container. After the specimen has been collected, it should be sent to the laboratory without delay.

A sample of blood is drawn during the urine collection period and sent to the laboratory with the timed urine specimen. The creatinine concentrations of both the urine and the serum are measured. The creatinine clearance is calculated by substituting into the following formula:

$$\text{Creatinine clearance (ml/min)} = \frac{U \times V}{S}$$

where U is milligrams of creatine per deciliter of urine; S is milligrams of creatinine per deciliter of serum; and V is milliliters of urine excreted per minute.

The normal range for creatinine clearance corrected to a surface area of 1.73 m² is 80 to 120 ml/minute. A creatinine clearance of 100 ml/minute means that in 1 minute the glomeruli in the kidneys are capable of clearing the creatinine from 100 ml of blood by filtration. Normal age-corrected creatinine clearance may be predicted by numerous formulas or normograms. One of the more popular formulas is:

$$\frac{\text{Creatinine}}{\text{clearance}} = \frac{(140 - \text{Patient's age}) \times \text{Body weight (kg)}}{72 \times \text{Serum creatinine}}$$

This formula is for men. The values for women are 85 percent of the predicted value for men.

Although the creatinine clearance may be reduced over a very broad range of renal damage, it is most useful as a prognostic device in patients with advanced renal insufficiency. Patients dying from chronic renal insufficiency usually have creatinine clearances of 10 ml/minute or less. When creatinine clearance is below 30 ml/minute serum electrolyte changes are usually evident.

Urine Concentration and Dilution Test. This test gives an estimate of the functional capacity of the renal tubules. On the day prior to the test the patient is given a usual breakfast. The patient is given no liquids for the remainder of the testing period. A dry lunch and dinner during the test period may include meat, potatoes, vegetables, pie, or gelatin. Oral medications may be taken with small amounts of water. At bedtime the patient must empty his or her bladder, discarding the specimen.

On the day of the test, after at least 14 hours of fluid deprivation, voided urine specimens are collected as follows: (1) contents of bladder on first voiding; (2) contents of bladder after 1 hour of bedrest; and (3) contents of bladder 1 hour later, after the patient has been ambulant.

All specimens are sent to the laboratory for specific gravity or osmolality determinations, care being taken to label each specimen with the time of collection. In addition the urine volume and protein content are measured.

For the urinary dilution portion of the test, the patient should be on bedrest during the entire period. Have the patient void, noting the time of voiding, and the drink 1200 ml of water (an occasional patient may vomit after drinking this much water). Collect urine specimens every hour for 4 hours and label each with the time voided. Send the specimens to the laboratory for specific gravity or osmolality determinations.

For urine concentrating ability it is preferable to measure the urine osmolality if this determination is available. Normally the urine osmolality is at least three times that of the plasma. This implies that the plasma osmolality must also be measured. It has been shown that if the urine osmolality is 850 mOsm/L or above, the concentrating ability is normal. A specific gravity of 1.025 or more in one of the specimens is accepted as evidence of normal concentrating ability. There are exceptions to this rule, however, and therefore, the osmolality is the preferred measurement.

With rehydration in the urinary dilution test, the specific gravity of the urine usually falls to 1.005 or less. If the specific gravity or osmolality is fixed, i.e., unchanging, this is taken as evidence of renal disease.

Acute Renal Failure

The causes of acute renal failure may be conveniently divided into prerenal, intrarenal, and postrenal. This classification is important as the diagnostic and therapeutic procedures for acute renal failure vary greatly depending on its cause. Prerenal azotemia develops as a result of decreased effective renal blood flow with resultant renal hypoperfusion. It is almost always due to hypotension or intravascular hypovolemia. Postrenal azotemia is due to obstruction of the urinary tract at any

TABLE 11-2. LABORATORY TESTS TO DIFFERENTIATE PRERENAL AZOTEMIA AND ACUTE TUBULAR NECROSIS

Determination	Urine and/or Serum Values	
	Prerenal	*ATN*
Urine sodium, mEq/L	<30	>30
Urine specific gravity	>1.018	<1.018
Urine osmolality	>400	<400
U/P osmolality ratio	1.2–3.0	0.9–1.2
U/P urea nitrogen ratio	>10	<10
U/P creatinine ratio	>30	<30
BUN:creatinine ratio (serum)	>10:1	10:1
FE_{Na}	<1.0	>1.0

U/P, urine/plasma; FE_{Na}, fractional excretion of sodium = (U/P) Na/(U/P) Cr × 100.

point along its course. Intrarenal azotemia is caused by pathology in the kidneys themselves. It is usually caused by acute tubular necrosis, but may be due to any one of a number of renal diseases.

The most common dilemma that arises clinically is whether acute renal failure is caused by prerenal azotemia or acute tubular necrosis. There are several laboratory tests that can be done to assist in this differentiation. They include urine sodium, urine specific gravity or osmolality, urine to plasma ratio of urea or creatinine, serum urea to creatinine ratio, and fractional excretion of sodium. Table 11–2 lists the findings in prerenal azotemia and acute tubular necrosis.

Chronic Renal Failure

Chronic renal failure leads to a number of laboratory abnormalities (Table 11–3). There is impairment of phosphorus ex-

TABLE 11-3. LABORATORY ABNORMALITIES IN UREMIA

Azotemia (increased blood urea, creatinine, uric acid)
Renal (or metabolic) acidosis
Hyperkalemia
Hypertension and myocardial failure
Anemia due to bone marrow suppression
Platelet dysfunction
Hypocalcemia, hyperphosphatemia, secondary hyperparathyroidism
Increased anion gap

TABLE 11–4. ABNORMALITIES OF RENAL TUBULAR FUNCTION

Substance Not Reabsorbed	Clinical Condition
Water	Nephrogenic diabetes insipidus (failure of tubule to respond to ADH)
Glucose (congenital)	Renal glycosuria
Hydrogen ion	Renal tubular acidosis
Phosphate	Vitamin D-resistant rickets
Cystine	Cystinuria
Amino acids, glucose, sodium, potassium, calcium, phosphate, bicarbonate, uric acid, protein	Fanconi's syndrome

cretion that results in chelation of calcium ions. This impairment combined with other factors leads to hypocalcemia and the development of secondary hyperparathyroidism. A normochromic, normocytic anemia is usually seen in chronic renal failure secondary to reduced erythropoietin production. There is a platelet dysfunction manifested by a bleeding tendency caused by impaired activation of platelet factor 3. Hyperkalemia can occur as the number of functional nephrons decrease. There is a metabolic acidosis caused by the impaired ability to excrete hydrogen ions and an increased anion gap caused by abnormal retention of phosphate, sulfate, and organic acid anions.

Inborn and Acquired Errors of Renal Tubular Function

A wide variety of tubular functional defects have been described, each defect having characteristic urinary and clinical features (Table 11–4). Although most of these syndromes are comparatively rare, some are quite important, if only from a differential diagnostic viewpoint.

Whereas these syndromes are primarily caused by defects within the renal tubules, an even larger group of inborn errors of metabolism are manifested by the appearance of amino acids or other metabolic products in the urine. These are, however, primarily diseases of the entire body, i.e., specific defects of protein or carbohydrate metabolism. This large group of diseases and their laboratory aspects is beyond the scope of this chapter.

SUGGESTED READINGS

Abuelo J: Proteinuria: Diagnostic principles and procedures. Ann Intern Med 98:186, 1983.

Abuelo J: The diagnosis of hematuria. Arch Intern Med 143:967, 1983.

Carson CC III, Segura JW, Greene LD: Clinical importance of microhematuria. JAMA 214:149, 1979.

Dunea G, Freedman P: Proteinuria. JAMA 203:973, 1968.

Dunea G, Freedman P: Renal clearance studies. JAMA 205:170, 1968.

Dunea G, Freedman P: Serum creatinine. JAMA 204:163, 1968.

Espinel C: The FE_{Na} test: Use in the differential diagnosis of acute renal failure. JAMA 236:579, 1976.

Greco F, Krumlovsky F: Role of the laboratory in management of acute and chronic renal failure. Ann Clin Lab Science 11:283, 1981.

Jacobson MH, Levy SE, Kaufman RM, et al.: Urine osmolality: A definitive test of renal function. Arch Intern Med 110:83, 1962.

Kopple JD, Coburn JW: Evaluation of chronic uremia. JAMA 227:41, 1974.

Kunin CM: Urinary tract infections—Flow charts (algorithms) for detection and treatment. JAMA 233:458, 1975.

Lubowitz H, Klahr S: Clinical estimation of functional nephron population. JAMA 203:657, 1968.

Miller T, et al.: Urinary diagnostic indices in acute renal failure. Ann Intern Med 89:47, 1978.

Oneson R, Groschel D: Leukocyte esterase activity and nitrite test as a rapid screen for significant bacteriuria. Am J Clin Pathol 83:84, 1985.

Pfallen M, Koontz F: Laboratory evaluation of leukocyte esterase and nitrite tests for the detection of bacteriuria. J Clin Microbiol 21:840, 1985.

Schrier R: Acute renal failure: Pathogenesis, diagnosis and management. Hosp Pract 16:93, 1981.

Ward P: Renal dysfunction: Proteinuria. Postgrad Med 69:91, 1981.

Ward P: Renal dysfunction: Urea and creatinine. Postgrad Med 69:93, 1981.

12
ACID-BASE DISORDERS

BASIC INFORMATION

Homeostasis

The primary homeostatic mechanisms for the regulation of the body pH within a rather narrow range are found in the buffer systems of the plasma and the erythrocytes. Two organs, the lungs and the kidneys, are secondarily involved. Many acute clinical conditions are associated with acid-base changes and are only partially corrected by the normal body systems. If the clinical condition directly involves either the lungs or the kidneys (or both organs) the resulting acid-base disturbances are magnified.

The relationships of the blood pH, PCO_2, and HCO_3^- (all reflect the acid-base status in the patient) are shown in Figure 12–1. The two coordinates show pH and HCO_3^-, whereas the partial pressure of carbon dioxide (PCO_2) at its normal level (40 mm Hg) is represented by the diagonal line sweeping from the upper right to the lower left. The normal condition is indicated by point A in the center of the figure.

The ratio of HCO_3^- to PCO_2 can change in four ways, i.e., HCO_3^- can increase or decrease and PCO_2 likewise can increase or decrease. Each of these four changes results in characteristic acid-base changes (Table 12–1), which are outlined in the following discussion.

Metabolic Acidosis

In metabolic acidosis, the primary change is a reduction of HCO_3^-, resulting in more acid pH (Fig. 12–1, point B). The HCO_3^- may decrease in many disorders, including uncontrolled diabetes or tissue hypoxia with lactic acidosis as, for

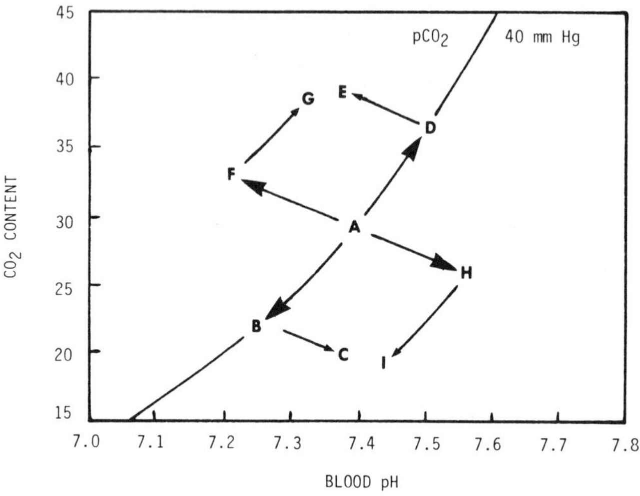

Figure 12–1. Blood pH, Pco_2, and HCO_3 relationships.

example, in shock. In this case, the respiratory system compensates by hyperventilation, which lowers the Pco_2 but raises the pH toward normal (Fig. 12–1, point C).

Metabolic Alkalosis

In metabolic alkalosis the primary change is elevation of HCO_3^- resulting in a more basic pH (Fig. 12–1, point D). This can be caused by uncompensated loss of acids (e.g., vomiting) or retention of bases. The respiratory system compensates by de-

TABLE 12–1. CHARACTERISTIC BLOOD CHANGES IN ACID-BASE DISORDERS*

Measurement	Mean Normal Value	Respiratory		Metabolic	
		Acidosis	*Alkalosis*	*Acidosis*	*Alkalosis*
Pco_2 (mm Hg)	40	↑	↓	N(↓)	N (↑)
HCO_3^- (mmol/L)	25	N(↑)	N(↓)	↓	↑
pH	7.40	↓	↑	↓	↑
Common causes		Hypoventilation	Hyperventilation	Diabetes, shock	Vomiting, excess alkali

N, normal; ↑, increased; ↓, decreased.
*Compensatory mechanisms in parentheses.

creasing pulmonary ventilation, which raises the P_{CO_2} and lowers the blood pH (Fig. 12–1, point E).

Respiratory Acidosis

In respiratory acidosis the primary change is an increase in P_{CO_2}, which results in a decrease in blood pH (Fig. 12–1, point F). The CO_2 retention that produces this change can be caused by hypoventilation or a ventilation–perfusion inequality. If the respiratory difficulties persist, the kidney compensates by the retention of HCO_3^- and the excretion of a more acidic urine, which tends to return the blood pH toward more normal levels, giving a compensated respiratory acidosis (Fig. 12–1, point G).

Respiratory Alkalosis

In respiratory alkalosis the primary change is a decrease in P_{CO_2} which results in an increased pH (Fig. 12–1, point H). Renal compensation occurs by an increased bicarbonate excretion, driving the pH back toward normal (Fig. 12–1, point I).

It is beyond the scope of this book to delve more deeply into the details of the pathophysiology of these conditions. Also, the therapy of the conditions will not be mentioned except as it relates to the monitoring of the effects of such therapy.

The initial study of these conditions lends itself admirably to the algorithmic or decision-tree approach, and such an approach will be used in the following discussion.

The reader is referred to a physiology textbook for review of the basic concepts of acid-base homeostasis as well as the pathophysiology of the common disorders. Finally, it must be pointed out that uncomplicated examples of these disorders are not always seen. For example, a metabolic acidosis superimposed on a chronic respiratory acidosis may at times be difficult to sort out.

The Anion Gap

The anion gap, also called the unmeasured anions, can be readily estimated from routine laboratory data. Although it is most useful in the diagnosis of the various types of metabolic acidosis, it may provide clues to other conditions. It is estimated using the following formula:

$$\text{Anion gap} = [Na^+ - (Cl^- + HCO_3^-)]$$

where the milliosmolar concentrations in the serum are substi-

TABLE 12–2. MEAN CONCENTRATIONS* OF ANIONS AND CATIONS

Measured cations		Measured anions	
Sodium (Na^+)	140	Chloride (Cl^-)	100
		Bicarbonate (HCO_3^-)	28
Unmeasured cations		Unmeasured anions	
Potassium (K^+)	4.5	Protein	15
Calcium (Ca^{2+})	5.0	Phosphate (PO_4^{3-})	2
Magnesium (Mg^{2+})	1.5	Sulfate (SO_4^{2-})	1
		Organic acids	5
Totals	151		151

*All measurements given in millimoles per liter.

tuted into the formula. A number of assumptions have been made in the use of this formula. One of the suggested readings listed at the end of this chapter (Oh and Carroll) discusses the concept in some detail. Nevertheless, the simplified formula given above provides very useful clinical information. In addition, the known interrelationships make the routine calculation of the anion gap a very useful quality control tool in the clinical laboratory (Table 12–2).

We know the following:

Total serum cations (151) = Total serum anions (151)

Substituting,

$$Na^+ + UC = Cl^- + HCO_3^- + UA$$

where UC denotes unmeasured cations and UA is unmeasured anions, or

$$140 + 11 = 100 + 28 + 23$$

Transposing to solve for $[Na^+ - (Cl^- + HCO_3^-)]$, i.e., the anion gap,

$$Na^+ - (Cl^- + HCO_3^-) = UA - UC$$

or

$$140 - 128 = 23 - 11$$
$$\text{Anion gap} = 12 \text{ mmol/L}$$

The normal range for the anion gap is from 8 to 16 mmol/L.

TABLE 12–3. CAUSES OF INCREASED ANION GAP

Decreased unmeasured cations
  Hypokalemia, hypocalcemia, or hypomagnesemia
Increased unmeasured anions
  Organic anions: lactate, keto acids
  Inorganic anions: phosphate, sulfate
  Protein: hyperalbuminemia (short-lived)
  Exogenous anions: salicylate, nitrate
  Medications: penicillin, carbenicillin
  Toxic agents: paraldehyde, etheylene glycol, methanol, salicylate
  Endogenous anions: uremia, hyperosmolar hyperglycemic nonketotic
    coma

Abnormalities of the Anion Gap

Unless there is some error in the measurement of Na^+, Cl^-, or HCO_3^-, any change in the anion gap must involve a change in the unmeasured anions or cations. The anion gap can be increased by two mechanisms: either a decrease in the unmeasured cations or an increase in the unmeasured anions. Table 12–3 catalogues some of the clinical conditions associated with an increased anion gap. In case of possibly decreased unmeasured cations, two of these cations (K^+ and Ca^{2+}) are almost routinely measured, and the third (Mg^{2+}) is readily measured in most laboratories. More commonly, an increased anion gap is attributable to an increased concentration of the unmeasured anions. Accumulations of organic acid, such as sulfate or phosphate in uremic acidosis, are common causes of an increased anion gap. Most of these substances are not readily measured; however, several (salicylate, methanol, and ethylene glycol) can be measured if necessary.

The anion gap can be decreased by two mechanisms: either an increase in the unmeasured cations or a decrease in the unmeasured anions. Causes of decreased anion gap are listed in Table 12–4. It is readily apparent that most of these specific causes can be easily measured in the laboratory. In fact, the routine measurements make the identification of these problems so straightforward that the general category of decreased anion gap is not usually even recognized as an entity.

The clinical usefulness of the anion gap lies primarily in its usefulness in the further delineation of the various causes of metabolic acidosis. Examples of this can be found in the section on metabolic acidosis.

TABLE 12–4. CAUSES OF DECREASED ANION GAP

Increased unmeasured cations
  Hyperkalemia, hypercalcemia, or hypermagnesemia
Retention of abnormal cations
  Myeloma globulins, Tris buffer, lithium
Decreased unmeasured anions
  Hypoalbuminemia

CLINICAL INVESTIGATION

Laboratory Studies

Screening Procedures

Electrolyte Panel. The measurement of electrolytes, i.e., sodium, potassium, chloride, and bicarbonate, is a readily available procedure and is widely and almost routinely ordered in many cases. A variety of abnormalities are seen clinically and are discussed throughout this book.

Definitive Procedures in Presumed Metabolic Acidosis

Blood pH. The measurement of blood pH is now almost always coupled with blood gas analyses. In metabolic acidosis the pH will give some quantitative measurement of the severity of the condition and will serve as a convenient benchmark for monitoring therapy. A pH of 7.1 or lower undoubtedly impairs cardiac and central nervous system functions and calls for prompt treatment. The P_{CO_2} will provide confirmatory evidence for the decreased bicarbonate concentration but is not of primary importance in the management of the uncomplicated case of metabolic acidosis.

Anion Gap. The calculation of the anion gap combined with data from the electrolyte panel, particularly the potassium levels, provides a valuable aid in the differentiation of acid-base disturbances (Table 12–5). The complete definition of these various forms of metabolic acidosis depends upon the clinical history or additional appropriate laboratory studies, or both, to confirm the presumed diagnosis.

TABLE 12–5. DEFINITIVE DIAGNOSIS OF METABOLIC ACIDOSIS

Normal Anion Gap		Increased Anion Gap
Low Potassium Concentration	*Elevated Potassium Concentration*	
Diarrhea	Chronic pyelonephritis	Diabetic ketoacidosis
Renal tubular acidosis (type 1 and 2)	Obstructive uropathy	Ketoacidosis with alcoholism
Carbonic anhydrase inhibitor medication	NH_4Cl medication	Renal failure
		Lactic acidosis, shock
		Toxins Methanol Salicylate Ethylene glycol Paraldehyde

Definitive Procedures in Presumed Metabolic Alkalosis

Blood pH. The blood pH gives some measure of the severity of the metabolic disorder and provides a convenient method for monitoring therapy.

Urine Chloride. The measurement of urine chloride provides a simple way to separate various causes of metabolic alkalosis (Table 12–6). Only a random sample is required. The decision level is around 10 mmol/L of chloride. This determination is also of prognostic value, indicating whether the condition will respond to chloride infusion.

TABLE 12–6. DEFINITIVE DIAGNOSIS OF METABOLIC ALKALOSIS

Low Urine Chloride (<10 mmol/L) (Salt-responsive)	High Urine Chloride (>10 mmol/L) (Salt-resistant)
Loss of gastric juice, vomiting	Hyperaldosteronism
Diuretic therapy	Cushing's syndrome
Posthypercapnea	Severe K^+ deficiency
Loss of Cl^- in diarrhea	Bartter's syndrome
	Licorice ingestion

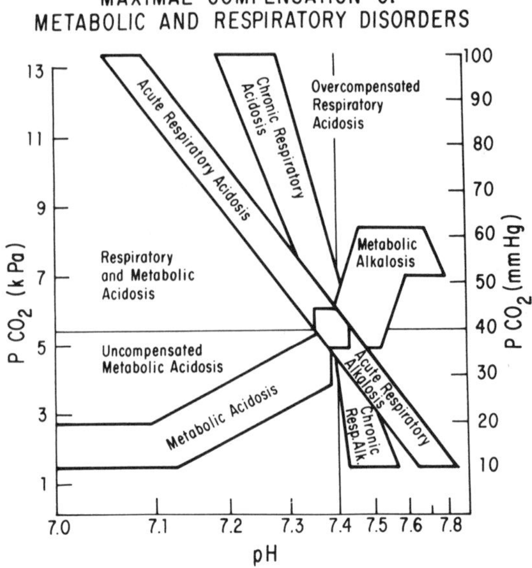

Figure 12–2. Maximal compensation of metabolic and respiratory disorders. (*Modified from Goldberg M, Green SB, Moss ML, et al.: Computer-based instruction and diagnosis—A systematic approach. JAMA 223:269, 1973.*)

Definitive Procedures in Respiratory Acidosis

Arterial Blood Gases. The measurement of PCO_2 and PO_2, usually in conjunction with the pH, provides a measurement of both the severity of the impairment of pulmonary function and the systemic effects of the pulmonary disease. In addition, monitoring the response to therapy with these measurements is most useful.

Blood gas and pH measurements are significantly different in acute, as compared with chronic respiratory acidosis. Figure 12–2 illustrates these changes.

Definitive Procedures in Respiratory Alkalosis

Arterial Blood Gases. The PO_2 and PCO_2 measurements, as well as arterial pH, are an indication of the severity of the acid-base disorder. The response to therapy is conveniently and directly measured by monitoring the blood gases. Some of the causes of respiratory alkalosis are listed in Table 12–7.

TABLE 12–7. CAUSES OF RESPIRATORY ALKALOSIS

Hyperventilation in:	
Pulmonary emboli	Salicylate poisoning
Bacteremia	Central nervous system disorders
Asthma	High altitudes
Hepatic disease	

Blood gas and pH measurements are significantly different in acute, as compared with chronic respiratory alkalosis. Figure 12–2 illustrates these changes.

SUGGESTED READINGS

Bear RA, Gribilk M: Assessing acid-base imbalances through laboratory parameters. Hosp Pract 9:157, 1974.

Coe FL: Metabolic alkalosis. JAMA 238:2288, 1977.

Emmett M, Narins R: Clinical use of the anion gap. Medicine 56:38, 1977.

Kassirer JP: Serious acid-base disorders. N Engl J Med 291:773, 1974.

Masoro E, Siegel P: Acid-Base Regulation: Its Physiology, Pathophysiology and the Interpretation of Blood Gas Analysis. Philadelphia, Saunders, 1977.

Newmark SR, Dluhy RG: Hyperkalemia and hypokalemia. JAMA 231:631, 1975.

Oh MS, Carroll HJ: The anion gap. N Engl J Med 297:814, 1977.

Tuller MA: Acid-Base Homeostasis and Its Disorders. Flushing, N.Y., Medical Exam Pub. Co., 1971.

West JB: Respiratory Physiology: The Essentials, 3rd ed. Baltimore, Williams & Wilkins, 1985.

13
ANEMIA

BASIC INFORMATION

Red Blood Cell Production

The circulating red blood cell is the final product of a series of divisions and maturation stages originating from a bone marrow stem cell. Coincidental with the cell divisions and maturation is the intracytoplasmic synthesis of hemoglobin. This production corresponds to the progression of cytoplasmic staining from the blue of immaturity to the red of the more mature forms. Hemoglobin production and the metabolic pathways for heme and globin biosynthesis are known in great detail.

Heme synthesis occurs in a series of steps beginning with the combination of succinyl-coenzyme A with glycine pyridoxal phosphate to form delta-aminolevulinic acid (ALA). Two molecules of ALA combine to form porphobilinogen (PBG), and four molecules of PBG subsequently combine to form uroporphyrinogen. This compound subsequently undergoes a series of internal structural changes, finally forming protoporphyrin, which combines with iron to form heme. Figure 13–1 illustrates these biosynthetic pathways and also illustrates where certain inborn and acquired errors of heme synthesis are accompanied by increases in some of these heme precursors.

Globin biosynthesis occurs simultaneously with heme production. Two different globin molecules (polypeptide chains) are synthesized. One, the alpha chain, consists of 141 amino acids and the other, the beta chain, contains 146 amino acids. The sequence of these amino acids is known. Deviation from the normal sequence are found in several inborn errors of

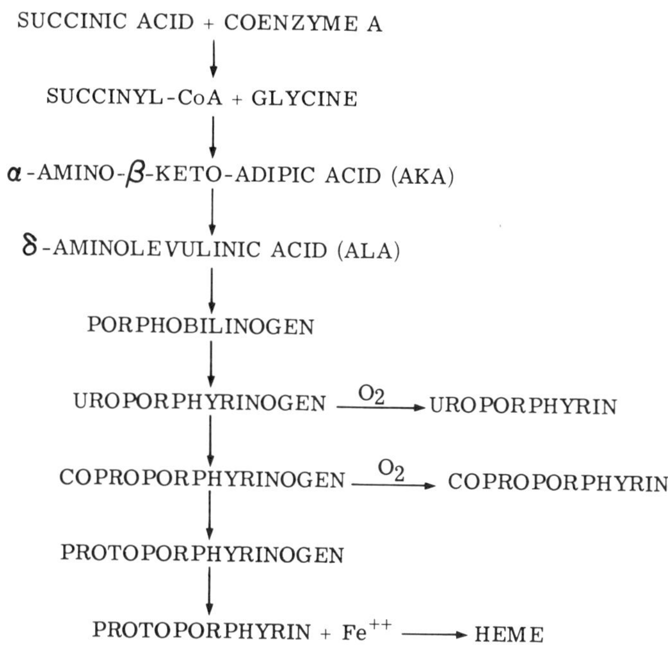

Figure 13–1. Heme biosynthesis. The reaction succinyl-CoA + glycine → AKA is inhibited in lead intoxication. Levels of ALA and PBG are increased in acute porphyria, whereas the level of protoporphyrinogen is increased in erythropoietic porphyria.

metabolism (e.g., Hb S, Hb C). An alpha and a beta chain combine to form a globin dimer, and then two globin dimers combine with four heme molecules to form a complete hemoglobin molecule.

Morpohologic Identification of Red Blood Cells

The identification of red blood cell precursors is primarily based on morphologic characteristics on bone marrow aspirate smear preparations stained with a Romanovsky stain such as a Wright or Giemsa stain. Other techniques as well as other stains are sometimes used. They are of limited importance except in the identification of other hematopoeitic cells (see Chap. 14). Table 13–1 summarizes some of the important features in determining the relative maturity of a hematopoietic cell, whether a white blood cell or red blood cell precursor. The following sections, and Figure 13–2, outline criteria for the more definitive identification of immature red blood cells.

TABLE 13–1. IMMATURE RED CELL IDENTIFICATION

	Immature	Mature
Cell Size	Larger	Smaller
Cytoplasm	Basophilic	Pink
Nuclear: cytoplasmic ratio	Larger	Smaller
Nucleus	Red-purple; fine Chromatin	Blue-black; coarsely clumped chromatin

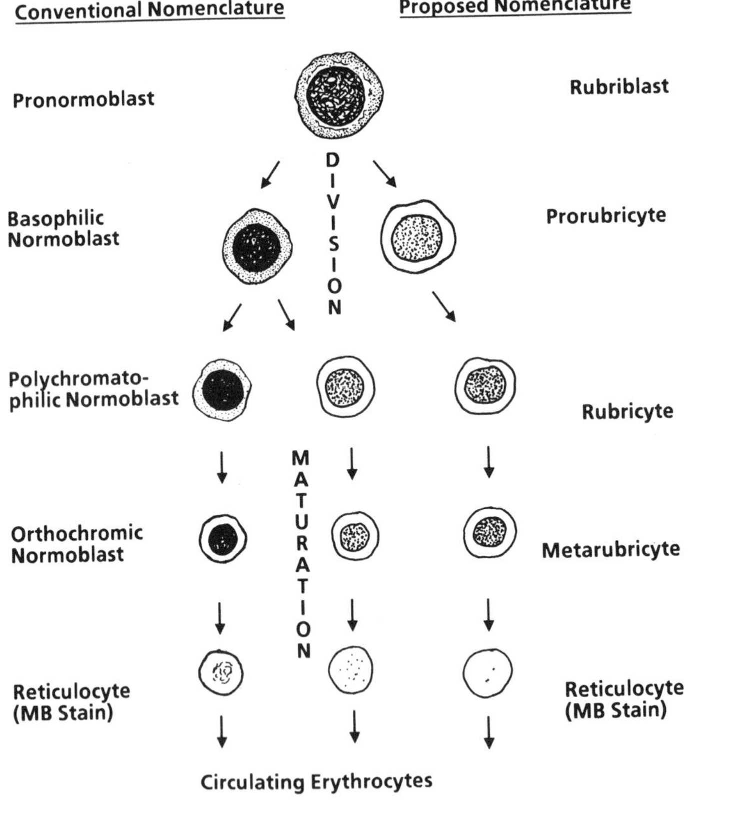

Figure 13–2. Erythropoiesis.

Types of Red Blood Cells

Rubriblast (Pronormoblast). The most immature red blood cell closely resembles the myeloblast. The more immature the cell, the more difficult it is to definitely identify. The rubriblast is characterized by a large, immature, centrally placed nucleus containing one or more prominent nucleoli. Nuclear chromatin is fine and delicate. The cytoplasm is blue, usually appearing to be bluer than that of a myeloblast. Occasionally there is a light blue halo around the nucleus, and at times cytoplasmic pseudopodia are seen.

Prorubricyte (Basophilic Normoblast). As the red blood cell precursor matures, both the cell and the nucleus become smaller. The nucleus loses its nucleolus, and the nuclear chromatin is more densely clumped. The cytoplasm in these cells is a paler blue than that of the rubriblast, but it remains definitely blue. No difficulty is encountered in distinguishing this and subsequent red blood cell precursors from other nucleated cells.

Rubricyte (Polychromatophilic Normoblast). As the cells mature, hemoglobinization of the cytoplasm becomes evident. The cytoplasm becomes blue-gray. The nucleus is smaller, and the nuclear chromatin is more densely clumped.

Metarubricyte (Orthochromic Normoblast). The last nucleated erythrocyte precursor has a dense nucleus. The cytoplasm stains in a manner similar to that of a mature erythrocyte.

Reticulocyte. This enucleated cell, somewhat larger than a mature erythrocyte, does not yet have the biconcave shape that is characteristic of the mature erythrocyte. Ribosomal RNA of reticulocytes may be aggregated by supravital stains, e.g., methylene blue. This is the stain used for the reticulocyte count.

Red Blood Cell Life Span

The mean life span of an erythrocyte is about 120 days. For experimental reasons it is more convenient to express red blood cell life span in terms of 50 percent survival or half-time ($\frac{1}{2}$T or T/2). Normally the mean half-time interval is 60 days. The most commonly available method for this measurement involves the use of sodium chromate labeled with Cr-51. The

TABLE 13–2. CAUSES OF EXCESSIVE HEMOLYSIS

Intravascular	Extravascular
Massive burns	Spherocytosis
Intravascular water	Sickle cell trait
(e.g., prostatic resection)	Thalassemia minor
Autoantibodies	Other hemoglobinopathies
Isoantibodies	Enzyme deficiencies
(hemolytic transfusion reactions)	(e.g., glucose-6-phosphate
Drug-induced hemolysis	dehydrogenase)
Paroxysmal nocturnal hemoglobinuria	
Sickle cell disease (occasionally)	
Thalassemia major (occasionally)	

normal marrow reserve can produce up to 10 times as many cells as are needed. In cases of accelerated destruction of erythrocytes, the erythrocyte survival time may be shortened to a T/2 of 6 days or less.

Intravascular and Extravascular Hemolysis

Toward the end of their life span, red blood cells lose the ability to maintain the biconcave disc shape. The senescent cell membrane is less able to maintain the sodium and potassium gradient across the membrane. Finally, the cell is phagocytized by the histiocytes of the reticuloendothelial system, primarily in the spleen. In the histiocyte the cell is destroyed; the globin portion is removed from the heme portion. The heme ring is broken, the iron is recycled, and the heme remenants are released into the plasma as bilirubin. The bilirubin, attached to albumin as a simple complex, is carried to the liver where it is subsequently conjugated to glucuronide. This process is called extravascular hemolysis and is the normal path for red blood cell removal.

In some cases (e.g., hemolytic transfusion reactions) excessive hemolysis may occur within the vascular compartment. In these cases red blood cell hemoglobin is released directly into the vascular space rather than traversing the reticuloendothelial cells. Up to 150 mg/dl of hemoglobin may be bound to haptoglobin, a normally occurring hemoglobin-binding protein. Hemoglobin in excess of this level is filtered through the renal tubules. Hemoglobin is then taken up by the tubular cells, which are subsequently sloughed into the urine. Urine

TABLE 13-3. ETIOLOGIC CLASSIFICATION OF ANEMIA

Type	Helpful Laboratory Tests
Anemia due to blood loss	Serum iron, TIBC, ferritin
Acute blood loss	
Chronic blood loss	
GI hemorrhage	
Menstruation	
Multiple pregnancies	
Anemia due to decreased production of red blood cells	
Nutritional	
Vitamin B_{12} deficiency	Serum B_{12}
Folate deficiency	Serum folate
Renal disease	BUN/creatinine
Bone marrow failure	
Idiopathic (aplastic anemia)	
Toxic (chemicals, drugs, irradiation)	Lead levels, etc.
Endocrine (myedema, adrenal)	Appropriate tests of endocrine function
Myelophthisis (myelofibrosis, leukemia myeloma, metastases)	Bone marrow examination especially biopsy
Anemia due to excessive destruction of red blood cells	
Hereditary	
Hereditary spherocytosis, elliptocytosis	Blood film examination, osmotic fragility
Enzyme deficiencies (e.g., G-6-PD deficiency, pyruvate kinase deficiency)	Screening enzyme tests
Hemoglobinopathies	Hemoglobin electrophoresis
Acquired	
Isoantibodies (transfusion, HDN)	Coomb's test
Autoantibodies (idiopathic, malignancy, CV disease)	Coomb's test
Drugs, chemicals (e.g., lead)	
Traumatic (mechanical)	
Infections	Cultures
Hypersplenism	
Paroxsymal nocturnal hemoglobinuria	Ham's test

hemosiderin is found only with intravascular hemolysis and is an important differential test in the study of hemolytic processes.

In the differential diagnosis of hemolytic anemia it is helpful, at times, to determine whether the hemolysis is intra- or

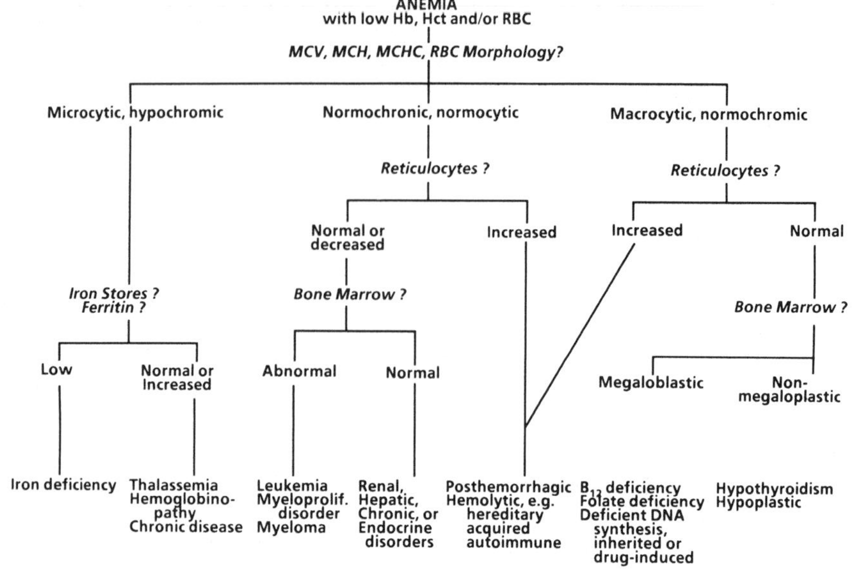

Figure 13–3. Classification of anemias based on morphology.

extravascular. Table 13–2 outlines these possibilities and divides various hemolytic syndromes on the basis of the location of the hemolysis.

CLASSIFICATION OF ANEMIA

There are two major ways to classify anemias. The first is based on the etiology of the anemia, e.g., blood loss, excessive destruction of red blood cells, or decreased production of red blood cells. This is the primary classification of the clinician (Table 13–3). The alternative is the morphologic classification. This is based primarily on the red blood cell indices and evaluation of the peripheral blood film. This is the primary classification of the clinical pathologist (Fig. 13–3). A blending of both systems provides the greatest amount of information for diagnosis and treatment and the maximal benefit to the patient.

CLINICAL INVESTIGATION

The clinical approach to an anemic patient begins with a good history and physical examination. Clues from the history and the physical examination will often save time, pain, and expense in obtaining the diagnosis.

History

The following are examples of topics that should be investigated.

- Diet. Alcoholics may develop folic acid deficiency anemia. Iron deficient diet can result in iron deficiency anemia.
- Drug ingestion and exposure to chemicals. Megaloblastic, hemolytic, and aplastic anemias may result from a variety of toxic agents.
- Occupation. People working in storage battery factories may develop anemia from lead poisoning.
- Bleeding history. Iron deficiency anemia can result from menorrhagia or multiple pregnancies.
- Ethnic and racial history. Sickle cell anemia in black patients; thalassemia in patients of Mediterranean descent; and pyruvate kinase deficiency in the Amish of central Pennsylvania.
- Neurologic symptoms. Patients with vitamin B_{12} deficiency commonly develop neurologic symptoms, such as distal parasthesias.
- Jaundice suggests hemolysis.
- History of other diseases producing anemias such as renal disease, liver disease, or chronic inflammatory diseases.

Physical Examination

A careful physical examination may reveal significant clues. Consider the following examples.

- Skin. Jaundice suggests hemolysis; dry skin, dry hair, and spooned nails suggest iron deficiency; leg ulcers suggest sickle cell disease.
- Eyes. Scleral icterus suggests hemolysis.
- Mouth. A dark line in the gums of the base of the teeth suggests lead poisoning; a smooth tongue and fissures at the corner of the mouth suggest a nutritional deficiency.
- Lymph nodes. Prominent lymphadenopathy in an anemic patient suggests lymphoma, leukemia, collagen vascular disease, infection, or sarcoidosis.
- Spleen. Mild splenomegaly may be seen in iron deficiency anemia and in some hemolytic anemias. Moder-

TABLE 13–4. HEMOGLOBIN—REFERENCE VALUES*

Group	Reference Range (Mean ± 2SD)	Significant Elevation	Significant Depression
Adult men	14–18	>19	<13
Adult women	12–16	>17	<11
Pregnant women (third trimester)	9–13	>14	<8
Newborns	19–23	>24	<17
Infants	10–14	>15	<9
Children	12–16	>17	<11

*All values given as grams per deciliter.

ate splenomegaly may be seen with chronic liver disease that is associated with red blood cell trapping and anemia. Massive splenomegaly is seen with the myeloproliferative disorders.

- Liver. Hepatomegaly may be seen in hemolytic anemia associated with Zieve's syndrome in the acute alcoholic. Nodular hepatomegaly may be seen with myelophthisic anemia such as carcinoma.
- Bones. Back pain and bone tenderness may be seen in the anemia secondary to myeloma.

Laboratory Examination

The initial laboratory evaluation of anemia should include a red blood cell count, hemoglobin, hematocrit, red blood cell indices, reticulocyte count, leukocyte count, and platelet count. It is also important to examine the peripheral blood film under the microscope.

Red Blood Cell Count, Hemoglobin, and Hematocrit

By definition, in anemia these counts are decreased. See Tables 13–4 and 13–5 for reference values for hemoglobin and hematocrit.

Red Blood Cell Indices

The calculations of the red blood cell indices using the red blood count, hemoglobin, and hematocrit can be very useful in approaching an anemia, as has been discussed earlier.

The mean corpuscular volume (MCV) represents the average volume of the red blood cell. It is calculated by the formula:

$$MCV = \frac{Hematocrit \times 10}{Red\ cell\ count\ (in\ millions)}$$

The mean corpuscular hemoglobin (MCH) is the average amount of hemoglobin in the red blood cell. It is calculated by the formula:

$$MCV = \frac{Hemoglobin \times 10}{Red\ cell\ count\ (in\ millions)}$$

The mean corpuscular hemoglobin concentration (MCHC) is the hemoglobin concentration of the average cell. It is calculated by the formula:

$$MCHC = \frac{Hemoglobin \times 100}{Hematocrit}$$

The normal values for the red blood cell indices are shown in Table 13–6.

Reticulocyte Count

The reticulocyte count allows a quick assessment of red blood cell production by simple and reliable techniques. One should always correct the reticulocyte count for the hematocrit:

$$\frac{Corrected}{reticulocyte\ count\ (\%)} = \frac{Actual}{reticulocyte\ count\ (\%)} \times \frac{Patient's\ hematocrit}{Normal\ hematocrit\ (i.e.,\ 0.45)}$$

Normal values for the reticulocyte count are about 1 ± 0.5 percent. Low corrected reticulocyte counts in the face of anemia suggest insufficient or inefficient erythropoiesis for any one of a number of reasons. An increased reticulocyte count suggests a hemolytic process or a recovering posthemorrhagic state.

Peripheral Blood Film

Examination of the peripheral blood film is one of the most important parts of the evaluation of anemia. There are a number of important observations that can be made concerning the erythrocytes, e.g., color, size, shape, and structure. These observations may give important clues as to the cause of a patient's anemia.

TABLE 13–5. HEMATOCRIT—REFERENCE VALUES*

Group	Reference Range (Mean ± 2SD)	Significant Elevation	Significant Depression
Adult men	0.40–0.50	>0.53	<0.37
Adult women	0.38–0.47	>0.52	<0.35
Pregnant women (third trimester)	0.30–0.40	>0.43	<0.27
Newborns	0.50–0.60	>0.63	<0.47
Infants	0.33–0.43	>0.46	<0.30
Children	0.35–0.45	>0.48	<0.32

*All values given as volume per volume (v/v).

Color. The depth of staining gives a rough guide to the hemoglobin content of the red blood cells. Normochromic cells have by definition a normal staining intensity. Hypochromic cells are paler with a larger central clear area. This is associated with a decreased amount of hemoglobin. Hyperchromic cells stain deeper and have less central pallor. This is associated with an increased hemoglobin content. Variation in color is anisochromia and is seen in sideroblastic anemia.

Size. Red blood cells may be abnormally small (microcytes), abnormally large (macrocytes), or show abnormal variation in size (anisocytosis). Anisocytosis is a rather nonspecific finding seen in a wide variety of anemias. (See Fig. 13–3 for anemias associated with various cell sizes.)

Shape. Red blood cells may vary in shape. This is called poikilocytosis. Any abnormally shaped cell is a poikilocyte. There

TABLE 13–6. RED BLOOD CELL INDICES—REFERENCE VALUES

Index	Reference Range (Mean ± 2SD)	Significant Increase	Significant Decrease
Mean corpuscular volume (MCV), Hct/RBC (fl)	82–97	>101	<78
Mean corpuscular hemoglobin (MCH), Hb/RBC (fmol)	27–32	>33	<26
Mean corpuscular hemoglobin concentration (MCHC), Hb/Hct (g/dl)	32–36	>37	<32

are a variety of poikilocytes that can be found and, if one variety is present in significant numbers, this can be a useful diagnostic finding.

Spherocytes are nearly spherical erythrocytes as compared to the normal biconcave disc. Smaller or microspherocytes are seen in hereditary spherocytosis; larger spherocytes are found in immune hemolytic anemias. Target cells are erythrocytes with a peripheral rim of cytoplasm and a dark central hemoglobin-containing area. They are seen in liver disease, after splenectomy, and in other hemoglobinopathies. Schistocytes are fragments of red blood cells that have been partially destroyed in such conditions as microangiopathic hemolytic anemia. Such shapes as helmets and triangles or blistered cells can be found.

Acanthocytes are red blood cells with irregular spicules whose ends may at times be bulbous or rounded. They are seen in liver disease abetalipoproteinemia, and other lipid metabolism disorders. Echinocytes (burr cells or crenated cells) are cells with an irregularly shaped periphery. They are seen in uremia, pyruvate kinase deficiency, and may be artifactual.

Teardrop cells with the characteristic shape that their name implies are seen in myelofibrosis, myeloid metaplasia, and thalassemia.

Structure. Basophilic stippling is characterized by the diffuse presence of irregular basophilic granules within the erythrocyte. Stippling is usually seen in anemias associated with disorders of hemoglobin synthesis, e.g., lead poisoning or thalassemia. Howell-Jolly bodies are smooth round nuclear remnants. Normally the spleen removes these remnants, hence, they can be seen in postsplenectomy patients. They are also seen in severe anemias.

Nucleated red blood cells are seen in the peripheral blood when the marrow is subjected to intense stimulation, e.g., acute hemorrhage, severe hemolytic anemia, or marrow replacement by metastatic carcinoma or leukemia.

Bone Marrow Examination

The aspiration of a bone marrow specimen should not be considered as a routine study in all patients with hematologic abnormalities. Rather, it should be done only after a consideration of the possible benefits to the patient and after a careful examination of the peripheral blood films and other laboratory data. Although local anesthetics or aspiration from the iliac crest (rather than the sternum) have eliminated much of the physical pain from the procedure, considerable psychic trauma precedes and accompanies marrow aspiration in most patients. The technique of marrow aspiration is outlined in Chapter 24.

After one arrives at a tentative diagnosis or differential diagnosis, a bone marrow examination may help establish or rule out a number of different diseases, as is summarized in Table 13–7. The figures in parentheses indicate the relative number of such cases in one university hospital hematology service. The remainder (approximately 40 percent) of the cases usually show nonspecific reactive changes as in granulocytic hyperplasia.

At times, a marrow aspiration may be indicated although no hematologic abnormalities are present. The evaluation of marrow cellularity before treatment by irradiation or chemotherapy would be such an indication. Following treatment for leukemia one or more marrow aspirates are necessary to permit adequate evaluation of the therapy. Occasionally, metastatic tumor or various storage disease may be present without hematologic abnormalities, and therefore such considerations may be an indication for marrow aspiration.

With the data accumulated from the history and the physical examination, as well as the initial laboratory evaluation, the physician is usually able to make a preliminary diagnosis of the cause of the anemia. After reaching a preliminary diagnosis based on these studies, the physician should then use specific diagnostic procedures to conclusively make the exact diagnosis.

TABLE 13–7. FINDINGS ON BONE MARROW EXAMINATION

Iron-deficiency anemia* (17%)	Lymphoma (3%)
Megaloblastic anemia (5%)	Plasma cell myeloma (1%)
Hypoplastic or aplastic anemia (9%)	Metastatic tumor ($<$1%)
Thrombocytopenia (4%)	Infectious granulomata ($<$1%)
Agranulocytosis or granulocytic hypoplasia (8%)	Reticuloendothelioses ($<$1%)
Leukemia (13%)	

*Evaluation of iron stores. Substitute serum ferritin.

IRON-DEFICIENCY ANEMIA

Iron Metabolism

Of all the trace metals iron is the most important because it is one of the integral building blocks of hemoglobin. The absorption of iron from the gastrointestinal tract is quite inefficient. Normally only about 10 percent is absorbed. The iron-poor diets of a large number of patients and the significant losses of iron caused by either pathologic or physiologic bleeding, e.g., in menstruation or pregnancy, result in large numbers of persons with varying degrees of iron deficiency, either latent or manifest.

Allocation of Body Iron

The body normally contains a total of about 3.5 g of iron. About 66 percent of the total body iron is bound to circulating hemoglobin; 30 percent is in iron stores (ferritin and hemosiderin); 3 to 5 percent is in myoglobin; 1 percent is in the iron containing enzymes (cytochromes, peroxidase, and catalase); and about 0.1 percent is circulating bound to specific iron-binding protein, i.e., transferrin.

Iron Absorption

The major absorption of iron occurs in the proximal small bowel. Gastric juice and gastric acidity enhance the absorption of inorganic iron. The small intestinal mucosa also influences the absorption of iron.

Food iron, reduced to the ferrous (Fe^{2+}) state, enters the mucosal cell, where it is combined with apoferritin to form ferritin. The iron is then transferred across the cell membrane and into the plasma, where it is carried by an iron-binding protein (transferrin or siderophilin) to the tissue iron receptors, chiefly the erythroid elements in the marrow.

The usual dietary intake of iron varies between 10 and 15 mg/day, about 10 percent of which is normally absorbed. In anemia of any type, iron absorption is increased. For instance, in iron-deficiency anemia, iron absorption may be increased up to 80 percent of the ingested amount. In pregnancy, absorption approaches 40 percent. Noniron-deficiency anemias also result in increased iron absorption. In hemochromatosis (presumably an inborn error of iron metabolism) there is apparently a slight but definite increase in iron absorption. Over many years greatly increased amounts of iron accumulate in the body in patients with this disease.

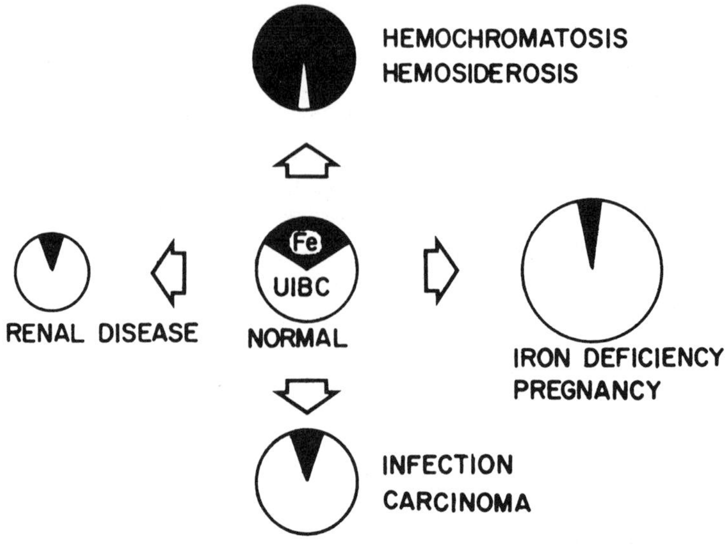

Figure 13–4. Serum iron and iron-binding capacity patterns. The size of the circles is proportional to the total iron-binding capacity, whereas the darkened areas represent the bound iron.

Transport of Iron Plasma

Iron is transported in the blood plasma bound to a specific iron-binding protein, a beta-1-globulin having a molecular weight of about 80,000 daltons. Each molecule of this globulin, known as transferrin or siderophilin, can combine with two atoms of ferric iron. Transferrin gives up the iron to the maturing cells for hemoglobin synthesis within these cells. Normally about one-third of plasma transferrin is bound with iron. The total capacity of transferrin for iron, called the total iron-binding capacity (TIBC), includes the yet unfilled iron-binding capacity designated the latent or unsaturated iron-binding capacity (LIBC or UIBC) plus the transferrin bound to iron.

Although the measurement of serum iron alone is of primary importance in the assessment of disorders of iron metabolism, the measurement of TIBC results in characteristic patterns in certain clinical conditions. For example, in iron-deficiency anemia the serum iron levels are quite low (<50 μg/dl), whereas the TIBC is characteristically though not invariably increased. The reason for this elevation is not known. In hemochromatosis the TIBC may be normal or at times even decreased, whereas the percentage of saturation with iron of the iron-binding protein approaches 100 percent. In renal diseases in which the iron-binding protein is lost into the urine, the TIBC falls to low levels. Figure 13–4 summarizes these characteristic changes.

There is a diurnal variation in serum iron levels; the concentration is greatest in the early morning and least in the afternoon. Total iron-binding capacity does not vary diurnally.

Iron Storage

Normally about 30 percent or 1.0 g of the total body iron is stored, primarily in the bone marrow, the liver, and the spleen. This storage iron can be easily visualized by staining tissues using a Prussian blue reaction, which stains the storage hemosiderin dark blue. Iron is also stored as ferritin (which is usually nonstainable), the distribution of which is quite similar to that of hemosiderin.

In iron deficiency, iron stores are completely depleted. In diseases characterized by increased absorption of iron (hemochromatosis) or by increased parenteral iron dosage (e.g., following numerous transfusions), the stores may be markedly increased. Occasionally up to 50 g of iron may be stored in the body.

Serum Ferritin

The detection in serum of minute levels of the storage form of iron, i.e., ferritin, has provided a very sensitive and practical method for the accurate determination of body storage iron. Ferritin levels are decreased when stores are depleted. The

TABLE 13–8. CAUSES OF IRON DEFICIENCY

Decreased Dietary Iron	Decreased Iron Absorption	Increased Losses
Decreased meat diet	Postgastrectomy state	Genitourinary or gastrointestinal tract hemorrhage, chronic
Vegetarians	Sprue	
Total milk diet in infants	Duodenal diverticulae	Pregnancies, multiple
	Blind loop syndrome	Excessive menstruation
	Myxedema	Parasitic infections, e.g., hookworm (rare)

correlation with marrow estimation of storage iron has been excellent.

Clinical Features

The causes of iron deficiency are multiple but may be grouped into three major categories as shown in Table 13–8. The patient will have signs and symptoms of anemia as well as from the predisposing causes of the particular anemia. In general, the patient complains of chronic fatigue and often also of weakness. With more severe anemia, dizzy spells, headache, palpitations, and paresthesias may occur. Although splenomegaly may be present, most clinicians believe that this is an uncommon finding. The stated characteristic clinical features associated with iron deficiency—koilonychia, stomatitis, and dysphagia—are so uncommon as to be of little use in most situations.

Laboratory Studies

Screening Procedures

Red Blood Cell Morphology. The morphology and staining of erythrocytes in iron deficiency of moderate severity are so characteristic that the finding of hypochromic (and microcytic) red blood cells, annulocytes, is almost diagnostic of the condition. However, several other anemias (sideroblastic anemia, thalassemia, and anemia of chronic disease) may have some similar features, and more definitive laboratory testing may be indicated.

Definitive Procedures

A number of laboratory determinations are quite helpful in the diagnosis of iron-deficiency and related anemias. Table 13–9 compares these studies for easier understanding. A number of parameters as well as good clinical judgment are necessary to differentiate iron-deficiency anemia from other microcytic hypochromic varieties.

Serum Iron and Iron Binding Capacity. The serum iron levels are significantly decreased below 50 μg/dl and frequently the iron concentration is below 15 μg/dl. Although characteristically the TIBC is increased, only about two of three iron-deficient patients may show this change. A characteristic decreased saturation of the iron-binding protein to below 15 per-

TABLE 13–9. MICROCYTIC HYPOCHROMIC ANEMIAS

	Normal	Latent Iron Deficiency	Iron-Deficiency Anemia	Thalassemia	Sideroblastic Anemia	Anemia of Chronic Disease
Anemia	Absent	Absent	Present	Present	Present	Present (mild)
Reticulocyte count	<1.5%	Normal	Normal	Increased	Decreased	Decreased
Serum iron	75–150 µg/dl	Slight decrease	Decreased	Increased	Increased	Decreased
Transferrin saturation (%)	30–45	Normal	<15	Increased	Near 100	Decreased
Serum ferritin	10–200 ng/ml	< 9 ng/ml	< 9 ng/ml	Increased	Increased	Increased
Marrow iron stores						
Hemosiderin	Normal	Reduced	Absent	Increased	Normal or increased	Normal or increased
Sideroblasts	Few	Normal	Absent	Increased	Normal or increased	—
Marrow cellularity	Normal	Normal	Variable	Increased	Increased	Variable
Response to iron therapy	No	Yes	Yes	No	No	Poor
Red cell morphology	Normal	Normal	Hypochromic, microcytic, anisocytosis, poikilocytosis	Targets	Hypochromic, microcytic, stippling Normal	Normal or nonspecific Targets

cent is probably the single most consistent abnormality in iron deficiency.

Marrow Iron Stores. In both latent and evident iron-deficiency anemia, bone marrow iron stores are markedly decreased or absent.

Serum Ferritin. This test, done on serum, provides a convenient measure of iron stores, avoiding a traumatic bone marrow examination. Ferritin levels are decreased in iron-deficiency states. Falsely elevated ferritin levels have been seen in rheumatoid disease, acute myocardial infarction, acute leukemia, hepatitis, and alcoholic cirrhosis, conditions that may therefore mask a depletion of iron stores.

BLOOD LOSS ANEMIAS

Clinical Features

Probably the most common cause of anemia is blood loss, either acute or chronic. Acute blood loss is discussed in Chapter 5, which examines hypotension and shock. This section discusses some ways in which the laboratory can help to diagnose anemia caused by chronic blood loss.

Chronic blood loss can, of course, occur from bleeding into any body cavity or into the gastrointestinal or genitourinary tract. Pregnancy is a common cause of anemia, usually caused by iron deficiency. The fetus is quite adept at acquiring iron for red blood cell production, even at the expense of the mother. Excessive menstruation also may lead to iron-deficiency anemia. Finally, excessive blood donations may result in anemia. Chronic blood loss usually results in iron-deficiency anemia, and all laboratory procedures directed toward that entity are applicable here.

Laboratory Studies

Testing for Occult Blood

The discovery of the bleeding site is at times very difficult. The examination of vomitus, stool, urine, or sputum for blood may be of help. The sensitivity of the test should be set so that the small amounts of meat myoglobin or vegetable peroxidase that may be found in such fluids do not yield false-positive results.

Iron Stains of Desquamated Cells

Occasionally the staining of desquamated cells for hemosiderin may be of benefit. Hemosiderin-laden macrophages may be seen in the sputum of patients with chronic pulmonary hemorrhage (hemosiderosis in Goodpasture's disease), or hemosiderin-filled renal tubular cells may be seen in patients with increased intravascular hemolysis and resulting chronic iron losses.

Serial Hemoglobin/Hematocrit Measurements

The interpretation of laboratory evidence of presumed blood loss, e.g., in bleeding peptic ulcer, must be modified by the knowledge of inherent variability of the procedures as well as the rates of fluid and blood replacement. A change of greater than 3 SD of the laboratory variability of the procedure is considered significant. In the case of hemoglobin, in most laboratories this would be a change greater than 1.0 g/dl and for the hematocrit, greater than 0.03.

MEGALOBLASTIC ANEMIA

Background Information

Megaloblastic anemias are most often caused by a deficiency of vitamin B_{12}, or folate, or both. It is important to realize that there are many causes of vitamin B_{12} deficiency and folate deficiency, e.g., inadequate intake, decreased absorption, or increased use. Vitamin B_{12} and folate are both involved in DNA synthesis.

Vitamin B_{12} is found in almost all animal tissues. It is absorbed in the terminal ileum after being complexed with an intrinsic factor that is secreted by the parietal cells of the stomach. One can imagine that there could be a number of causes of vitamin B_{12} deficiency; e.g., inadequate intake (vegetarians); lack of intrinsic factor secondary to gastric atrophy with loss of gastric secretions (pernicious anemia) or postgastrectomy; or lack of absorption secondary to ileal diseases such as sprue or ileitis. Normally the body stores a several years' supply of vitamin B_{12}.

Folate is found in many foods, especially green leafy vegetables. It is absorbed in the proximal jejunum. It does not require an intrinsic factor for absorption. There are also a number of causes of folate deficiency; e.g., inadequate intake associated with alcoholism; lack of absorption secondary to ileal diseases such as sprue or ileitis; or increased requirements such as pregnancy. Normally the body stores less folate (only a several months' supply) than vitamin B_{12}, therefore megaloblastic anemia is more common secondary to folate deficiency rather than to vitamin B_{12} deficiency.

Clinical Findings

Patients usually complain of fatigue and weakness secondary to the anemia. They may also have glossitis or gastrointestinal symptoms such as abdominal pain, constipation, or diarrhea. In addition patients with vitamin B_{12} deficiency, but not folate deficiency, may manifest neurologic signs and symptoms such as distal paresthesias, loss of position or vibratory sense, weakness, or spasticity. On physical examination the patient may appear pale and slightly icteric. The degree of anemia varies from mild to severe.

Laboratory Studies

Screening Procedures

Red Blood Cell Morphology. Here again, the simplest test to screen for megaloblastic anemia is the well-stained peripheral blood film. The macrocytes have a characteristic oval or "Irish potato" appearance as opposed to the more rounded macrocytes seen in liver disease. In addition, there usually are many bizarre poikilocytes. Howell-Jolly bodies may be found in occasional red blood cells. Finally, the observation of hypersegmented polymorphonuclear leukocytes (six or more lobes) is characteristic of megaloblastic anemia.

Lactate Dehydrogenase. As with the bilirubin measurement, lactate dehydrogenase levels are frequently markedly elevated in the megaloblastic anemia apparently due to ineffective erythropoeisis in this disease. The lactate dehydrogenase (LD) isoenzymes LD-1 and LD-2 are responsible for the increase.

Bilirubin. Because there is also a mild hemolytic component (intramedullary hemolysis), the nonspecific laboratory tests for hemolysis (unconjugated bilirubin or urobilinogen) may show elevated values.

Haptoglobin. Again because of the mild hemolysis, serum haptoglobin is decreased.

Bone Marrow. The bone marrow is megaloblastic and hypercellular with an increase in the erythroid elements. Megaloblasts are red blood cell precursors that are larger than normal and have a finer, more delicate, chromatin pattern than normal. The granulocytic series shows giant forms. The most characteristic is the giant band cell.

Definitive Procedures

Serum Vitamin B_{12} and Folate Concentrations. The measurement of serum vitamin B_{12} or folate levels is a convenient and simple way to diagnose deficiencies of these substances. There are two major types of assays, microbiologic assays and radioimmunoassays. The microbiologic assays are more reliable but take longer to perform. Because some patients may have low but still normal levels of vitamin B_{12} when assayed using the newer radioimmunoassay procedures, caution is advised in the interpretation of these tests.

Therapeutic Trials

Vitamin B_{12}. The patient is given low doses of vitamin B_{12} (1 μg) and observed for a hematologic response. No reticulocyte response should be seen in patients with folate deficiencies, whereas patients with vitamin B_{12} deficiencies should have a reticulocytosis about 5 to 7 days after therapy.

Folate. The patient is given low doses of folate (50 to 200 μg/day) and observed for a hematologic response. Patients deficient in folate should develop a reticulocytosis after 5 to 7 days, whereas patients deficient in vitamin B_{12} should not.

Tests Useful to Determine the Cause of Vitamin B_{12} Deficiency

Gastric Analysis. The absence of gastric acidity may be of help in diagnosing pernicious anemia. The test must be done with histamine stimulation before it is decided that the patient is truly achlorhydric. A significant number of elderly patients have achlorhydria that responds to histamine stimulation.

Schilling Test. The Schilling test is less popular than it was previously. However, it does allow for the definitive diagnosis of vitamin B_{12} malabsorption. In this test the patient is given an oral dose of radioactive vitamin B_{12} and then a large flushing parenteral dose of nonradioactive vitamin B_{12}. This test measures the patient's ability to absorb (and subsequently excrete)

TABLE 13–10. CHARACTERISTIC RESULTS OF SCHILLING TESTS

	Normal	Pernicious Anemia, Postgastrectomy	Malabsorption
Vitamin B_{12} alone	5%	0–3%	0–3%
Vitamin B_{12} + intrinsic factor	5%	>5%	0–3%

radioactive vitamin B_{12}. Care must be taken to obtain complete collections of urine. In patients with urinary retention, catheterization or prolonged (>24 hour) collection periods may be necessary to rule out the possibility of malabsorption. Measuring plasma levels of radioactive vitamin B_{12} avoids the difficulties associated with 24-hour urine collection. Vitamin B_{12} with intrinsic factor is given as a confirmatory procedure. Typical excretion results for the Schilling test are in Table 13–10.

One significant advantage of the test is that it will be abnormal in all patients with the disease even when hemoglobin and serum vitamin B_{12} levels are normal.

ANEMIA OF CHRONIC DISEASE

Clinical Features

The anemia of chronic disease is seen in a variety of chronic disorders such as chronic infections, chronic noninfectious inflammations (systemic lupus erythematosus or rheumatoid arthritis), and malignant diseases. The anemia is usually mild to moderate and is overshadowed by the signs and symptoms of the underlying disease.

Laboratory Studies

Screening Procedures

Perpheral Film. The red blood cells are usually normochromic and normocytic, though they may be hypochromic or microcytic. The leukocytes and platelets are morphologically normal.

Reticulocyte Count. The reticulocyte count is normal or reduced.

Serum Iron and Total Iron Binding Capacity. These studies are both decreased. The percent iron saturation is usually decreased (15 to 30 percent) though not as low as in iron-deficiency anemia.

Bone Marrow. The bone marrow is usually normal. Iron stains reveal decreased sideroblastic iron but increased storage iron.

ANEMIA OF RENAL FAILURE

Clinical Features

There is a positive correlation between the severity of the anemia in renal disease and the blood creatinine level. Several factors are involved in this anemia. First, there is a decreased erythropoeitin production by the damaged kidney. Second, the uremic environment shortens the red blood cell life span. Third, the uremic serum appears to contain inhibitors to red blood cell production.

Laboratory Studies

Screening Procedures

Peripheral Film. The red cells are usually normochromic and normocytic. Numerous burr cells are seen. The leukocytes and platelets are usually normal.

Reticulocyte Count. The reticulocyte count is usually normal or decreased.

Definitive Procedures

Laboratory tests used in evaluating renal disease are discussed at length in Chapter 11.

ANEMIA OF LIVER DISEASE

Clinical Features

Many patients with liver disease also have anemia, the cause of which is not completely understood. It is known, however, that there are significant hemolytic, deficiency, and toxic components present in variable combinations. In addition, gastrointestinal bleeding from varices or a peptic ulcer may complicate the picture.

Because of the widespread incidence of liver disease, this type of anemia is much more common than most of the other anemias discussed in this chapter. The clinical aspects are those of the primary hepatic disease.

Laboratory Studies

Screening Procedures

Peripheral Blood Film. Again, the peripheral blood smear is quite helpful in diagnosing this type of anemia. There is most often a moderate macrocytosis, but these red blood cells are round as compared with the oval macrocytes of megaloblastic anemia. Target cells, stomatocytes, or acanthocytes may occasionally be seen. If there is a significant splenomegaly with hypersplenism, there may also be thrombocytopenia and granulocytopenia.

Definitive Procedures

Other than measurement of folate levels, no definitive laboratory procedures are presently available. Laboratory procedures are still done to rule out other causes of anemia. Chemical measurements are chiefly a reflection of primary hepatic disease and are treated at length in Chapter 9, which discusses the problem of jaundice.

HEMOLYTIC ANEMIAS

General Considerations

Hemolytic anemias are anemias secondary to shortened red blood cell life span. There are a number of different causes for hemolytic anemias. They can be caused by a defect of the red blood cell itself or by factors outside the red blood cell. Red blood cell defects can be divided into membrane, metabolic, or hemoglobin defects. Examples of each of these are discussed. An example of a hemolytic anemia caused by factors outside the red blood cell is discussed, i.e., autoimmune hemolytic anemia.

General Laboratory Findings

Peripheral Blood Film

The morphologic features of the peripheral film will often suggest the possible diagnosis. These are discussed for each particular diagnosis.

Reticulocyte Count

The reticulocyte count is usually elevated in hemolytic anemias reflecting the compensatory increase in erythropoeisis by the bone marrow. The normal corrected reticulocyte count is 0.5 to 1.5 percent. In hemolytic anemias it is frequently increased to 10 to 20 percent.

Serum Haptoglobin

Serum haptoglobins are $alpha_2$-glycoproteins that can combine with hemoglobin. The normal range is 50 to 150 mg/dl. Hemolysis leads to formation of hemoglobin–haptoglobin complexes. Thus, a decrease in the serum haptoglobin levels is suggestive of hemolysis.

Bilirubin

Increased unconjugated (indirect) serum bilirubin is usually seen in hemolysis. This is a rather nonspecific finding but can be useful.

Serum Lactate Dehydrogenase

LD is elevated in patients with hemolysis, more so with intravascular hemolysis than extravascular hemolysis.

These are the general laboratory findings seen in most cases of hemolytic anemias. More specific laboratory findings are discussed with each particular diagnosis.

HEMOLYTIC ANEMIAS ASSOCIATED WITH RED BLOOD CELL MEMBRANE DEFECTS

There are a number of hemolytic anemias associated with red blood cell membrane defects. Two will be discussed: hereditary spherocytosis and paroxysmal nocturnal hemoglobinuria.

HEREDITARY SPHEROCYTOSIS

Clinical Features

Hereditary spherocytosis is a hereditary hemolytic disorder characterized by microspherocytic anemia, intermittent jaundice, red blood cell membrane defects, splenomegaly, and a good response to splenectomy. It is inherited as an autosomal dominant trait. The exact molecular abnormality of the red blood cell membrane defect is not known. The hemolytic process is variable in severity.

Laboratory Studies

Screening Procedures

Red Blood Cell Morphology. The search for microspherocytes on a well-prepared and carefully stained blood film may reveal only very few such cells, but they are almost diagnostic when found. As other conditions give rise to spherocytes (usually larger), such information must be properly interpreted. Conditions that are associated with larger spherocytes include burns, other autoimmune anemias, and hemolytic disease of the newborn.

Definitive Procedures

Osmotic Fragility Studies. The careful measurement of erythrocyte osmotic fragility is the procedure of choice. It measures the ability of the red blood cell to withstand graded hypotonic saline solutions. Because the spherocyte has a low surface area to volume ratio, it is unable to withstand exposure to hypotonic solutions and ruptures in higher concentrations of saline. About 25 percent of affected persons have normal unincubated tests, therefore, an incubated osmotic fragility should be done if the unincubated test is normal.

PAROXYSMAL NOCTURNAL HEMOGLOBINURNIA

Clinical Features

Paroxysmal nocturnal hemoglobinurnia (PNH) is a disease in which the patient's red blood cells are unusually sensitive to complement. It is probably related to a defect in the red blood cell membrane. PNH usually occurs in young adults and is characterized by chronic intravascular hemolysis with or without hemoglobinuria although hemosiderinuria is usually present. The episodic intravascular hemolysis may initiate intravascular coagulation, and thrombic episodes are at times associated with this disease. Platelets and neutrophils also appear to be sensitive to complement, leading to thrombocytopenia and leukopenia.

Laboratory Studies

Screening Procedures

Red Blood Cell Morphology. The peripheral film usually shows a normocytic anemia with polychromatophilia and occasionally nucleated red blood cells. One may also observe leukopenia and thrombocytopenia.

Reticulocyte Count. The reticulocyte is increased as one would expect in a hemolytic anemia.

Serum Haptoglobin. Serum haptoglobin is decreased as one would expect in a hemolytic anemia.

Definitive Tests

Sucrose Hemolysis Test. This test is based on the fact that sucrose provides a medium of low ionic strength which promotes the binding of complement to red blood cells. The patient's cells are mixed with a source in complement (fresh serum) and sucrose. The amount of hemolysis is then observed. In PNH hemolysis is usually greater than 10 percent. Suspicious results (5 to 10 percent hemolysis) may be obtained in some other hematologic diseases such as megaloblastic anemia or autoimmune hemolytic anemia.

Acidified Serum Test (Ham Test). In acidified serum, complement is activated by the alternative pathway, binds to red blood cells and lyses PNH cells that are unusually sensitive to complement. In PNH, 10 to 50 percent of the cells are lysed. A positive Ham test will occur in congenital dyserythropoeitic anemia, type II (or HEMPAS), but in HEMPAS the sucrose hemolysis test is negative.

HEMOLYTIC ANEMIAS SECONDARY TO ABNORMAL RED BLOOD CELL METABOLISM

BASIC INFORMATION

The primary function of the red blood cell is to carry oxygen to the cells of the body. To accomplish this, this anuclear cell must maintain the integrity of the cell membrane and the intracellular hemoglobin in a functional state. This requires energy that is derived from glucose metabolism. Glucose metabolism in the red blood cell involves two major enzyme pathways. The first is the Embdem–Meyerhof pathway, which is primarily concerned with generation of ATP used to maintain the integrity of the red blood cell membrane. The second is the hexose monophosphate pathway, which is primarily concerned with maintaining glutathione in the reduced state, which is necessary to protect hemoglobin from oxidative denaturation. Each metabolic step is catalyzed by an enzyme with or without a coenzyme. In recent years a large number of inborn errors of erythrocyte metabolism have been elucidated, each characterized by a deficiency of a specific enzyme. The clinical expression of these enzyme deficiencies is a congenital hemolytic anemia. Two of these enzyme deficiencies, pyruvate kinase deficiency and glucose-6-phosphate dehydrogenase deficiency, are discussed.

PYRUVATE KINASE DEFICIENCY

Clinical Features

Pyruvate kinase (PK) deficiency is the most common red blood cell enzyme deficiency involving the Embden-Meyerhof pathway. It is inherited as an autosomal recessive trait and is particularly frequent among the central Pennsylvania Amish. The anemia is variable in severity.

Laboratory Studies

Screening Procedures

Red Blood Cell Morphology. The red blood cells are usually normochromic and normocytic or macrocytic. Anisocytosis and poikilocytosis, polychromasia and nucleated red blood cells may be seen.

Reticulocyte Count. The reticulocyte count is increased as one would expect in a hemolytic anemia.

Serum Haptoglobin. Serum haptoglobin is decreased as one would expect in a hemolytic anemia.

Fluorescent Screening Test. This test depends on the fact that PK catalyzes the following reaction:

$$\text{Phosphoenolpyruvate (PEP)} + \text{ADP} \longrightarrow \text{Pyruvate} + \text{ATP}$$

The above reaction can be coupled to the following reaction:

$$\text{Pyruvate} + \text{NADH} \longrightarrow \text{Lactate} + \text{NAD}^+$$

The NADH is fluorescent under UV light but NAD is not. Thus, if fluorescence remains after the patient's red blood cells are combined with PEP, ADP, and NADH, then the patient is PK deficient.

Definitive Procedures

Qualitative Assays. Assays of PK can be done using spectrophotometric techniques. This procedure is usually available only in reference laboratories.

GLUCOSE-6-PHOSPHATE DEHYDROGENASE DEFICIENCY

Clinical Features

Glucose-6-phosphate dehydrogenase (G-6-PD) deficiency is the most common metabolic disorder of red blood cells. This enzyme catalyzes the first step in the hexose monophosphate shunt. The gene for G-6-PD is located on the X chromosome, therefore, the deficiency is mainly found in the male hemizygote though it may be partially expressed in women (recall the Lyon hypothesis regarding inactivation of one of the two X chromosomes in the woman). The most common clinical presentation is a self-limited episode of hemolytic anemia after an oxidant stress, be it drug, infection, or fava beans. Recall that the hexose monophosphate pathway is primarily concerned with protecting hemoglobin from oxidant stress. In the face of an oxidant stress, such as antimalarial drugs, a red blood cell deficient in G-6-PD cannot protect its hemoglobin, the hemoglobin precipitates (seen as Heinz bodies in the peripheral blood film), leading to increased cell rigidity, which leads to hemolysis.

Laboratory Studies

Screening Procedures

Red Blood Cell Morphology. The morphology will be normal except during a hemolytic episode when fragmented red blood cells and spherocytes may be seen.

Reticulocyte Count. The reticulocyte count will usually be increased several days after the hemolytic episode.

Heinz Body Preparation. As discussed above, when hemoglobin precipitates it forms Heinz bodies. These can be seen in blood films stained with vital stains such as methyl violet or crystal violet. It should be noted that Heinz bodies may also be seen in patients with unstable hemoglobins or thalassemia.

Fluorescent Screening Test. This test resembles the PK fluorescent spot test described previously. In G-6-PD deficiency the principle reaction is:

$$\text{G-6-P} + \text{NADP} \xrightarrow{\text{G-6-PD}} \text{6-P-Glucose} + \text{NADPH}$$

In this case the normal test is fluorescent, whereas the red blood cell deficient in G-6-PD shows little or no fluorescence.

Definitive Procedures

Quantitative assays of G-6-PD can be done using spectrophotometric techniques. This procedure is usually done only in reference laboratories.

HEMOLYTIC ANEMIAS SECONDARY TO HEMOGLOBIN DISORDERS

Background Information

Hemoglobin is composed of four heme groups and two pairs of polypeptide chains (globin). Hemoglobin A, normal adult hemoglobin, is composed of two alpha and two beta chains.

Hemoglobin F, the major fetal hemoglobin, is composed of two alpha and two gamma chains. Hemoglobin A_2, found in small amounts in normal adults, is composed of two alpha and two delta chains. In hemoglobinopathies the structure of one of the polypeptide chains is abnormal, usually due to a single amino acid substitution. A number of hemoglobinopathies have been described, the most common is hemoglobin S or sickle cell hemoglobin. Hemoglobin S is identical with hemoglobin A except that there is a single amino acid substitution in the beta chain (valine for glutamic acid at the sixth position).

In thalassemias the globin chains are usually of normal structure but they are produced at decreased rates.

Clinical Features

Patients with abnormal hemoglobin in their erythrocytes may or may not have a significant hemolytic anemia. This is a matter of the amount as well as the type of abnormal hemoglobin. Persons who are homozygous for sickle or thalassemic hemoglobin usually become severely anemic early in life and are faced with a life of chronic illness. On the other hand, if the person is a heterozygous carrier of an abnormal hemoglobin, only mild and at times even undetected problems may be present. In recent years many abnormal hemoglobins have been discovered and characterized.

Any black person with anemia should be suspected of having sickle cell anemia until proven otherwise. Likewise, people of southern European extraction have a high incidence of thalassemia.

The clinical picture is primarily related to the degree of anemia. However, in addition, because of anoxia, secondary organ dysfunction may be present. Many patients with severe hemolytic anemia develop severe hemosiderosis in tissues because of both multiple transfusions and the characteristic increased iron absorption associated with these diseases. Focal organ infarction (e.g., the spleen in sickle cell disease) may further complicate the clinical picture.

Laboratory Studies

Screening Procedures

Red Blood Cell Morphology. The peripheral blood film morphology is helpful in diagnosing these diseases. Significant numbers of target cells (e.g., >20 percent) are usually seen in

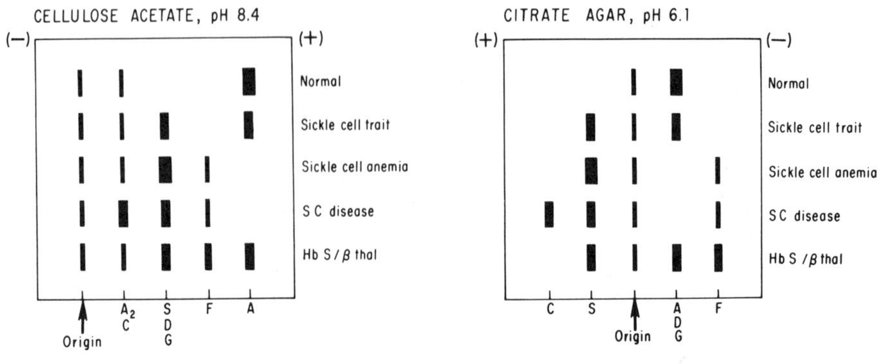

Figure 13–5. Comparison of electrophoretic mobilities of major hemoglobin types at pH 8.4 versus 6.1.

thalassemia major and hemoglobin C disease, and further definitive procedures are indicated. A few target cells can be noted in almost any anemia, and thus few numbers are of little significance.

Although sickled cells are almost invariably present on the peripheral blood film in homozygous sickle cell disease (Hb SS), sickle cells are usually not seen on blood smears in patients with the sickle cell trait (Hb AS). In hemoglobin C disease, crystals of C hemoglobin may be found in occasional red blood cells.

Hemoglobin Solubility. This has become the most popular method to screen for the presence of sickle hemoglobin. He-

TABLE 13–11. COMMON HEMOGLOBIN ELECTROPHORETIC PATTERNS

Major Components	Minor Component	Diagnosis
AA	F (<2%) A$_2$ (<3%)	Normal adult
F (75%)	A (25%)	Newborn
A and S (<50%)	F (<2%)	Sickle cell trait
S and S (>75%)	F (2–25%)	Sickle cell anemia
A and C	F (<2%)	AC hemoglobinopathy
S and C	F (<10%)	SC hemoglobinopathy
S and D	F (<2%)	SD hemoglobinopathy
A and F or A$_2$ (10–90%)		Thalassemia major
S	A$_2$ or F (<18%)	S-thalassemia
A	F or A$_2$ (2–10%)	Thalassemia trait

moglobin S is relatively insoluble in the buffered salt solution, whereas normal Hb A as well as most abnormal hemoglobins are quite soluble in the testing system.

Sickle Cell Preparation. Only in sickle cell disease (SS) are sickle cells seen on the routine peripheral film. In sickle cell trait (AS) or combinations of sickle hemoglobin with other abnormal hemoglobins (C,D, Thal) a special sickle cell preparation is necessary to bring out the sickling phenomenon. The preparations must be checked for up to 1 hour before they are reported as being negative. Pseudosickling is sometimes seen at the edges of the preparation, apparently because of some evaporation.

Definitive Tests

Hemoglobin Electrophoresis. This procedure is now widely available and provides exact answers for identification of hemoglobin. The test is done at pH 8.4 on cellulose acetate. Electrophoresis on citrate agar gel at pH 6.0 may be useful in separating materials that migrate with hemoglobin S or hemoglobin C. Figure 13–5 shows a comparison of electrophoretic migration patterns of various hemoglobins on cellulose acetate and citrate agar. Table 13–11 catalogues the most common electrophoretic patterns.

AUTOIMMUNE HEMOLYTIC ANEMIA

Clinical Features

Autoimmune hemolytic anemias (AIHA) are disorders in which red blood cell survival is decreased because of the deposition of immunoglobulins or complement, or both, on the red blood cell membrane. They can be classified according to serologic or clinical characteristics. About 70 percent of AIHA are mediated by antibodies (usually IgG) that have maximal activity at 37C, the warm reacting antibodies. The antibodies are often directed against the Rh complex. Most cases (40 to 50 percent) of warm AIHA are idiopathic. Secondary cases are usually associated with lymphoid malignant diseases, collagen vascular disorders, or drug reactions. About 30 percent of AIHA are mediated by antibodies (usually IgM) that have maximal activity at 4C, the cold reacting antibodies. They usually

TABLE 13–12. SEROLOGIC FINDINGS IN AUTOIMMUNE HEMOLYTIC ANEMIAS

Hemolytic Anemia	Direct Antiglobulin Test	Immunoglobulin Type	Specificity
Warm AIHA (most common type of AIHA)	IgG only IgG and complement Complement (no IgG)	IgG	Usually within Rh system
Cold agglutinin syndrome	Complement alone	IgM	Usually anti-I but can be anti-i
Paroxsysmal cold hemoglobinuria	Complement alone IgG cold antibody eluted from RBCs at 37°C or even at room temperature	IgG	Anti-P

have anti-I specificity but can have anti-i or anti-Pr. Most cases of cold AIHA are idiopathic, but they can be associated with mycoplasma pneumonia, infectious mononucleosis, or lymphoma. Paroxysmal cold hemoglobinuria is an interesting AIHA associated with a cold antibody. It is an IgG with biphasic activity that fixes complement to the red blood cell in the cold, e.g., in the peripheral circulation. When the blood is warmed (e.g., returns to the central circulation) the remainder of the complement proteins are activated and hemolysis occurs. Table 13–12 summarizes the serologic finding in the autoimmune hemolytic anemias.

Laboratory Studies

Screening Procedures

Antihuman Globulin Test. A positive direct antihuman globulin (Coomb's) test using broad-spectrum antiserum (anti-IgG and anti-C3) indicates antibody coating of the patient's red blood cells. The test can be performed with only anti-IgG and only anti-C3 to determine whether the erythrocytes are coated with IgG or complement or both. An effort must be made to ensure that no transfused cells are in the test system because the patient may normally coat these cells with antibody or complement, which may invalidate the test.

Definitive Procedures

A positive Coomb's test can be studied using a variety of temperatures and reagents. This information can be useful in the study of immune hemolytic anemia.

Definitive Antibody Identification. Occasionally a specific antibody can be identified. For example, anti-I or anti-Rh antibodies may be found sometimes. If a specific antibody is found, it may aid in the choice of blood for transfusions. Except in the most grave situations, however, transfusions are contraindicated. Packed or washed red blood cells are the component of choice.

Donath-Landsteiner Test. This test is useful when a diagnosis of paroxysmal cold hemoglobinuria is considered. It demonstrates hemolysis in a blood sample that is chilled in ice water and then warmed to 37C.

TABLE 13–13. DRUGS ASSOCIATED WITH UNEXPECTED BLOOD DYSCRASIAS (MEDIUM- AND SHORT-TERM USAGE)*

Drug	Agranulocytosis	Thrombocytopenia	Aplastic Anemia	Hemolytic Anemia	Megaloblastic Anemia
Antimicrobials					
Ampicillin	X	⊗	⊗		
Cephalothin	X	X		⊗	
Chloramphenicol	⊗	⊗	⊗		
Methicillin	X		X		
Nitrofurantoin	X			⊗	
Penicillin	X	X	X	⊗	
Rifampicin		X			
Sulfonamides	⊗	X	X	⊗	
Trimethoprim (sulfa-methoxazole)	⊗	⊗	⊗	⊗	X
Cardiac					
Heparin		X			
Methyldopa		⊗		X	
Procainamide	⊗				
Quinidine	X	⊗	X		
Diuretics					
Acetazokamide		X	X		
Furosemide		⊗			
Hydrochlorothiazide		X		⊗	

*X Indicates known associations; ⊗ denotes most important drugs in terms of number of cases.
Modified from de Gruchy GC: Drug-induced Blood Disorders. Oxford, Blackwell Scientific Publ., 1975.

TABLE 13–14. DRUGS ASSOCIATED WITH UNEXPECTED BLOOD DYSCRASIAS (CHRONIC USAGE)*

Drug	Agranulocytosis	Thrombocytopenia	Aplastic Anemia	Hemolytic Anemia	Megaloblastic Anemia
Antidepressants (tranquilizers)					
Chlorpromazine	Ⓧ		X		
Imipramine	X	X			
Meprobamate	X	X	X		
Phenobarbital			Ⓧ		Ⓧ
Prochlorperazine			X		
Antiepileptics					
Mesatoin			X		X
Phenytoin	X		Ⓧ		Ⓧ
Antirheumatics					
Acetylsalicylic Acid		Ⓧ	X	X	
Allopurinol			Ⓧ		
Gold			Ⓧ		
Indomethacin	Ⓧ	Ⓧ	Ⓧ	Ⓧ	
Phenylbutaxone and oryphenbutazone	Ⓧ	Ⓧ	X		
Antidiabetics					
Chlorpropamide	X	Ⓧ	X		
Tolbutamide	X		X		
Antithyroid					
Thiouracils	X		X		

*X Indicates known associations; Ⓧ denotes most important drugs in terms of number of cases.
Modified from de Gruchy GC: Drug-induced Blood Disorders. Oxford, Blackwell Scientific Publ., 1975.

ANEMIA OF BONE MARROW FAILURE

Clinical Features

Bone marrow failure may be associated with a variety of diseases. It may also follow apparent bone marrow injury after exposure to toxic drugs or chemicals (Tables 13–13 and 13–14). An idiopathic category including a premalignant variant completes the picture. This group of anemias is poorly understood, and therefore, the diagnosis is usually made by exclusion of the more common causes of anemia. Therapy is likewise empiric.

The degree of marrow failure is variable. The apparent cellularity may not reflect the functional state of the marrow as, for example, in maturation defects with hyperplasia but deficient production of circulating cells. Marrow failure may only be evident during times of stress, when increased demands for hematopoietic cells are made.

The body compensates for the loss of blood cell production in the marrow spaces by a process called extramedullary hematopoiesis. Certain tissues (nodes, liver, and in particular the spleen) undergo a process called myeloid metaplasia, i.e., the tissues revert to their fetal function of myelopoiesis and erythropoiesis. The cells produced by these tissues and released into the circulation tend to be poorly formed (teardrop erythrocytes, giant platelets) or immature (myelocytes, myeloblasts, nucleated red cells).

Laboratory Studies

Peripheral Blood Film

The blood film is consistent with anemia, leukopenia, or thrombocytopenia. These impressions should be confirmed with a quantitative blood count. Occasional red blood cells may show a teardrop shape and nucleated red cells may be found. In cases with myeloid metaplasia, immature leukocytes, both lymphocytic and neutrophilic, may be seen.

Reticulocyte Count

The reticulocyte count, both relative and absolute, is decreased or even nonexistent.

Bone Marrow Examination

The examination of the bone marrow is of great importance in separating the various types of marrow failure. Even a dry tap

TABLE 13–15. BONE MARROW FAILURE

Type	Marrow Histology	Cause
Aplastic	Fibrous or fatty with scattered lympho-cytes and stromal cells	Idiopathic; viral infection (?); irradiation, drugs, or chemicals
		Endocrine (thymic tumors, myxedema, pituitary failure)
		Chronic disease (renal, hepatic, infectious)
Hypoplastic	Hypoplasia of normal elements (relative and/or absolute) increased stromal elements	As for aplastic marrow
Myelophthisic	Marrow replaced by tumor, granulo-mata, or microabscesses	Metastatic malignancy; leukemia, lymphoma, infection
Maturation defect	Characteristically hyperplastic; may have ringed sideroblasts	Usually associated with deficiency of essential metabolite or blockage of heme or globin synthesis

marrow aspiration, when attempted by an experienced physician, can provide valuable information for diagnosis. Table 13–15 compares various types of marrow failure including characteristic marrow pictures.

SUGGESTED READINGS

Bonnet J: Normocytic normochromic anemia. Postgrad Med 61:139, 1977.

Bothwell TH, Finch CA: Iron Metabolism. Boston, Little, Brown, 1962.

Callender ST: Iron deficiency and iron overload. In: Clinics in Haematology, vol 2-2. London, Saunders, 1974.

Casale T: Aplastic anemia. Postgrad Med 71:59, 1982.

Chaplin H: Autoimmune hemolytic anemia. Arch Intern Med 137:346, 1977.

Cook J: Clinical evaluation of iron deficiency. Semin Hematol 19:6, 1982.

Dacie JV, Lewis SM: Practical Haematology, 6th ed. London, J & A Churchill Livingstone, 1984.

de Gruchy GC: Drug-induced Blood Disorders. Oxford, Blackwell Scientific Publ, 1975.

Forget B: Hemolytic anemias, congenital and acquired. Hosp Pract 15:67, 1980.

Glader BE: Perinatal haematology. In: Clinics in Haematology, vol 7-1. London, Saunders, 1978.

Green J: Macrocytic anemias. Postgrad Med 61:155, 1977.

Herbert V: The nutrional anemias. Hosp Pract 15:65, 1980.

Hillman R, Finch C: Red Cell Manual. Philadelphia, Davis, 1985.

Koepke JA (ed): Laboratory Hematology. New York, Churchill Livingstone, 1984.

McDowell GA, Dodds TC, Cruickshank B: Atlas of Haematology, 4th ed. New York, Churchill Livingstone, 1978.

Miale JB: Laboratory Medicine—Hematology, 6th ed. St. Louis, C. V. Mosby, 1982.

Prankerd TAJ, Bellingham AJ: Haematolytic anemia. In: Clinics in Haematology, vol 4-1. London, Saunders, 1975.

Reeves W, Haurani F: Clinical applicability and usefulness of ferritin measurements. Ann Clin Lab Sci 10:529, 1980.

Schumacher H, Garvin D, Triplett D: Introduction to Laboratory Hematology and Hematopathology. New York, Alan Liss, 1984.

Weatherall DJ: Abnormal haemoglobins. In: Clinics in Haematology, vol 3-2. London, Saunders, 1973.

Williams WJ, Beutler E, Erlev AJ, Rundles RW. (eds): Hematology. New York, McGraw-Hill, 1972.

Wintrobe M, et al.: Clinical Hematology, 8th ed. Philadelphia, Lea & Febiger, 1981.

14
LEUKEMIA AND LEUKEMOID DISORDERS

BASIC INFORMATION

Leukocyte Count

After the routine urinalysis and the hemoglobin or hematocrit determination, probably the most commonly performed laboratory test is the white blood cell or leukocyte count. Both the enumeration and the differential counting of white blood cells are of considerable importance to the physician. Almost all acute illnesses in some way affect the white blood cell count. Although these changes are often rather nonspecific, the count can be very helpful in distinguishing one disease from another, and at times the white blood cell count and differential count can be diagnostic of an illness.

Essentially, there are two methods of counting leukocytes. In one method, which uses a counting chamber (hemocytometer) and diluting pipettes, a direct visual count is made with the aid of a microscope. A more accurate method is now available, using automated counting instruments. This newer method has resulted in more precise as well as accurate white counts. In addition, the laboratory staff can do many more counts because of the speed of these machines. These instruments do, however, require continual checks of their performance and preventive maintenance to keep them operating at top efficiency. In a good laboratory a hand count can be guaranteed to be only within ±5 percent of the true mean value. A machine count is usually within ±2.5 percent of the true value. Table 14–1 shows the normal total white blood cell count at different ages.

The white blood cell count can change for three major reasons. First, the white blood cell count may rise because of a

TABLE 14–1. REFERENCE TOTAL WHITE BLOOD CELL COUNT*

	Reference Range (Mean ± 2 SD)	Significant Elevation	Significant Depression
Adults	4.0–12.0	>14.0	<2.0
Children	4.5–13.5	>16.0	<2.0
Infants	6.0–17.5	>20.5	<3.0

*All counts given as leukocytes × 10^9/L.

physiologic (e.g., exercise) or pathologic (e.g., infection) stimulus to white blood cell production. Second, the white blood cell count may increase or change in character as a result of neoplastic white blood cell production (e.g., leukemia). Finally, the white blood cell count may fall because of a decrease in production of white blood cells. This situation may follow a toxic depression of the marrow cells or a replacement of the functioning marrow by fibrosis or tumor.

In addition to changes in the total number of white blood cells, significant changes can also occur in the number and proportion of the individual types of white blood cells. In general terms there are two major types of white blood cells, granulocytes and lymphocytes. Other cell types, such as monocytes, usually comprise less than 10 percent of the peripheral white blood cells. A change in the total white blood cell count usually results from a significant increase or decrease in lymphocytes or granulocytes. Various combinations of changes are possible, which result in relative or absolute changes in the white blood cell count (Table 14–2). To avoid confusion, the reporting of differential counts only in absolute terms appears to have considerable merit.

The manual leukocyte differential count is done on a blood film using a microscope. One hundred cells are counted. The physician must appreciate the sampling variability of such a count, or any apparent differences from one count to the next may be overinterpreted. Table 14–3 gives the statistically derived variability, as well as some indication of changes that can be considered significant.

The increasing number of automated differential counters that are being used will have a considerable effect on the sampling variability of differential counts. In the pattern recognition instruments 200, 400, and 500 cells are usually counted. The cytochemical instruments count 10,000 cells per channel, and the precision is, therefore, considerably improved.

Whether the increased precision is clinically useful has not yet been determined.

Morphologic Identification of White Blood Cells

As with the red blood cell series, white blood cell identification is based on morphology as seen on Romanovsky-stained film preparations (Fig. 14–1). Cell maturity criteria are also similar to the red blood cell standards.

Myeloblast

This is an immature cell with a large nucleus that has a fine chromatin pattern. Usually one or more nucleoli are present. There is a scanty amount of blue cytoplasm that may contain a few nonspecific granules. Cells of blast morphology found in association with promyelocytes should be tentatively classified as myeloblasts.

Promyelocyte

This cell has a nuclear chromatin that is more coarse than that of a blast cell. Discernible prominent red or purple (nonspecific or azurophilic) granules are seen in the cytoplasm, which is pale blue or gray. Nucleoli are uncommon or absent.

Myelocyte

This cell has a round or oval nucleus. It is distinguished from the promyelocyte by the loss of large granules and from the metamyelocyte by the absence of indentation in the nucleus. It is noticeably smaller than a promyelocyte. It is at this stage that specific neutrophilic, basophilic, or eosinophilic granules can first be seen.

TABLE 14–2. CHARACTERISTIC WHITE BLOOD CELL COUNT CHANGES

| | Mean WBC | Lymphocyte Count | | Granulocyte Count | |
		Relative (%)	*Absolute**	*Relative (%)*	*Absolute**
Normal	6.0	40	2.4	60	3.6
Bacterial pneumonia	24.0	10	2.4	90	21.6
Viral infection	12.0	70	8.4	30	3.6
Agranulocytosis	2.5	96	2.4	4	0.1

*All absolute counts given as leukocytes $\times$ 10^9/L.

TABLE 14–3. CONFIDENCE LIMITS FOR THE REAL PERCENTAGE OF BLOOD CELLS OF A GIVEN TYPE IF a% CELLS OF THIS TYPE HAVE BEEN OBSERVED AMONGST n DIFFERENTIATED CELLS

a	$n = 100$	$n = 200$	$n = 500$	$n = 1000$	$n = 10,000$
0	0–4	0–2	0–1	0–0.4	0–0.1
1	0–6	0–4	0–3	0.4–1.9	0.8–1.3
2	0–8	0–6	0–4	1.2–3.1	1.7–2.3
3	0–9	1–7	1–5	2.0–4.3	2.6–3.4
4	1–10	1–8	2–7	2.8–5.5	3.6–4.5
5	1–12	2–10	3–8	3.7–6.6	4.5–5.5
6	2–13	3–11	4–9	4.6–7.7	5.5–6.5
7	2–14	3–12	4–10	5.4–8.8	6.5–7.6
8	3–16	4–13	5–11	6.3–9.9	7.4–8.6
9	4–17	5–14	6–12	7.2–11.0	8.4–9.6
10	4–18	6–16	7–13	8.2–12.1	9.4–10.7
15	8–24	10–21	11–19	12.8–17.4	14.3–15.8
20	12–30	14–26	16–24	17.5–22.7	19.2–20.8
25	16–35	19–32	21–30	22.3–27.9	24.1–25.9
30	21–40	23–37	26–35	27.1–33.0	29.1–31.0
35	25–46	28–43	30–40	32.0–38.1	34.0–36.0
40	30–51	33–48	35–45	36.9–43.2	39.0–41.0
45	35–56	37–53	40–50	41.8–48.2	44.0–46.0
50	39–61	42–58	45–55	46.8–53.2	49.0–51.0
55	44–65	47–63	50–60	51.8–58.2	54.0–56.0
60	49–70	52–67	55–65	56.8–63.1	59.0–61.0
65	54–75	57–72	60–70	61.9–68.0	64.0–66.0
70	60–79	63–77	65–74	67.0–72.9	69.0–70.9
75	65–84	68–81	70–79	72.1–77.7	74.1–75.9
80	70–88	73–86	76–84	77.3–82.5	79.2–80.8
85	76–92	79–90	81–89	82.6–87.2	84.2–85.7
90	82–96	84–94	87–93	87.9–91.8	89.3–90.6
91	83–96	86–95	88–94	89.0–92.8	90.4–91.6
92	84–97	87–96	89–95	90.1–93.7	91.4–92.6
93	86–98	88–97	90–96	91.2–94.6	92.4–93.5
94	87–98	89–97	91–96	92.3–95.4	93.5–94.5
95	88–99	90–98	92–97	93.4–96.3	94.5–95.5
96	90–99	92–99	93–98	94.5–97.2	95.5–96.4
97	91–100	93–99	95–99	95.7–98.0	96.6–97.4
98	92–100	94–100	96–100	96.9–98.8	97.7–98.3
99	94–100	96–100	97–100	98.1–99.6	98.7–99.2
100	96–100	98–100	99–100	99.6–100	99.9–100

*Given as 95% limits.

(Modified from Rümke CL: Variability of results in differential cell counts on blood smears. Trangle, Sandoz Journal of Medical Science 4(4):156, 1960, copyright Sandoz Ltd, Basle, Switzerland.)

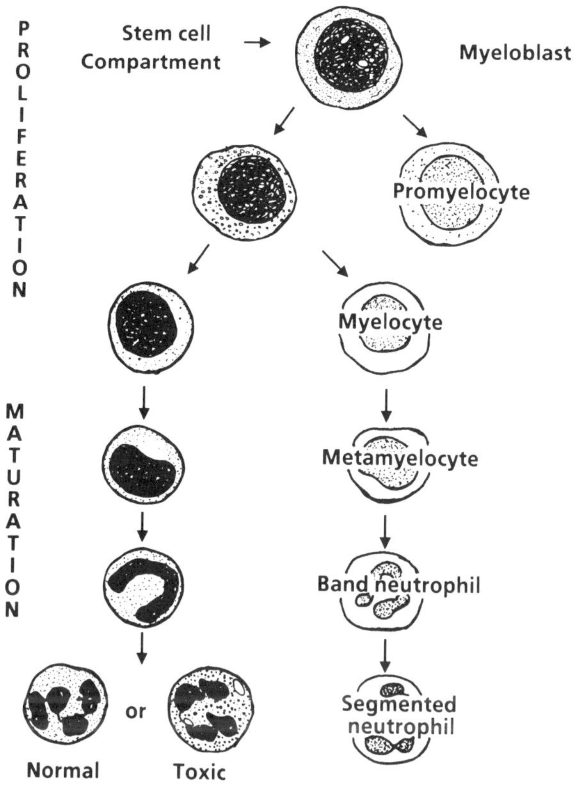

Figure 14–1. Myelopoiesis.

Metamyelocyte

Any cell of the granulocytic series that has specific granules in the cytoplasm and a nucleus intermediate in shape between that of the myelocyte and the band cell is labeled a metamyelocyte. The nucleus has an indented oval shape, resembling a kidney bean. The adjacent cytoplasm may present a halo or dawn appearance.

Band Neutrophil

A band cell has a nucleus with parallel sides that may be curved or coiled. If the indentation does not completely segment the nucleus into lobes connected by a thin filament, it is still classified as a band form. It is differentiated from the metamyelocyte by an appreciable length of the nucleus having parallel sides, and from the segmented neutrophil by having no indentation that could be described as a filament. The cytoplasm has definite specific granules.

Segmented Neutrophil or Polymorphonuclear (PMN) Leukocyte

A segmented cell has a lobated nucleus, each lobe connected by a filament, which is defined as a threadlike structure. At times, it is impossible to be certain whether two parts of the nucleus are connected by a filament or a band of chromatin. These cells are arbitrarily placed in the segmented category.

Mature Lymphocytes

The mature lymphocyte may vary considerably in size, with large forms more common in the blood of children and infants. The nucleus is round or oval, may be slightly indented, and shows a characteristic smeary chromatin. Generally no nucleoli are seen. The cytoplasm is typically sky blue and occasionally may contain red granules (Fig. 14–2). The blood of children contains a higher proportion of lymphocytes than does that of adults. In addition, lymphocytes in children tend to be larger than those in adults.

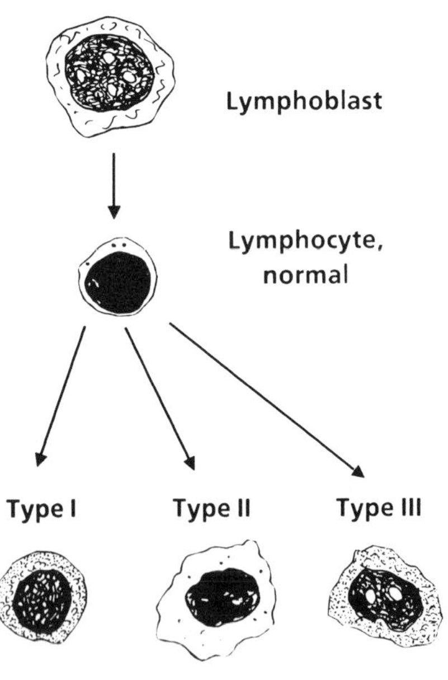

Figure 14–2. Lymphocyte morphology.

Monocytes

These large circulating phagocytic cells are characterized by their large irregular cell morphology. The cytoplasm is usually gray, at times containing evident debris. The nuclei are large and have an irregular shape, which occasionally appears to be forming irregular lobes. Nucleoli are not seen.

CLINICAL INVESTIGATION OF THE PATIENT WITH ABNORMAL WHITE BLOOD CELLS

The benefits of a combined clinical and laboratory approach to the diagnosis of disease is nowhere better illustrated than in the study of patients with abnormalities of the white blood cells. The clinical picture helps to interpret the laboratory findings and vice versa. At times there are barely discernible differences between benign and malignant white blood cells or between lymphoblasts and myeloblasts or other immature forms. Every available aid must be used to arrive at a diagnosis. In essence, the physician or the hematologist is faced with several questions. Are the white blood cell changes caused by a benign or malignant process? If benign, what is the cause of the reaction? If malignant, what is the type of the malignant cells?

From the laboratory viewpoint, it is useful to consider two general classes of white blood cell changes. One is the group of myeloproliferative responses, and the second is a somewhat less complex group called the lymphoproliferative responses. In the broadest terms, the responses may be either benign (reactive) or malignant (disorder). Figure 14–3 illustrates these relationships.

Myeloproliferative Responses

A myeloproliferative response can be defined as the proliferation of myeloid tissue caused by a stimulus that usually results in the outpouring of abnormal numbers or types of white blood cells into the peripheral circulation. The process may be benign or malignant. It may involve any or all of the myeloid elements: granulocytic, megakaryocytic, and erythrocytic. The apparent process as well as the type of myeloid element involved may significantly change as the disease progresses. Only the bone marrow seems to participate in many processes, especially early in the course of the disease. But myeloid tissues including the extramedullary elements (liver and spleen)

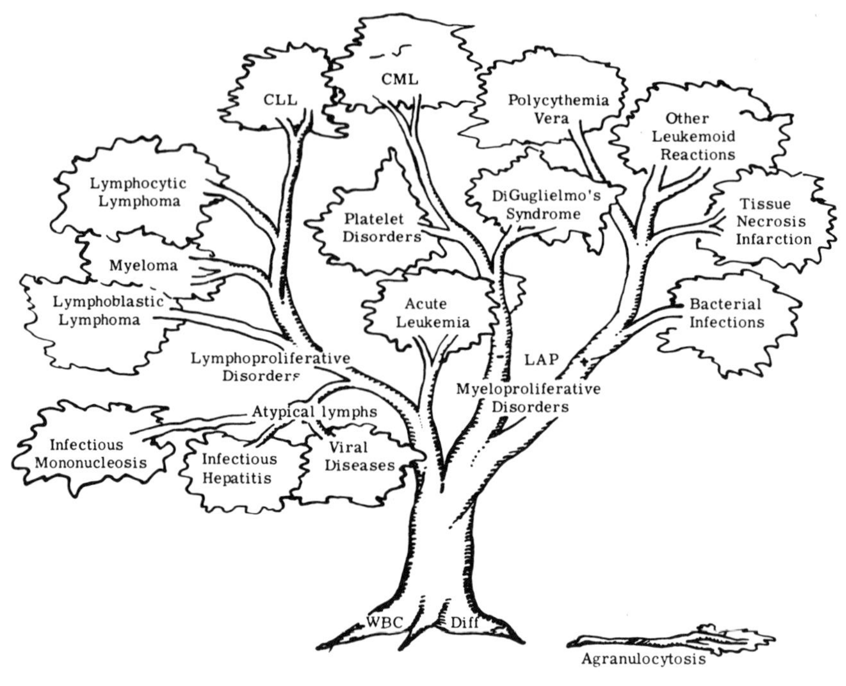

Figure 14–3. Disorders of white blood cells. This tree shows the relationships between many of the common white cell abnormalities, both benign and malignant, including myeloproliferative and lymphoproliferative processes.

may participate in this proliferation. The later reaction most often indicates progression of the malignant process.

Lymphoproliferative Responses

Lymphoproliferative responses, on the other hand, are diseases and conditions that have an associated proliferation of lymphoid tissue, usually with abnormal numbers of types of lymphoid elements circulating in the peripheral blood. The primary lymphoid tissue proliferation is found in lymph nodes, but lymphoid tissue in spleen, liver, and even bone marrow may also participate in this process. Again the proliferation may be benign or malignant. These lymphoproliferative responses may involve primarily the tissue (lymphoma) with little if any peripheral blood involvement or they may be manifested primarily by peripheral blood changes (leukemia) (Table 14–4).

TABLE 14–4. MALIGNANT WHITE BLOOD CELL DISORDERS

White Blood Cell Element	Tissue Phase	Leukemic Phase
Granulocyte	Chloroma*	Myelocytic
Lymphocyte	Lymphoma	Lymphocytic
Plasma cell	Plasmacytoma* and multiple myeloma	Plasma cell*
Monocyte or histocyte	Histocytic lymphoma	Monocytic

*A rare disease.

Several concepts are particularly useful in understanding the problem of variation in the laboratory picture of lymphoproliferative responses of the malignant variety (lymphoproliferative disorder). This includes appreciation of a continuum between a pure lymphocytic leukemia and a pure tissue lymphoma; all gradations in between are found. In addition, lymphomas often change into leukemias. These variations are understandable if one appreciates the broad scope of the term lymphoproliferative disorder. Thus, there can be an apparent change in the disease process so that primary tissue involvement may progress to a frank leukemia. This should not be considered an unusual change; in fact, this is frequently seen in clinical practice.

It may be difficult to decide from examination of the peripheral blood whether the proliferating cells are of myeloid or lymphoid origin. The blastic leukemias are examples of this problem. Studies involving special stains are sometimes helpful; experience and expert judgment are of more help, but in other cases the question will be answered only with time.

The decision tree in Figure 14–3 illustrates some of the important clinical entities involving the white blood cells and will serve as a general outline for the short discussions that follow. As was mentioned, essentially four groups of white blood cell responses are seen clinically: benign and malignant myeloproliferative processes and benign and malignant lymphoproliferative processes. A small but important transition branch includes the acute leukemias.

Clinical Features

The clinical history of patients with white blood cell changes may often correlate with the abnormalities of the white blood cell count. For instance, in patients with pneumonia there is a stimulus to white blood cell production. The leukemia patient, in contrast, usually cannot point to a time after which he or she was sick. This disease slowly becomes manifest with anemia or bleeding tendencies, both reactions being secondary to the primary leukemic process. The patient with agranulocytosis often is not able to recall exposure to potentially toxic drugs or chemicals.

The primary physical findings of greatest importance in these patients include the size and consistency of the lymph nodes and the size of the liver and the spleen. Lymphadenopathy (palpable lymph nodes) may be generalized or localized, and the nodes may be described as matted, tender, shotty, or even suppurative. Hepatic enlargement and splenic enlargement also provide clues to the cause of the white blood cell changes. Examples of various combinations of organ enlargement are found in Table 14–5.

Clinical evidence of anemia and thrombocytopenia usually indicate significant bone marrow replacement by neoplastic cells. Thrombocytopenia without significant evidence of anemia is characteristic of acute and rapid growth of neoplastic cells in the marrow.

Laboratory Studies

Complete Blood Count

Initially a complete blood count should be done on the patient. This includes a hemoglobin, hematocrit, red blood cell count, total white blood cell count, differential white blood cell count, and a platelet count. A most important study is the thorough search of a well-prepared blood film for abnormal leukocytes. One searches both for normal cells ordinarily not found in the peripheral circulation (e.g., normoblasts, plasma cells, myelocytes) and for frankly abnormal cells (e.g., blasts, bizarre primitive cells, or unusual lymphocytes).

At this point a diagnosis may be quite unequivocal and no further diagnostic studies may be necessary. The typical pattern of chronic lymphocytic leukemia (mild anemia and markedly elevated white blood cell count with a large majority of mature-appearing lymphocytes) and chronic myelogenous leukemia (markedly elevated white blood cell count with all varieties of granulocyte precursors, especially myelocytes or more mature varieties) would be examples of such cases.

TABLE 14–5. ORGAN ENLARGEMENT IN SELECTED DISEASES

Disease	Lymphadenopathy		Hepatomegaly	Splenomegaly
	Localized	*Generalized*		
Infections, systemic	0	+	±	±
Leukemia				
Acute	0	+ + +	+	+
Chronic myelocytic	0	±	+ +	+ + +
Chronic lymphocytic	0	+ +	+	+ +
Hodgkin's disease	+	±	+ +	+ + +
Lymphoma	+ +	+ +	+ +	+

TABLE 14–6. INDICATIONS FOR BONE MARROW EXAMINATION IN WHITE BLOOD CELL PROLIFERATIVE DISORDERS

Peripheral Blood Abnormality	Primary Diagnostic Consideration	Considerations in Differential Diagnosis
Myeloproliferative		
Agranulocytosis	Marrow aplasia, especially granulocytic elements	Aleukemic leukemia
Thrombocytopenia	See differential diagnosis	Idiopathic thrombocytopenia Acute leukemia Marrow aplasia
Immature granulocytes	Myelocytic leukemia	Disseminated tuberculosis
Left shift granulocytosis	Granulocytic leukemia	Bacterial infection
Normoblasts	Metastic tumor	Severe anemia Other malignancies
Lymphoproliferative		
Immature lymphs	Lymphocytic leukemia, acute lymphoma	Infectious mononucleosis
Lymphocytosis	Lymphocytic leukemia	Viral disease
Plasma cells	Myeloma	Chronic infection
Myeloproliferative versus lymphoproliferative		
Blasts	Acute leukemia	Infectious mononucleosis

Bone Marrow Examination

More often than not the diagnosis may still be in doubt. In these cases the next logical step is to obtain a sample of the bone marrow. A detailed description of this procedure is found in Chapter 24. The following remarks are directed primarily to bone marrow studies in diseases of the white blood cells.

When abnormal kinds or numbers of white blood cells are found in the peripheral blood, the bone marrow examination may be helpful in the conditions noted in Table 14–6. After these initial clinical and laboratory examinations have been done, the physician is in a position to make a tentative diagnosis or, if that is not possible, at least a reasonable differential diagnosis. These diagnoses may at times be quite specific, whereas at other times only a general diagnostic category may be under consideration.

The following discussion suggests ways to corroborate or to rule out the diagnosis in question and in this manner arrive at the correct diagnosis.

BENIGN MYELOPROLIFERATIVE OR LYMPHOPROLIFERATIVE REACTIONS

LEUKEMOID REACTIONS

White blood cell proliferation is an almost universal reaction to acute disease. Thus, it is nonspecific. Also, there is usually no difficulty in distinguishing reactive or regenerative white blood cell proliferation from malignant proliferation. There are cases, however, in which the proliferative reaction is of such a magnitude or type that the differentiation from leukemia may be difficult. This is called a leukemoid reaction and may be defined as a reaction in which the total white blood cell count is greater than $50 \times 10^9/L$ or blast forms are found in the peripheral circulation. In this definition circulating nucleated red blood cell precursors are included as blast forms.

Many different processes can result in a leukemoid reaction, and therefore the clinician is interested in pinpointing the cause. Some of these processes are discussed in the following sections. One major cause of leukemoid reactions is infection. Although bacterial infections usually result in myeloproliferation with a left shift in the granulocytic differential count, viral infections (unless complicated by secondary bacterial infection) characteristically have a lymphoproliferation with abnormal or atypical lymphocytes.

Clinical Features

Infections

Infections are usually accompanied by fever as well as local effects that depend on the location of the infectious process. Laboratory studies are directed toward finding the site of infection, isolating the offending organism, and initiating appropriate therapy. Chapter 20, which deals with unexplained fever, provides additional information.

Tuberculosis

One infection, disseminated tuberculosis, deserves special mention in any discussion on leukemoid reactions because this disease may closely mimic various malignant myeloproliferative disorders. Immature myelocytes and even myeloblasts (rarely containing Auer rods) may be seen in the peripheral blood in miliary tuberculosis. Leukopenia may also be present, suggesting an aleukemic phase of leukemia. The marrow may be hyperplastic and quite immature, at times even difficult to aspirate (packed marrow?). Accompanying anemia is the rule.

Because the hematologic picture resembles acute leukemia in so many ways, the possibility of disseminated tuberculosis must always be kept in mind. Bone marrow tissue sections examined for early granulomata and stained for acid-fast organisms are extremely helpful. Cultures of marrow are less helpful because of the time delay before this organism will grow in cultures.

Tumor Infiltration of Marrow

Malignancy with, or at times even without, marrow metastases may have an associated leukemoid reaction. Carcinoma of the breast, lung, and thyroid as well as myeloma and Hodgkin's disease are associated with leukemoid reactions. Marrow metastases are often associated with the presence of nucleated red blood cells in the peripheral circulation. If such cells are found without obvious cause, metastatic malignancy should be seriously considered. Marrow aspiration clot preparations processed as tissue sections should be examined carefully for clumps of metastatic tumor cells.

Hemolysis and Hemorrhage

Sudden severe hemolytic episodes as well as severe hemorrhages may be associated with a leukemoid reaction and the outpouring of nucleated red blood cells into the peripheral circulation.

Toxic Reactions

Reactions to burns or poisoning (e.g., mercury) or eclampsia also may have associated leukemoid reactions. The clinical status of the patient leaves no doubt as to the cause of leukemoid reactions in such cases.

Myeloid Metaplasia

In cases of myeloid metaplasia with myelofibrosis or myelosclerosis, immature myelocytic and normoblastic elements are commonly found in the peripheral circulation, presumably associated with their production and release from extramedullary hematopoietic sites such as spleen and liver. The fibrotic or sclerotic marrow picture may presage the development of frank leukemia. This illustrates the pattern of a seemingly benign myeloproliferation changing into a malignant variant.

Infectious Mononucleosis and Hepatitis

The foregoing remarks have been primarily concerned with benign myeloproliferative reactions presenting as a leukemoid reaction. Benign lymphoproliferative disorders that may masquerade as leukemia include those diseases associated with variant (atypical) lymphocytes, primarily infectious mononucleosis and infectious hepatitis. The clinical manifestations of mononucleosis include a prodromal stage resembling an upper respiratory infection followed by prostration and a wide variety of signs and symptoms including rash, splenomegaly, and hepatic involvement. A variety of complications may occur including hemolytic anemia. Infectious hepatitis may occur as frankly icteric hepatitis or subclinical variants in which only biochemical (i.e., enzyme) or immunologic (i.e., HBsAg) evidence of hepatic involvement is found. Both diseases may be followed by prolonged convalescence. In addition, complications of chronic active hepatitis or even postnecrotic cirrhosis may follow the episode of acute hepatitis.

Laboratory Studies

Screening Procedures

Differential White Blood Cell Count. Evidence of the bacterial origin of a leukocytosis may become evident with a thorough study of the peripheral blood film. There may be an evident shift to the left in the granulocytic differential count, i.e., there are some immature granulocytic cells in the peripheral circulation. This concept originated with the method of Schilling for reporting the differential white blood cell count. Table 14–7 illustrates several typical patterns. Although rare, the Pelger-Huet anomaly, a genetic defect, results in an apparent left shift of hyposegmentation of mature granulocytes. It is included for comparison and represents the normal differential count for these individuals.

Although these patterns seem clear-cut, occasional patients present with hybrids that are difficult to interpret. In

TABLE 14–7. CHARACTERISTIC DIFFERENTIAL WHITE BLOOD CELL COUNTS*

Characteristics	Blasts	Promyelocytes	Myelocytes	Metamye-locytes	Band Neutrophils	Segmented Neutrophils	Other Cells
Normal	—	—	—	—	3	60	Normal
Left shift due to infection	—	Occasional	4	6	20	50†	Normal
Pelger-Huet anomaly	—	—	—	3	58	2	Normal
Leukemic hiatus	22	5	—	—	3	50	Normal
Chronic lymphocytic leukemia	—	—	—	—	2	10	Lymphocytes
Chronic granulocytic leukemia	Occasional	8	28	20	6	10	Normal
Leukemoid reactions Tuberculosis, disseminated	Occasional	Occasional	5	10	20	40	Normal
Tumor infiltration of marrow	—	—	—	—	3	60	Nucleated RBCs
Hemolysis/hemorrhage	—	—	—	—	10	70	Normal
Toxic reaction	—	—	—	5	10	70†	Normal
Myeloid metaplasia	Occasional	5	10	20	25	20	Nucleated RBCs
Infectious mononucleosis/ hepatitis	—	—	—	—	10	30	Variant lymphs

*All values given as percent of white cells, if present.
†Toxic granulation.

addition, some cases of myelocytic leukemia may have a prominent left shift with immature granulocytes circulating in the peripheral blood.

The finding of toxic neutrophils points toward an infectious or other toxic cause for the myeloproliferation rather than a malignant cause. A toxic neutrophil is one showing toxic granules and vacuoles in the cytoplasm, as well as condensation of the nuclear chromatin. The grading of the severity of toxic changes depends more on the degree of change than on the percentage of cells involved. Occasionally Döhle bodies may be seen in these cells. These are clear, light blue areas usually in the periphery of the cytoplasm (Fig. 14–1).

Another variety of atypical or abnormal cell, i.e., the variant (or atypical) lymphocyte, may point to the cause of the leukocytosis or leukemoid reaction. Variant lymphocytes may also be thought of as turned on lymphocytes that have begun to respond immunologically to a viral infection. Variant lymphocytes are found in infectious mononucleosis, but they are also seen in a variety of viral diseases, especially viral hepatitis.

Downey described three types of variant (atypical) lymphocytes. Type I lymphocytes are the smallest of the three types. Their nuclei are frequently lobulated or clefted. They have moderate amounts of basophilic frothy cytoplasm (Fig. 14–2, left). Type II lymphocytes, the most common variant in infectious mononucleosis, are larger than type I cells. They have smudgy chromatin and pale-blue watery cytoplasm. They occasionally contain scattered granules (Fig. 14–2, middle). Type III lymphocytes are also larger cells. They have clumped blocky chromatin and often nucleoli. Their cytoplasm is very basophilic (Fig. 14–2, right).

Infestations with parasitic worms and protozoans may have an associated eosinophilia, which varies considerably depending on the reaction of the patient. Eosinophilia is most prominent during the visceral phase of the infestation, but tends to disappear with chronic infections. Numerous other diseases also may have an associated eosinophilia, as listed in Table 14–8.

Definitive Procedures

Leukocyte Alkaline Phosphatase. Special stains for white blood cell enzymes are sometimes of help in differentiating between benign and malignant myeloproliferation. The leukocyte alkaline phosphatase procedure was the most widely

TABLE 14–8. SOME CAUSES OF EOSINOPHILIA

Parasitic diseases	Blood diseases
Trichinosis	Chronic myelocytic leukemia
Hookworm infestation	Polycythemia vera
Strongyloidiasis	Leukemia, eosinophilic
Ascariasis	Miscellaneous
Visceral larva migrans	Serum sickness
[Toxocara]	Ulcerative intestinal disease
Amebiasis	Periarteritis nodosa
Allergic conditions	Dermatomyositis
Hay fever	X-ray therapy
Asthma	Drug reactions
Certain skin diseases	

available in the past. In this procedure the granulocytes are specially stained for alkaline phosphatase activity. One hundred granulocytes (segmented, band, or metamyelocyte forms) are examined, and the relative amount of alkaline phosphatase activity is estimated from none (score zero) to a full complement (score 4). The cumulative score of these 100 cells is determined. Although most benign processes and leukemias other than myelocytic have normal or elevated scores, myelocytic leukemias (acute or chronic) have low scores, as indicated in Table 14–9.

Infectious Mononucleosis Tests. As noted above, variant lymphocytes, although usually associated with infectious mononucleosis, may also be found in patients with infectious hepatitis or other viral diseases.

The laboratory confirmation of infectious mononucleosis is by serologic procedures. Rapid slide tests are widely available to detect the heterophil antibodies that occur in infectious

TABLE 14–9. TYPICAL LEUKOCYTE ALKALINE PHOSPHATASE SCORES*

Condition	Score
Normal	50–125
Pregnancy	250–280
Chronic myelocytic leukemia	1–25
Polycythemia vera	200–300
Leukemoid reactions	275–325

*Method of Kaplow.

mononucleosis. These tests are highly specific as well as sensitive. False-positive results are very rare. False-negative results may occur in young children who produce heterophil antibodies in low concentrations. Epstein-Barr virus-specific serologies may be used to diagnose heterophil–antibody-negative infectious mononucleosis. These tests will be negative in hepatitis.

Transaminases. The most sensitive indicator of hepatic cell necrosis is the measurement of serum transaminase levels, either AST or ALT. This is an especially sensitive procedure in subicteric or subclinical hepatitis. Other liver function tests, e.g., bilirubin and alkaline phosphatase, may also be helpful in differentiating hepatitis from mononucleosis.

Hepatitis Serologies. These tests may be useful for diagnosing hepatitis A or B. They are discussed at length in Chapter 9.

Viral Isolation Studies. Few laboratories are currently able to offer the services of a viral diagnostic laboratory. Therefore, the diagnosis of a viral disease associated in the present discussion with atypical or abnormal lymphocytes, is usually made on clinical evidence alone. It is hoped that there will be continued advancement in this area so that contemporary viral studies will be available and thus immediately helpful to the patient.

MALIGNANT PROLIFERATIVE DISEASES

LEUKEMIA

Leukemia is a generalized neoplastic proliferation or accumulation of leukopoietic cells with or without evidence in the peripheral blood. Leukemias may be divided into acute and chronic forms. The acute leukemias are usually fatal within 3 months, if no remission is induced. The bone marrow contains a very high proportion of immature cells of the hematopoietic series involved. Patients with chronic leukemias usually live longer than 1 year even if no remission is induced. The malignant cells tend to be more mature than in acute leukemias. Leukemias are also classified according to cytologic characteristics and there are two major cytologic categories, lymphocytic and nonlymphocytic (myelocytic).

ACUTE LEUKEMIA

Clinical Features

Acute leukemias present with a variety of symptoms linked to the loss of normal marrow function (i.e., thrombocytopenia, granulocytopenia, or anemia) and to signs or symptoms associated with leukemic infiltration of tissues (lymphadenopathy, hepatosplenomegaly, and possibly gingival or skin manifestations). Sometimes signs and symptoms are minimal or even completely absent, as, for example, in preleukemia or smoldering leukemia.

Laboratory Studies

Screening Procedures

Complete Blood Count. Anemia, thrombocytopenia, and leukopenia may be evident to variable degrees. Immature blast cells may or may not be found, although they invariably occur as the disease progresses.

Bone Marrow. The marrow is hypercellular, having increased numbers of immature white blood cells. Normal elements are consequently decreased. Although the marrow is usually easily aspirated, the marrow space is sometimes so packed with leukemic cells that marrow particles cannot be obtained (a dry tap).

Although the type of leukemic cell can be determined from the marrow smears stained with a Romanovsky stain (e.g., Auer rods in acute myelogenous leukemia), at times the immaturity of the cells is such that even the differentiation of acute lymphocytic leukemia (ALL) from acute nonlymphocytic leukemia (ANLL) cannot be made. In these cases special procedures are of help (discussion follows).

Definitive Procedures

Leukemic Cell Cytochemistry. A variety of cytochemical procedures are now widely used to aid in the differentiation of the acute leukemias. The interpretation of these tests is summarized in Figure 14–4. The interpretation of these studies must be modified by the realization that the incidence of false-negative results is substantial. Only positive reactions can be

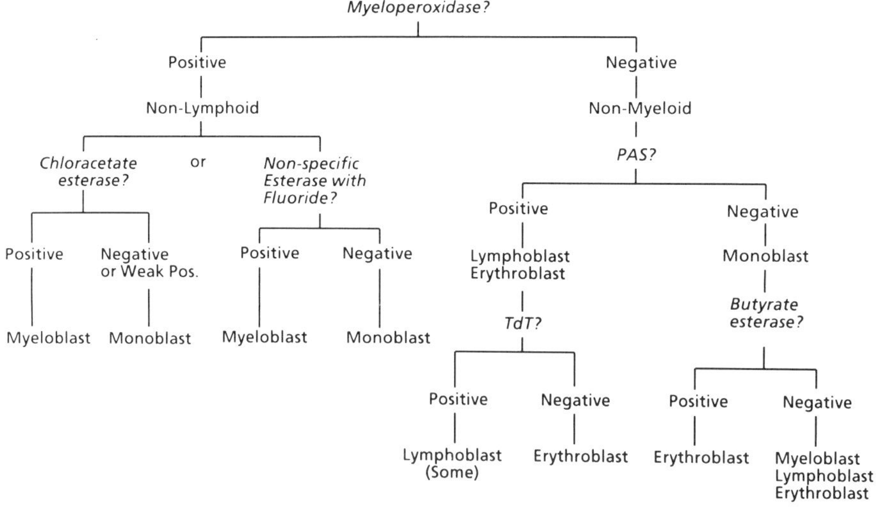

Figure 14–4. Cytochemical analysis of leukemic blasts. PAS, Periodic Acid-Schiff; TdT, Terminal deoxynucleotidyl transferase.

TABLE 14–10. FRENCH-AMERICAN-BRITISH (FAB) CLASSIFICATION OF THE ACUTE MYELOID LEUKEMIAS

Granulocytic component predominant

M1: Myeloblastic without maturation
($>$3% of blasts are peroxidase positive; or blasts with azurophilic granules or Auer rods)

M2: Myeloblastic with maturation
(maturation at or beyond promyelocyte)

M3: Hypergranular promyelocytic
(majority of cells abnormal promyelocytes)

Monocytic component predominant

M4: Myelomonocytic
($>$20% of cells are promonocytes and monocytes and $>$20% of cells are myeloblasts and abnormal granulocytic precursors)

M5: Monocytic
(almost complete replacement of marrow by abnormal monocytoid cells; $<$20% abnormal granulocytic precursors)

Erythropoietic component predominant

M6: Erythroleukemia
($>$50% of cells are abnormal erythroid precursors; or $>$30% of cells are precursors and 10% are bizarre erythroid cells)

Modified from Bennett JM, et al.: Proposals for the classification of the acute leukemias. Br J Haematol 33:451, 1976.

TABLE 14–11. FRENCH-AMERICAN-BRITISH (FAB) CLASSIFICATION OF THE ACUTE LYMPHOBLASTIC LEUKEMIAS

Cytology	L1	L2	L3
Nucleus			
Size	Small	Large	Large and homogeneous
Chromatin	Homogeneous	Variable	Finely stippled
Shape	Regular	Irregular	Oval to round
Nucleoli	Rare	Present	1–3
Cytoplasm			
Amount	Scanty	Moderate	Moderate
Basophilia	Moderate	Variable	Intense
Vacuolation	Variable	Variable	Often prominent

From Bennett JM, et al.: Proposals for the classification of the acute leukemias. Br J Haematol 33:451, 1976.

used as evidence of the definitive identification of immature leukemic cells.

Acute Myelogenous Leukemia

A French-American-British (FAB) Cooperative group has published proposals for the classification of acute leukemias. The classification is based on the morphology of cells in blood and marrow films and certain cytochemical reactions. According to their criteria there must be at least 30 percent blasts in the marrow for a diagnosis of acute leukemia to be made. They have described six types of acute myeloid leukemia (AML) (Table 14–10).

Acute Lymphoblastic Leukemia

The FAB group has divided lymphoblastic leukemia into three types (Table 14–11) based on morphology of the blast cell.

ALL can also be divided into five subtypes depending on the reaction of the blasts with lymphocyte cell marker assays (Table 14–12).

CHRONIC LEUKEMIA

Chronic Myelocytic Leukemia

Clinical Features

Chronic myelocytic leukemia (CML), usually insidious in onset, is practically asymptomatic in its early stages. Subse-

TABLE 14–12. CLINICAL FEATURES AND MARKERS OF DIFFERENTIATION IN RECOGNIZED SUBGROUPS OF ACUTE LYMPHOCYTIC LEUKEMIA

ALL Subtype	Percentage of Cases	Markers						
		TdT	*CALLA*	*Ia*	*ER*	*TAg*	*SIg*	*CIg*
Common (non-T, non-B)	60	+	+	+	−	−	−	−
Pre-B	~10	+	+	+	−	−	−	+
Null	~10	+	−	+	−	−	−	−
T	20	+	±	−	+	+	−	−
B	2	−	±	+	−	−	+	−

TdT, terminal deoxynucleotidyl transferase; CALLA, common ALL antigen; Ia, immune-associated antigen; ER, sheep erythrocyte rosette; TAg, T cell antigen; SIg, surface immunoglobulin; CIg, cytoplasmic immunoglobulin.

quently signs and symptoms are often secondary to anemia or thrombocytopenia caused by a displacement of the normal marrow by the proliferating leukemic cells. Late in the disease leukemic infiltration of many organs, particularly the liver and the spleen, results in clinical and laboratory changes owing to these complications. Bleeding caused by thrombocytopenia or vascular infiltration, or both, and lowered resistance to infection because of a decrease in normal phagocytes are almost invariable consequences of the disease.

The clinical course in chronic myelocytic leukemia may be compatible with several years of symptom-free life while the patient undergoes periodic courses of therapy.

Laboratory Studies

Screening Procedures

Complete Blood Count. The peripheral blood film in CML is almost diagnostic with a granulocytic leukocytosis. This is evident as a complete spectrum of granulocytic cells from myeloblasts to mature neutrophils. The more mature cells are present in the greatest number and the less mature in diminishing frequency. Basophilia is consistently present. Anemia is usually present.

Bone Marrow. The marrow is markedly hypercellular, primarily attributable to granulocytic proliferation with all stages represented. Sufficient specimen must be obtained to rule out leukemoid reactions, myelofibrosis, or metastatic carcinoma. Red blood cell precursors and megakaryocytes are typically decreased, but occasionally early in the disease they may be normal or increased.

Definitive Procedures

Leukocytic Alkaline Phosphatase. The assessment of the myelocytic cells for alkaline phosphatase activity may be very helpful in differentiating chronic myelocytic leukemia from leukemoid reactions that mimic this condition. The alkaline phosphatase activity in mature granulocytes is uniformly low in myelocytic leukemia, i.e., less than 25 (see Table 14–9).

Philadelphia Chromosome. Chromosome cultures with identification of the abnormal Philadelphia chromosome (Ph') are now believed to be pathognomonic of the common variety of chronic myelocytic leukemia. The Philadelphia chromosome is a small piece of chromosome 22 that has translocated to chromosome 9. It is found in 85 to 95 percent of patients with typical chronic myelogenous leukemia. Failure to find this abnormal chromosome leads to a diagnosis of an atypical myelocytic leukemia.

CHRONIC LYMPHOCYTIC LEUKEMIA

Clinical Features

Chronic lymphocytic leukemia (CLL) is a disease of older individuals with a median age of onset of 65 years. The disease is characterized by a slowly progressive accumulation of lymphocytes in the peripheral blood, bone marrow, lymph nodes, spleen, and liver. The onset of the disease is insidious and it is usually discovered by chance during investigation for another problem. The patient presents with lymphadenopathy and splenomegaly caused by an accumulation of lymphocytes. In advance stages of the disease there can be anemia and thrombocytopenia from bone marrow failure. The average life expectancy is 6 to 7 years from the onset of the disease. Laboratory predictors of poor prognosis at diagnosis include: anemia, thrombocytopenia, diffuse extensive marrow involvement, increased prolymphocytes and blasts, and possibly large cell size.

Laboratory Studies

Complete Blood Count. The absolute lymphocyte count is usually greater than $15 \times 10^9/L$ with the median in the 30 to 40 $\times$ $10^9/L$ range. The great majority of these lymphocytes are similar and appear normal, although the nuclear chromatin may be more coarsely condensed with a more distinct separation of the chromatin and parachromatin than normal. Anemia and thrombocytopenia usually develop as the disease progresses.

Bone Marrow. The marrow shows a lymphocytosis. The lymphocyte percentage is between 40 and 100 percent, but is most often between 60 and 80 percent. The infiltrative pattern can be focal, diffuse, or a combination of both.

Immunologic Studies. Over 95 percent of cases of CLL are of B cell lineage, less than 5 percent are of T cell origin.

TABLE 14–13. HISTOLOGIC CLASSIFICATION OF HODGKIN'S DISEASE

Subtype	Major Morphologic Alteration	Percentage of Cases	Incidence of Bone Marrow Involvement
Lymphocyte predominant	Usually diffuse, sometimes vaguely nodular pattern, abundant lymphocytes, few Reed-Sternberg cells, no fibrosis	7	0
Nodular sclerosis	Nodular pattern formed by birefringent collagen bands; moderate number of lymphocytes, eosinophils, plasma cells, lacunar variant of Reed-Sternberg cells	68	2–10
Mixed cellularity	Diffuse involvement, numerous Reed-Sternberg cells, moderate number of lymphocytes, eosinophils, plasma cells	23	5–20
Lymphocyte depletion	Diffuse involvement, decreased cellularity, occasionally numerous bizarre-shaped Reed-Sternberg cells	2	45–75

MALIGNANT LYMPHOMA

Malignant lymphoma is a neoplastic proliferation of one of the cell types of the lymphopoietic–reticular system. The disease usually begins in lymph nodes although it may also arise in the spleen or the gastrointestinal tract. As the disease progresses, it spreads to lymphoid tissue beyond the site of origin and may also involve most any organ in the body. Patients with malignant lymphoma can present with asymptomatic enlarged lymph nodes or fever, night sweats, weight loss, and pruritis. Lymphomas are divided into Hodgkin's disease and non-Hodgkin's lymphomas.

Hodgkin's Disease

Hodgkin's disease may occur from early childhood to old age with increased frequency in the second and third decade of life and after age 50. The hallmark of Hodgkin's disease is the Reed-Sternberg cell, which is a large binucleated cell with each nucleus having a prominent nucleolus. The current histologic classification scheme is that of the Rye conference (Table 14–13).

Laboratory Studies

Complete Blood Count. About 50 percent of cases have a normocytic anemia. The leukocyte and platelet counts can be normal, reduced, or elevated.

Bone Marrow. A bone marrow biopsy is clearly superior to aspirate preparations in detecting malignant lymphoma. The

TABLE 14–14. CLINICAL STAGING OF LYMPHOMAS

Stage	Description	Five-Year Survival (%)
I	Single lymph node group or contiguous lymph node on same side of diaphragm	90
II	Two or more lymph node groups or lymphatic tissues on same side of diaphragm	70
III	Involvement of lymphatic tissue on both sides of diaphragm	40
IV	Involvement of extranodal sites, e.g., bone marrow, liver, lung, skin	20

patterns of bone marrow involvement are focal paratrabecular, focal nonparatrabecular, and diffuse. The incidence of bone marrow involvement varies depending on the histologic type of Hodgkin's disease (Table 14–13). It must be remembered that small, benign lymphoid follicles may be found in normal marrow, especially in elderly patients. Benign lymphoid aggregates are usually well circumscribed, round, focal, nonparatrabecular, and contain mature-appearing lymphocytes with a few admixed histiocytes, plasma cells, and mast cells.

Clinical Staging

Clinical staging is used to determine the extent of disease at the time of diagnosis. Workup usually includes a history and physical examination, radiographic studies, complete blood count, erythrocyte sedimentation rate, neutrophil alkaline phosphatase, bone marrow biopsy, liver function tests, urinalysis, and skin tests for delayed hypersensitivity. Using this information, patients are divided into one of four stages (Table 14–14). The stages are additionally divided into A, if systemic symptoms are absent, or B, if systemic symptoms are present. The staging system is very useful in guiding the therapeutic approach to a particular patient.

Non-Hodgkin's Lymphomas

Non-Hodgkin's lymphomas (NHL) are a heterogeneous group of lymphoreticular neoplasms and many classification systems have been proposed. The Rappaport classification has been widely used. It classifies non-Hodgkin's lymphomas on the basis of cell size and the pattern of nodal involvement, i.e., nodular or diffuse (Table 14–15). Studies have shown that this classification system has clinical relevance. It was subsequently recognized that cells originally designated as histiocytic in the Rappaport classification were, in fact, lymphocytic. This led to other classification systems. Because of the confusion created by the multiple classification systems, a multi-institutional review of a large number of lymphomas led to a new classification system called the Working Formulation (Table 14–16). This system appears to be reproducible, clinically relevant, and uses functionally relevant terminology.

Laboratory Studies

Complete Blood Count. Peripheralization of lymphoma cells is a relatively common finding in NHL. Anemia, neutropenia,

TABLE 14–15. REVISED RAPPAPORT CLASSIFICATION FOR NON-HODGKIN'S LYMPHOMA

Histiocytic Subgroups	Relative Incidence (%)	Five-Year Survival (%)
Nodular pattern		
Lymphocytic, well differentiated	1–2	75
Lymphocytic, poorly differentiated	15–20	70
Mixed lymphocytic-histiocytic	15–20	50
Histiocytic	4–7	70
Diffuse pattern		
Lymphocytic, well differentiated (with or without plasmacytoid features)	2–3	65
Lymphocytic, poorly differentiated (with or without plasmacytoid features)	8–15	40
Mixed lymphocytic–histiocytic	8–12	35
Histiocytic (with or without sclerosis)	28–35	40
Undifferentiated	1–2	<10
Burkitt's tumor	1–2	<5
Lymphoblastic (with or without convoluted cells)	2–3	30
Unclassified		

From Golomb H, Gams R, Hoppe R: Hematology. Education Program, American Society of Hematology, 1981.

TABLE 14–16. WORKING FORMULATION OF NON-HODGKIN'S LYMPHOMA FOR CLINICAL USAGE WITH RELATIVE FREQUENCY BY MORPHOLOGY TYPE

Type of Non-Hodgkin's Lymphoma	Overall Incidence	Incidence of Bone Marrow Involvement	Five-Year Survival (%)
Low grade			
ML, small lymphocytic consistent with CLL plasmacytoid	4	71	59
ML, follicular predominantly small cleaved cell, diffuse areas, sclerosis	23	51	70
ML, follicular mixed small cleaved and large cell, diffuse areas, sclerosis	8	30	50
Intermediate grade			
ML, follicular predominantly large cell, diffuse areas, sclerosis	4	34	45
ML, diffuse small cleaved cell, sclerosis	7	32	33
ML, diffuse mixed small and large cell, sclerosis, epithelioid cell component	7	14	38
ML, diffuse large cell, large cleaved cell, large non-cleaved cell, sclerosis	20	10	35
High grade			
ML, large cell, immunoblastic plasmacytoid clear cell, polymorphous epithelioid cell component	8	12	32
ML, lymphoblastic convoluted cell, nonconvoluted cell	4	50	26
ML, small noncleaved cell, Burkitt's follicular areas	5	14	23
Miscellaneous Composite Mycosis fungoides Histiocytic Extramedullary plasma-cytoma Unclassified Other	10	—	—

ML, malignant lymphoma; CLL, chronic lymphocytic leukemia.

and thrombocytopenia may be present in patients with bone marrow involvement.

Bone Marrow. The incidence of bone marrow involvement in NHL varies depending on the morphologic type of the tumor (Table 14–16). As with Hodgkin's disease the pattern of involvement may be focal paratrabecular, focal nonparatrabecular, or diffuse. Again, biopsy specimens are superior to aspirates.

Clinical Staging

The clinical staging criteria for NHL are similar to those used for Hodgkin's disease (discussed previously).

MULTIPLE MYELOMA

Clinical Features

Multiple myeloma is a neoplastic proliferation of plasma cells that almost always has an associated monoclonal gammopathy. The median age at the time of diagnosis is 62 years. The bone marrow and skeletal infiltrates result in bone pain, fractures, and cytopenias. The protein abnormalities can result in renal failure, infection, and hyperviscosity.

Laboratory Studies

Complete Blood Count

There is usually a normochromic normocytic anemia. Normoblasts may be present in the blood. The leukocyte count is usually normal and an occasional immature myeloid cell may be found. There is usually red blood cell rouleaux formation secondary to the increased immunoglobulins.

Bone Marrow

The bone marrow shows an increased number of plasma cells. The percentage of plasma cells required for the diagnosis varies depending on the associated findings (Table 14–17). The plasma cells can appear normal; but usually they show some abnormality such as immaturity, frank malignancy, or appearance in sheets.

TABLE 14–17. CLINICAL PATHOLOGIC CRITERIA FOR THE DIAGNOSIS OF PLASMA CELL MYELOMA

Criteria	Expected Finding
Plasmatocytosis	
Peripheral blood	>0.5 × 109/L plasma cells
Bone marrow*	5–30% plasma cells
Abnormal plasma cells	Present in marrow aspirate
Monoclonal gammopathy	
Increased immunoglobulins*	>3.5 g/dl γG, or >2.0 g/dl γA, or >1.0 g/day κ, or λ chains in urine
Suppressed normal immunoglobulins	< 600 mg/dl γG, or < 100 mg/dl γA, or <50 mg/dl γM
Evidence for plasmacytoma (single or multiple)	
Palpable tumor	Physical examination
Biopsy	Plasma cell infiltrate
Radiographic*	Osteolytic lesions

*Important diagnostic features.

Immunoglobulins

Serum protein electrophoresis will usually (80 percent of the time) show a monoclonal peak that is located in the gamma region, although it is occasionally in the beta region. The protein is identified using immunoelectrophoresis. The monoclonal protein is IgG in over one-half of the cases, IgA in about one-fifth of the cases, only light chains in about one-fifth of cases, and IgD, IgM, or IgE only rarely.

Proteinuria is common in multiple myeloma. About 50 percent of patients have Bence Jones protein in their urine. This can eventually result in renal failure. Testing for Bence Jones protein in the urine is widely available. A routine urinalysis with an absence of proteinuria (when tested with sulfosalicylic acid) rules out the possibility of this protein. The widely used urine dipsticks are not satisfactory for ruling out Bence Jones protein. Immunoelectrophoretic procedures to identify the kappa and lambda light chains of Bence Jones protein are now widely available.

X-ray Studies

Roentgenographic evidence of multiple punched-out lesions in the bones of the skull or pelvis is extremely helpful in making the diagnosis of myeloma.

AGRANULOCYTOSIS AND GRANULOCYTOPENIA

Clinical Features

Although not a malignant disease of the bone marrow, agranulocytosis is frequently fatal. A wide variety of drugs, chemicals, or physical agents, such as irradiation, may destroy or inhibit the granulocytic marrow either alone or in combination with the erythroid and megakaryocytic elements (see Chap. 13). It is also believed that certain as yet unnamed viruses may cause temporary or permanent marrow aplasia. Sometimes granulocytopenia also is noted in early stages of leukemia, the so-called aleukemic leukemia. Finally, the term idiopathic aplasia is reserved for those cases in which no presumed cause can be discovered. Absence or shortage of granulocytes results in increase susceptibility to bacterial infection. If antibiotic therapy is successful in preventing bacterial infection, mycotic infections usually supervene.

Laboratory Studies

Screening Procedures

Complete Blood Count. The blood count indicates a marked decrease (granulocytopenia) or even total absence (agranulocytosis) of granulocytes in the peripheral blood. If other marrow elements are also involved, anemia or thrombocytopenia, or both, may also be manifest (see also Chap. 13 on anemia).

Definitive Procedures

Bone Marrow Examination. Marrow biopsy reveals only a fatty acellular stroma without appreciable numbers of granulocytes. Erythroid elements or megakaryocytes, or both, may also be absent. Only scattered lymphocytes, plasma cells, and, at times, hyperplastic stromal cells remain in the marrow.

SUGGESTED READINGS

Bennett J, et al.: Proposals for the classification of the acute leukemias. Br J Haematol 33:451, 1976.

Colby T, et al.: Hodgkin's disease: A clinicopathologic study of 569 cases. Cancer 49:1848, 1981.

Foon K, et al.: Immunologic classification of acute lymphoblastic leukemia: Implications for normal lymphoid differentiation. Blood 56:1120, 1980.

Foucar K: Acute leukemias: Part 1. Acute lymphoblastic leukemias. Lab Med 12:404, 1981.

Foucar K: Acute leukemias: Part 2. Acute nonlymphocytic leukemias. Lab Med 12:473, 1981.

Foucar K, Goeken J: Clinical application of immunologic techniques to the diagnosis of lymphoproliferative and immunodeficiency disorders. Lab Med 13:403, 1982.

Glick A: Acute leukemia of adults. Am J Clin Pathol 73:459, 1980.

Humphrey G: Cell surface markers in acute lymphoblastic leukemia. Ann Clin Lab Sci 10:169, 1980.

Kobrinsky N, et al.: Acute non-lymphocytic leukemia. Pediatr Clin North Am 27:345, 1980.

Koepke JA (ed): Laboratory Hematology. New York, Churchill Livingstone, 1984.

Miller D: Acute lymphoblastic leukemia. Pediatr Clin North Am 27:269, 1980.

Parker JA: A new look at malignant lymphomas. Diagn Med 3(6):77, 1981.

Pedraza M, et al.: Acute leukemias: Ultrastructural, cytochemical, and immunologic diagnostic approaches. Lab Med 14:45, 1983.

Schroff R, et al.: Immunologic classification of lymphocytic leukemias based on monoclonal antibody-defined cell surface antigens. Blood 59:207, 1982.

Ward P: The lymphoid leukocytoses. Postgrad Med 67:217, 1980.

Weitzman, M: Diagnostic utility of white blood cell and differential cell counts. Am J Dis Child 129:1183, 1975.

15

ABNORMAL BLEEDING

BASIC INFORMATION

Hemostasis

Hemostasis is conveniently divided into three interdependent components, vascular, platelet, and coagulation protein system. A common misconception regarding patients who have a bleeding disorder is that coagulation and hemostasis are one and the same process. By definition, hemostasis is the stopping of bleeding, whereas coagulation includes only the clotting of plasma with the formation of fibrin.

In the laboratory, we can easily study the plasma coagulation process, the platelet contribution with some difficulty, and the vascular phase only in very rudimentary ways. But until better methods become available we are tied to available procedures, although they have some serious shortcomings.

Vascular Component

Of the three components of the hemostatic system, the vascular component is the least understood. Initially, it was thought that the vascular function in hemostasis involved only vasoconstriction. However, recent research indicates that the vascular system contributes more than vasoconstriction to normal hemostasis. For example, the endothelial cells (1) synthesize prostacyclin (a potent inhibitor of platelet aggregation and vasodilation), (2) contain a cofactor for activation of protein C (an inhibitor of coagulation), (3) contain plasminogen activator (an enzyme involved in fibrinolysis), and (4) are a site of von Willebrand factor synthesis.

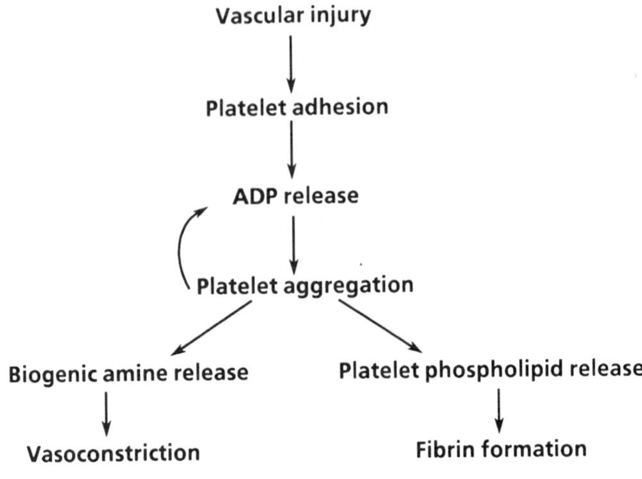

Figure 15–1. Platelet response to vascular injury.

Platelet Component

In vivo, the response of platelets to vascular injury is adhesion to the damaged vessel wall. This results in release of ADP from the platelets leading to platelet aggregation. This process proceeds in a cascading fashion that results in the release of compounds that interact with both the vascular component and the coagulation protein component of the hemostatic system. Biogenic amines (e.g., serotonin and bradykinin) are released, inducing vasoconstriction, and platelet phospholipids (e.g., platelet factor 3) are released, interacting with the coagulation protein system to produce fibrin formation (Fig. 15–1).

Screening for quantitative disorders of platelets is simple because accurate platelet counts are now widely available. In the case of low platelet counts a bone marrow examination is useful in distinguishing between decreased production or increased destruction of platelets. With a normal platelet count, the bleeding time is a good indicator of qualitative platelet defects. In the case of a prolonged bleeding time, platelet aggregation studies are useful in classifying the qualitative platelet defect.

Coagulation Protein Component

A familiarity with the coagulation process is necessary for the proper interpretation of results from the coagulation laboratory as applied to the care of patients either under treatment with

TABLE 15–1. COAGULATION FACTORS

Factor	Name	Factor	Name
I	Fibrinogen	IX	Christmas factor, plasma thromboplastin component (PTC)
II	Prothrombin	X	Stuart-Prower factor
III	Thromboplastin, tissue factor	XI	Plasma thromboplastin antecedent
		XII	Hageman factor
IV	Calcium	XIII	Fibrin stabilizing factor (FSF)
V	Labile factor, proaccelerin	—	Prekallikrein (Fletcher factor)
VII	Stable factor, proconvertin	—	High molecular weight kininogen (HMWK) (Fitzgerald factor)
VIII	Antihemophilic factor (AHF)		

anticoagulants or under substitutional therapy for plasma coagulation factor deficits. Although it is generally agreed that the coagulation process proceeds in a series of individual steps (the cascade theory), it is nevertheless useful to consider coagulation as occurring in three major steps or stages. These stages, which parallel several of the coagulation tests used in the laboratory, are as follows:

Stage I   Activation of factor X
Stage II   Thrombin formation
Stage III   Fibrin formation

In the normal sequence of events, the fibrin is subsequently dissolved by fibrinolysins. It is helpful to include this final step for a better understanding of intravascular coagulation disorders and abnormal fibrinolysis and their effect on hemostatic mechanisms.

The known coagulation factors are listed in Table 15–1 along with some of the common synonyms. Factor VI in the original listing was subsequently found to be activated factor V and was therefore removed from the list. Names, rather than numbers of the first four factors, are still used with the common practice of using only Roman numeral designations for the remaining procoagulants.

Most of these coagulation factors, or procoagulants, circulate in an inactive form. When coagulation is initiated by the

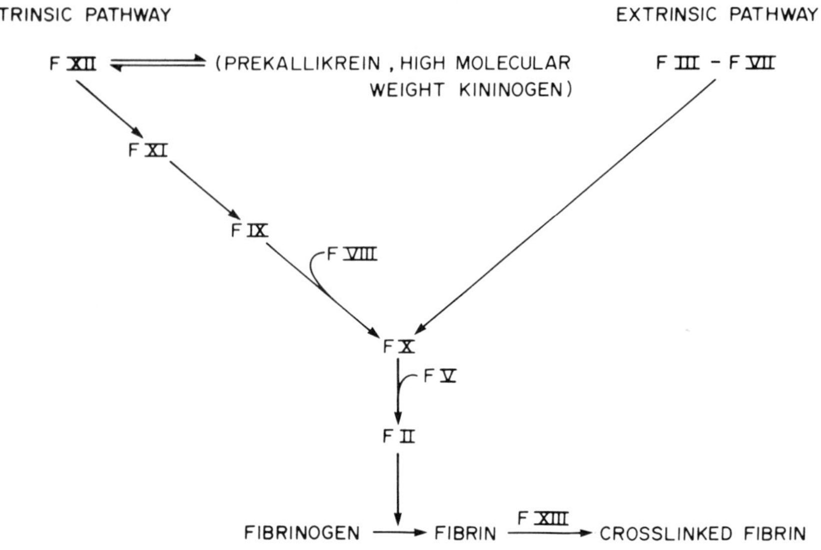

Figure 15–2. Schematic diagram of coagulation cascade indicating order of the activation reactions. *(From Pizzo SV: An overview of coagulation. In Koepke JA (ed): Laboratory Hematology. New York, Churchill Livingstone, 1984, p 506.)*

action of platelet phospholipids and calcium, the inactive factors are individually activated or transformed into serine proteases, which allow the coagulation cascade to proceed.

Figure 15–2 outlines the normal coagulation schema. Several points are worthy of special mention. Deficiencies of the stage I factors include the hemophilias (VIII, IX), and XI deficiency. In stage II, prothrombin is converted to thrombin. The important factors in this reaction (prothrombin, VII, IX, and X) are usually combined as the prothrombin complex. Deficiencies in these factors are most often acquired either secondary to liver disease with decreased production of the prothrombin complex factors or as a result of anticoagulant therapy (coumarin derivatives). Stage III defects are also generally acquired, frequently associated with intravascular coagulation, abnormal fibrinolysin formation, shock, or hemolytic transfusion reactions.

One final point regarding the coagulation schema should be mentioned. There is an alternative mechanism, the extrinsic

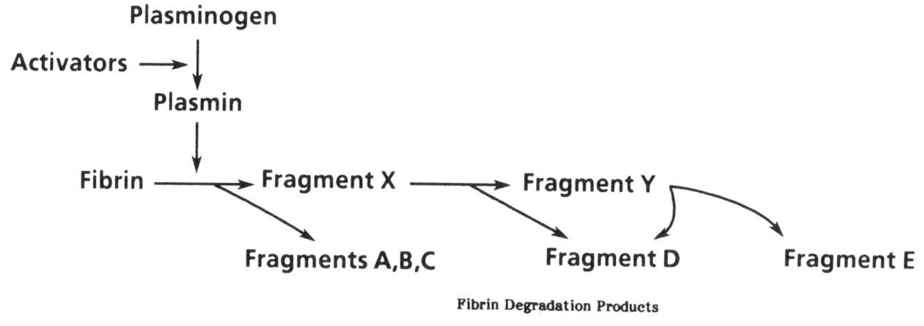

Figure 15–3. Fibrinolytic pathways showing the lysis of fibrin to form the several fibrin degradation products.

system (i.e., tissue juice), for the activation of factor X. Substances possessing thromboplastic activity are widely distributed throughout the body. For example, brain and lung tissues are the usual sources of laboratory thromboplastin preparations. If a venipuncture is traumatic, thromboplastic substances in the perivascular tissues may be introduced into the blood specimen being drawn for coagulation studies and clotting may be initiated in the specimen. This makes the specimen unsuitable for accurate determinations.

Fibrinolysis is the final step in the coagulation process. Indeed, the generation of fibrin sets in motion the mechanisms that are capable of lysing the clot. Plasmin is the major fibrinolytic enzyme. It circulates in plasma in its inactive form, plasminogen. There are several activators that enhance the conversion of plasminogen to plasmin (Fig. 15–3).

There are certain clinical situations where the fibrinolytic system is activated at an accelerated rate. For example, in disseminated intravascular coagulation there is excessive thrombin and plasmin formed. This leads to excessive formation and degradation of fibrin. Eventually, because of increased consumption of fibrinogen, hypofibrinogenemia develops. At this point widespread bleeding can occur.

CLINICAL INVESTIGATION

As noted earlier, the physician must keep in mind all the causes of defective hemostasis. Inquiry and examination for

TABLE 15–2. TYPE OF HEMORRHAGE VERSUS HEMOSTATIC DEFECT

Type of Hemorrhage	Vascular Defect	Platelet Deficiency	Intrinsic System Deficiency	Prothrombin Deficiency
Petechiae and ecchymoses	Common	Common	Rare	Rare
Epistaxis	Common	Common	Rare	Rare
Hemarthroses	Rare	Rare	Common	Rare
Postoperative	Common	Less Common	Common	Common

possible vascular, platelet, or plasma coagulation defects should be done.

Clinical History

Bleeding is a normal physiologic process following trauma, and one must first determine at what point the patient's bleeding is excessive. Bleeding that persists more than 12 to 14 hours is a convenient starting point. A basic point that usually can be determined by incisive questioning is whether the bleeding has been present for the lifetime of the patient (congenital) or has become manifest later in life (acquired). Usually, this point can be established easily. On occasion, however, certain types of stress may activate or uncover a previously unknown congenital abnormality.

The inquiry into possible abnormal bleeding following the stress of trauma or operation (including dental manipulation) is quite important in the interview. Did abnormal bleeding occur following circumcision, tonsillectomy, dental extractions, a major operation, or trauma? Does the patient suffer spontaneous hemorrhages into the skin (ecchymoses and petechiae), respiratory mucous membranes, including nasal membranes (epistaxis), or the joints (hemarthroses)? The answers must always be interpreted in the full clinical context. Remember, patients with completely normal hemostasis can also develop bleeding peptic ulcers, have nose bleeds, and can bleed following tonsillectomy. Easy bruising, especially in women, is so common as to be considered almost normal.

The type of bleeding may be characteristic of the type of deficiency. As indicated in Table 15–2 the details of bleeding may provide valuable clues to the definitive diagnosis.

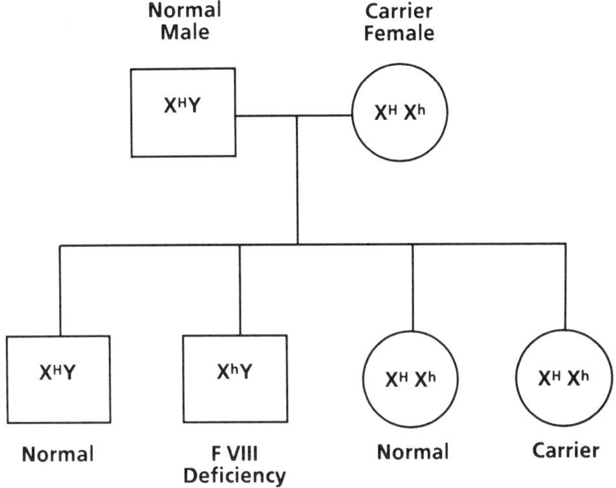

Figure 15–4. Hemophilia pedigree. This diagram illustrates the possible offspring of a female carrier of the hemophilia gene. The pattern is similar for factor IX deficiency.

Family History and Genetics

The importance of the close examination of the family history of a bleeder is stressed because a distinctive and at times diagnostic history may be uncovered. The genetics of factor VIII deficiency has been worked out completely and is worthwhile reviewing as an example of a sex-linked disease or inborn error of metabolism. The pedigree is illustrated in Figure 15–4. This figure shows that only a male offspring will be affected with hemophilia. The X^h (hemophilia) gene is suppressed and nonfunctional when present in conjunction with a normal X^H gene. When in combination with a Y gene, X^h becomes manifest as clinical hemophilia. Female carriers do not have bleeding abnormalities. However, factor VIII levels are mildly decreased in carriers, but not to the level (<30 percent) that would lead to spontaneous hemorrhage.

Examination of the second pedigree (Fig. 15–5) reveals why it is impossible for a hemophiliac father to sire affected sons, although carrier daughters may be produced.

The family history in Christmas disease (factor IX deficiency) is quite similar to that of factor VIII deficiency, and it is impossible to make the differential diagnosis between factor VIII and factor IX deficiency on historical grounds alone. Von

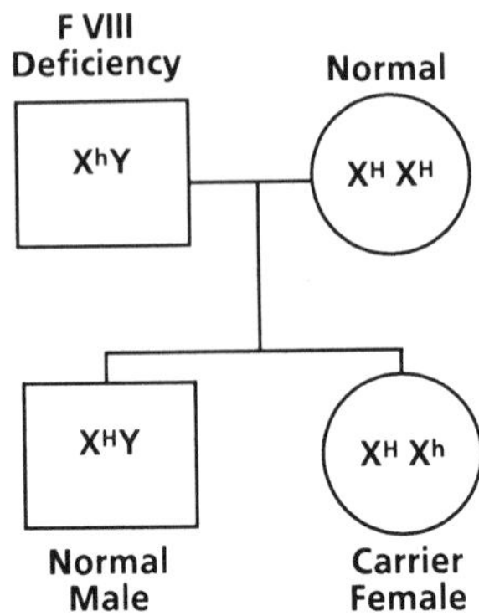

Figure 15–5. Hemophilia pedigree. The diagram illustrates how a hemophiliac man can sire only normal sons and carrier daughters but no affected children. The pattern is similar for factor IX deficiency.

Willebrand's disease is usually inherited as an autosomal dominant trait. Thus, a relative with a documented coagulation problem may provide valuable information. At times the family history may be completely negative, indicating the possible occurrence of mutations resulting in these diseases.

TABLE 15–3. ACQUIRED COAGULATION DISORDERS

Defect	Cause
Platelet deficiency	Aplastic anemia
	Leukemia
	Myelophthisic states
	Hypersplenism
Intrinsic system defects	
Factor VIII deficiency	Intravascular coagulation
Prothrombin complex deficiency	Hepatic disease
	Anticoagulant therapy
	Malabsorption of vitamin K
Fibrinogen deficiency	Defibrination syndrome
Fibrinolysins	Shock
	Carcinoma
	Extensive surgery, especially prostatic surgery
Coagulation factor inhibitors	Replacement therapy in hemophilia
Combined defects	Defibrination syndrome
	Intravascular coagulation

Differentiating Congenital from Acquired Coagulation Disorders

The laboratory diagnosis of a congenital coagulation disorder is almost invariably associated with the deficiency of a single procoagulant. An acquired bleeding disorder secondary to different diseases or conditions is a more common problem. Table 15–3 explains this point. The tip-off that one is dealing with an acquired defect is the presence of significant abnormalities in a number of the coagulation tests that measure different stages of the coagulation process. The good example of this type of disorder is disseminated intravascular coagulation, which is discussed more completely later in this chapter.

LABORATORY INVESTIGATION

Coagulation Panel

A great variety of laboratory tests have been used in the study of bleeding disorders. All these procedures must be carefully performed by well-trained technologists. Experience is needed for interpreting the tests. The panels of tests shown in Table 15–4 have been satisfactory in many laboratories.

Some of the panel tests are precise and accurate (e.g., fibrinogen or prothrombin time), whereas others are only semiquantitative or qualitative at best (e.g., bleeding time and clot retraction). Any results as well as day-to-day changes seen

TABLE 15–4. HEMOSTASIS PANELS

Test	Bleeding	Consumption	Platelet	Normal
Prothrombin time	+	+	+	12–14 seconds
Partial thromboplastin time	+	+	+	23–39 seconds
Fibrinogen	+	+	+	0.15–0.4 g/L
FDP		+		<10 µg/ml
D-dimer		+		<200 ng/ml
Platelet count	+	+	+	150–400 $\times$ 10^9/L
Bleeding time			+	<8 minutes
Platelet aggregation			+	Positive
Platelet adhesiveness			+	25–60%
Clot retraction			+	50–100%

in each different test must be interpreted with these facts in mind.

Coagulation Screening Tests

Two tests listed in Table 15–4 are of special importance in the laboratory diagnosis of coagulation disorders. These are the prothrombin time (one stage) and the partial thromboplastin time. Discussions of these two keystone tests follow.

Prothrombin Time (PT). This is the most important laboratory test to screen for defects in the extrinsic coagulation pathway. With the addition of a complete tissue factor or thromboplastin (rabbit brain extract) to the patient's plasma in the presence of calcium, normal patient plasma will clot in 12 to 14 seconds.

Factors from patient's plasma (fibrinogen, prothrombin, factors V, VII, and X) $+$ Tissue factor from reagent (complete thromboplastin) $\xrightarrow{\text{Ca}^{2+}}$ Clot (9 to 11 seconds)

The source and the quality of the thromboplastin reagent represent the most important variable factors in the test. Thromboplastin reagents from different sources may give markedly different prothrombin times. Thus, unless the test is standardized, the particular laboratory system reference values should be known to the physician.

The prothrombin time will be prolonged when factors V, VII, or X are significantly decreased (e.g., 20 to 25 percent of normal). Prothrombin and fibrinogen must be even more decreased (e.g., 10 to 15 percent) for the prothrombin time to be prolonged.

Appropriate substitution tests that use the prothrombin time as an indicator system can permit differentiation of deficiencies of single procoagulants (Table 15–5). However, this maneuver is no longer commonly done.

Partial Thromboplastin Time (PTT). A more recent addition to the coagulation laboratory's battery of tests has been the PTT test. It is also commonly known as the activated partial thromboplastin time or aPTT. Appropriate preparation of a partial thromboplastin reagent makes the test system sensitive to deficiencies of intrinsic system procoagulants. The PTT will be prolonged when factors XII, XI, IX, VIII, X, or V are significantly decreased (e.g., 20 to 25 percent of normal). As with

TABLE 15–5. PATTERNS OF COAGULATION TEST CORRECTION

Factor Deficiency	Prothrombin Time	PTT	Abnormal Test Corrected with Adsorbed Plasma	Abnormal Test Corrected with Serum
Intrinsic system				
Factor VIII (AHF)	Normal	Abnormal	Yes	No
Factor IX (PTC)*	Normal	Abnormal	No	Yes
Factor XI (PTA)	Normal	Abnormal	Partially	Partially
Prothrombin complex				
Prothrombin*	Abnormal	Normal	No	Partially
Factor VII (stable)	Abnormal	Normal	No	Yes
Factor V (labile)	Abnormal	Abnormal	Yes	No
Factor X*	Abnormal	Normal	No	Yes
Anticoagulants or fibrinolysins	Normal or abnormal	Abnormal	No	No

*Vitamin K dependent.

the PT, prothrombin and fibrinogen must be even more decreased (e.g., 10 to 15 percent of normal) for the PTT to be prolonged. Also, as with the prothrombin time test, there is much interlaboratory variability in the PTT test.

$$\text{Factors from patient's plasma (All coagulation proteins except factor VII)} + \text{Platelet phospholipid reagent (partial thromboplastin)} + \text{Activator} \xrightarrow{\text{Ca}^{2+}} \text{Clot (23 to 34 seconds)}$$

Appropriate substitution of whole plasma, reagent factor VIII, and factor IX as well as cross-correctional experiments that use plasmas with known deficiencies allow for the definitive diagnosis of single coagulation deficiences (Table 15–5). As with deficiences of the extrinsic system, this method is not often used and is replaced by specific factor assays (discussion follows). Therefore, multiple deficiencies yield results that are more difficult to interpret.

Coagulation Factor Assays. The specific measurement of coagulation factor levels is the preferred method to diagnose coagulation factor deficiencies. It is a procedure now available in many hospital laboratories. This procedure is also of use in following replacement therapy of hemophiliacs, although serial PTT studies may sometimes be adequate.

THE HEMOPHILIAS AND OTHER COAGULATION DISORDERS

HEMOPHILIA CAUSED BY FACTOR VIII OR FACTOR IX DEFICIENCY

Clinical Features

Hemophilia A (classic hemophilia or factor VIII deficiency) and hemophilia B (Christmas disease or factor IX deficiency) are congenital bleeding disorders. Factor VIII deficiencies account for about 70 percent of all inherited deficiencies of coagulation factors, whereas factor IX deficiencies account for about 12 percent.

A carefully taken, accurate, and complete medical history is of prime importance in the evaluation of hemophilia, whether caused by factor VIII or factor IX deficiency. Although laboratory studies are also important, they must be integrated into the historical evaluation of the patient to be interpreted in a meaningful manner. Two points relative to this statement are important. First, patients with mild to moderately severe hemophilia may have normal values with some of the screening tests for hemophilia (e.g., whole blood clotting time or prothrombin consumption). Second, mildly affected patients, unless carefully questioned, may be thought to have no disease, and only when they are subjected to surgical procedures or major trauma will the bleeding disorder become manifest. In these instances more sensitive laboratory testing is necessary.

The previous discussion implies the existence of several levels of severity of hemophilia; this is useful to keep in mind because diagnosis and treatment correlate with this arbitrary division (Table 15–6).

Children with hemophilia, because of the relative protection from injury before they begin to walk, usually do not sustain hemorrhages before that time, and it is only when they are 2 or 3 years old that they develop hemarthroses.

Family History

The sex-linked recessive mode of inheritance of both factor VIII and factor IX deficiency has already been covered. However, one should keep in mind that a few cases of hemophilia may arise spontaneously, presumably due to gene mutations. Therefore, an entirely negative family history does not necessarily rule out this disease.

TABLE 15–6. CORRELATION OF HEMORRHAGIC MANIFESTATIONS WITH FACTOR VIII LEVELS

Severity of Hemophilia	Type of Hemorrhage	Factor VIII Levels (% of Normal)
Severe	Spontaneous, into joints and muscles; major hemorrhage after trauma	<0.5
Moderate	Only after minor trauma or surgery	1–5
Mild	Only after major trauma or surgery	5–35
Normal	None	>50

Laboratory Studies

Screening Procedures

The Lee-White clotting time and the skin bleeding time are *not* adequate screening tests for hemophilia because these tests are abnormal in only about one-half of the affected persons. An inadequate test is worse than none at all because it gives the patient, the family, or the physician a false sense of security.

Partial Thromboplastin Time. PTT has provided a powerful tool for hemophilia screening as well as for monitoring therapy. The cross-correction procedures with additions of fresh plasma, adsorbed plasma, and serum may be adequate for diagnosis. In mild deficiency, however, equivocal results may be obtained.

Definitive Procedures

Factor VIII (or IX) Assay. Levels of factor VIII (or IX) will be decreased. As was stated earlier, the factor VIII level correlates with the hemorrhagic manifestations of the disease. Direct assays are much more useful than the substitution procedure described earlier.

Therapy of Hemophilia

In the therapy of coagulation deficiencies, missing factors are supplied by the transfusion of the deficient component or factor. Thus, the exact diagnosis of the coagulant deficiency (i.e., factor VIII or factor IX deficiency) is a prerequisite to rational therapy. There are several preparations available for the treatment of hemophilia. They contain differing amounts of the various coagulation factors (Table 15–7).

TABLE 15–7. PREPARATIONS FOR TREATMENT OF HEMOPHILIA

Product	Amount of Factor VIII	Amount of Factor IX
Fresh frozen plasma	+	+
Cryoprecipitate	+ +	None
Factor VIII concentrate	+ + +	None
Prothrombin complex concentrates (factor II, V, VII, and IX)	None	+ + +

Fresh frozen plasma (FFP), by definition, contains 1 unit/ml of both factor VIII and factor IX. Its usefulness in treatment of hemophilia is limited by the fact that to achieve hemostatic factor levels, very large volumes of FFP are required. To avoid the problem of volume overload, concentrates have been developed. Cryoprecipitate, prepared in blood banks, contains approximately 100 units of factor VIII activity per bag (approximately 5 to 15 ml). It does not contain significant amounts of factor IX. Commercial factor VIII concentrates have been developed that are prepared from pooled human plasma and are about 150 times purified. The factor VIII activity of the concentrate has been assayed and the amount is indicated on the label of each bottle. Factor IX concentrates, as opposed to factor VIII concentrates, are not pure concentrates. Rather, factor IX concentrates contain concentrated activities of all four vitamin K dependent factors, i.e., II, VII, IX, and X. DDAVP (1-deamino-8-D-arginine-vasopressin), a synthetic analog of antiduretic hormone, has been used recently in treatment of mild classic hemophiliacs. It produces a twofold or greater rise in factor VIII levels. The mechanism is not well understood and it is only effective in mild classic hemophiliacs, not severe classic hemophiliacs or any factor IX deficient patients.

When treating bleeding episodes in hemophiliacs several factors have to be considered. One must realize that there are different critical levels of factor VIII (or IX) that must be obtained to stop bleeding from different locations. For example, factor levels of only 10 to 15 percent are needed to control epistaxis, whereas factor levels of greater than 80 percent are necessary if the patient is to undergo major surgery. The critical factor level desired influences the type of replacement chosen, e.g., minor bleeding episodes may be treated with FFP or cryoprecipitate whereas major bleeding episodes require commercial concentrates. The choice of therapy may also depend on severity of the patient's hemophilia. For example, a patient with mild classic hemophilia with a mild bleeding episode may require only DDAVP for therapy. One must also consider that the type of bleeding episode will dictate the length of replacement therapy, e.g., dental extractions may require only one dose whereas major surgery may require 10 days of therapy. One further consideration: there is risk of hepatitis or acquired immune deficiency syndrome (AIDS) from the various preparations. Commercial concentrates have a greater risk than cryoprecipate because they are prepared from large pools whereas DDAVP has no such risks. Recent studies indicate that heat treatment of factor VIII concentrates destroys the HTLV III virus, the apparent etiologic agent for AIDS.

The usual method of replacement consists of giving a loading bolus followed by maintenance doses at 12- to 24-hour intervals. One should obtain pre- and posttransfusion factor VIII (or IX) levels to monitor therapy. Table 15–8 summarizes one of the many schemes used in the treatment of bleeding episodes in classic hemophiliacs. The optimal postinfusion factor levels are also applicable to factor IX deficient patients. The dosage and dosing interval is somewhat different than for factor VIII patients in that the volume of distribution of factor IX is twice as large as factor VIII and the plasma half-life of factor IX is twice as long as factor VIII.

Inhibitors to Factor VIII

Clinical Features

Factor VIII inhibitors arise in approximately 10 to 15 percent of patients with severe classic hemophilia and in patients with a number of other conditions, e.g., postpartum women, patients with allergic reactions to drugs, collagen–vascular diseases (e.g., SLE and rheumatoid arthritis), neoplasms, inflammatory bowel disease, and in elderly patients for no apparent cause. These inhibitors are antibodies to factor VIII that are time, temperature, and pH dependent.

Clinically, as the patient develops an inhibitor, he or she requires increasing amounts of cryoprecipitate or concentrates, at times resulting in an almost complete lack of response to massive doses of procoagulants. The treatment of these patients is very complex and should be directed by specialists.

TABLE 15–8. TREATMENT OF BLEEDING IN HEMOPHILIACS

Bleeding Episode	Optimal Posttransfusion Factor VIII Level (%)	Factor VIII Dosage (units/kg)	Number of Doses
Superficial cuts, epistasis	10–15	7–10	1–2
Hemarthroses	~ 30	20	1–2
Gastrointestinal bleeding	~ 50	30	3–5
Dental extraction	~ 50	30	1
Surgery, central nervous system trauma	~ 100	60	6–20

Several therapeutic options have been tried: (1) high dose of factor VIII concentrate; (2) porcine factor VIII; (3) prothrombin complexes in an attempt to bypass the need for factor VIII in the coagulation cascade; (4) exchange transfusions to lower the antibody level; and (5) immunosuppressive therapy to decrease the production of the inhibitor.

Laboratory Studies

Screening Procedures

Inhibitor Sereening Test. This is an in vitro test for inhibitors where mixtures of normal and patient plasma are studied using the PTT technique. The most sensitive technique uses a mixture of four parts patient plasma to one part normal plasma incubated for 2 hours at 37C. Normally the PTT on this mixture is within 5 percent of the normal control. In the presence of an inhibitor the mixture will be prolonged greater than 10 percent over that of the control.

Definitive Procedures

Bethesda Inhibitor Assay (BIA). This is a standard method for quantitating factor VIII inhibitor levels. One Bethesda unit is the amount of antibody that will inactivate 50 percent of the factor VIII activity in 1 milliliter of plasma. The test is done by incubating equal amounts of normal plasma and patient plasma for 2 hours at 37C. The residual factor VIII activity is then measured and compared with a control.

VON WILLEBRAND'S DISEASE

Clinical Features

Von Willebrand's disease is a bleeding disorder characterized by a complex hemostatic defect. It accounts for about 8 percent of all hereditary coagulation disorders. The abnormalities in von Willebrand's disease seem to arise from a quantitative or qualitative abnormality in the von Willebrand's factor, a large multimeric glycoprotein that circulates in the blood complexed with the factor VIII procoagulant protein. The bleeding in von Willebrand's disease usually involves the mucous membranes (e.g., epistasis, easy bruising, menorrhagia, and gastrointestinal bleeding) as opposed to hemophilia, which usually involves joints and muscles. Diagnosis of von Willebrand's disease involves a careful history and physical examination coupled with a detailed laboratory evaluation.

Family History

Von Willebrand's disease is usually inherited as an autosomal dominant gene, although autosomal recessive patterns have been described. This is in contrast with hemophilia, which is a sex-linked recessive trait.

Laboratory Studies

Screening Procedures

Bleeding Time. The skin bleeding time is characteristically prolonged in von Willebrand's disease in contrast with hemophilia where it is normal.

Definitive Procedures

Factor VIII Procoagulant Assay (VIII:C). This is an assay of the protein that corrects the coagulation abnormality in classic hemophilia. VIII:C levels in von Willebrand's disease are usually decreased, but can be normal. The levels in a particular patient can be variable over time.

Factor VIII Related Antigen (VIII R:Ag). This is a measure of the antigenic expression of the von Willebrand's factor. It is an immunologic, not a functional assay. The VIII R:Ag level is usually decreased in von Willebrand's disease, but as with VIII:C levels it can be variable in a particular patient over time.

Ristocetin Cofactor Activity (VIII R:RCo). Platelets from healthy persons agglutinate when they are exposed to the drug ristocetin. Platelets from most patients with von Willebrand's disease fail to agglutinate in the presence of ristocetin. As with the other assays in von Willebrand's disease, it may vary in a particular patient over time.

Multimeric Structure. It appears as if the von Willebrand's factor circulates in the blood as a series of multimers. Analysis of the multimeric composition in patients with von Willebrand's disease allows one to subclassify these patients. This is a reference laboratory procedure.

OTHER CONGENITAL COAGULATION DISORDERS

Other congenital coagulation disorders are also seen in clinical practice, but they are relatively rare. All are autosomal recessively inherited, in contrast with the hemophilias. A complete discussion of each is beyond the scope of this book. In this introduction to the clinical laboratory, they need be remembered as a group only, as they are so rare. Table 15–9 may be of some aid in this regard.

THROMBOCYTOPENIA

Clinical Features

Thrombocytopenia may be associated with a variety of diseases and may occur following the use of drugs, chemicals, or irradiation, which depress platelet production by the megakaryocytes. Therefore, one should usually consider thrombocytopenia as evidence of underlying difficulties rather than as a primary disease. The exception to this is the condition known as idiopathic or immune thrombocytopenic purpura (ITP), which often appears to be a disease of megakaryocytes and platelets in which autoimmune substances that cause thrombocytopenia and purpura are produced.

As with anemia, there are a variety of conditions that result in thrombocytopenia. This discussion is directed toward providing guidelines regarding the groups of etiologic factors, rather than cataloging the many different conditions associated with thrombocytopenia. The effects of thrombocytopenia are superimposed on the clinical manifestations of the disease that caused the thrombocytopenia.

Bleeding because of thrombocytopenia is unusual with platelet counts above $20 \times 10^9/L$ unless there is concomitant vascular injury or impaired vascular integrity. Apparently this occurs because the platelet count is really only an indirect measure of platelet function. Platelets can be thought of as existing in several different compartments as illustrated in the schema

$$\text{Marrow} \rightarrow \text{Circulating blood} \rightarrow \text{Endothelium.}$$

It is only when the number of functional platelets in the endothelial compartment is critically reduced that petechial hemorrhages occur. Therefore, a low plasma platelet count per se

TABLE 15-9. UNCOMMON CONGENITAL COAGULATION DISORDERS

Deficient Factor	Major Clinical Features	Laboratory Investigation
Fibrinogen	Similar to factor VIII deficiency but less severe; no residual disabilities	Fibrinogen
Prothrombin	Hematomas; menorrhagia; mucosal bleeding	Prothrombin time; prothrombin assay
Factor V (labile)	Epistaxis; bruising; menorrhagia	Prothrombin time PTT; factor V assay
Factor VII (stable)	Articular hemorrhage; mucosal bleeding, menorrhagia	Prothrombin time; factor VII assay
Factor X (Stuart-Prower)	Mild bleeding disorder	Prothrombin time; PTT; factor X assay
Factor XI (PTA)	Epistaxis; bleeding following trauma	PTT; factor XI assay
Factor XII (Hageman)	No bleeding tendency; test-tube bleeder	PTT; factor XII assay
Factor XIII (FSF)	Bleeding from umbilicus in newborns; poor wound healing after surgery	Urea solubility; factor XIII assay
Preallikrein (Fletcher)	No bleeding tendency; test-tube bleeder	PTT
HMWK (Fitzgerald)	No bleeding tendency; test-tube bleeder	PTT

may not necessarily be associated with bleeding. The platelet count merely reflects the status in the vascular compartment. Accordingly, it is not appropriate to treat the platelet count in a patient with thrombocytopenia, but rather to treat the patient, supplying platelets only when hemorrhage due to platelet deficiency occurs. Furthermore, the transfusion of viable platelets sooner or later results in the production of platelet antibodies, after which even massive platelet transfusions are of no use.

Laboratory Studies

Screening Procedures

Platelet Count. Although there may be technical difficulties with platelet counting, this measurement is now widely avail-

TABLE 15–10. PLATELET ESTIMATIONS

Platelets on Blood Film (avg no./oil immersion field)	Platelet Count ($\times$ 10⁹/L)
0–1	5
1–5	10–50
6–10	60–100
>10	100+

able. Precision varies at ±10 percent at best. A well-prepared peripheral blood film is invaluable in an evaluation of both platelet number and probable function. A comparison of the film examination and actual platelet count is given in Table 15–10. In fact, this comparison is a routine part of the platelet count procedure. On the film the platelets should be evenly distributed and not clumped. If the film is inadequate, another film must be prepared, either from a new fingerprick or from an adequately mixed tube of blood with EDTA anticoagulant. This estimate, as expected, is related to the size of microscopic field, which varies from one microscope to another and must be checked.

The morphology of the individual platelets can be a rough indicator of platelet function. Extreme platelet anisocytosis is characteristic of leukemias, with or without therapy. These findings probably are even better visualized in the counting chamber preparations that use phase-contrast illumination. Loss of tentacles is usually associated with poor function.

Bone Marrow. The bone marrow examination is of great importance in the evaluation of thrombocytopenia. Its usefulness is in determining the number and apparent age of the mega-karyocytes. Two patterns are commonly found (Table 15–11).

TABLE 15–11. MARROW MEGAKARYOCYTES IN THROMBOCYTOPENIA

Type of Thrombocytopenia	Marrow Megakaryocytes	Comment
Primary	Decreased or absent	Bone marrow failure, idio-pathic or following drugs or irradiation (± fibrosis)
Secondary	Increased, immature	Increased peripheral destruc-tion of platelets, e.g., ITP

The implications insofar as therapy is concerned are obvious. Primary thrombocytopenia may be treated by platelet transfusion. This method is often unsatisfactory, especially if attempted over an extended period of time because of antiplatelet antibody formation. In secondary thrombocytopenia, therapy is usually directed toward the primary disease or toward elimination or neutralization of antiplatelet antibodies.

DISSEMINATED INTRAVASCULAR COAGULATION

Clinical Features

Acute disseminated intravascular coagulation (DIC) is a pathologic condition caused by the presence of thrombin in the systemic circulation leading to initiation of clotting. This results in a decrease of the coagulation factors that are usually consumed during blood clotting. DIC is not a primary event, but occurs secondary to many different triggering conditions. The final common pathway of all causes of DIC is the formation of thrombin and plasmin. All the clinical and laboratory manifestations of DIC are a result of the actions of thrombin and plasmin. Figure 15–6 illustrates some of these relationships.

Chronic DIC may be seen in patients with malignancy and is characterized by much milder clinical and laboratory findings. Clinically, the manifestations of DIC are diverse. The patient may have some or all of the following signs and symptoms: fever, hypotension, acidosis, hypoxia, and proteinuria. The patient may also manifest some or all of the following more specific signs: petechiae, purpura, wound bleeding, oozing from venipuncture sites, and gastrointestinal tract bleeding. A significant number of microvascular thromboses or emboli may occur in DIC. This can result in significant end organ damage as shown in Figure 15–6.

Laboratory Studies

Screening Procedures

Prothrombin Time. The PT is usually prolonged because of the presence of fibrin degradation products that act as inhibitors, or decreases in factors I, II, V, or X.

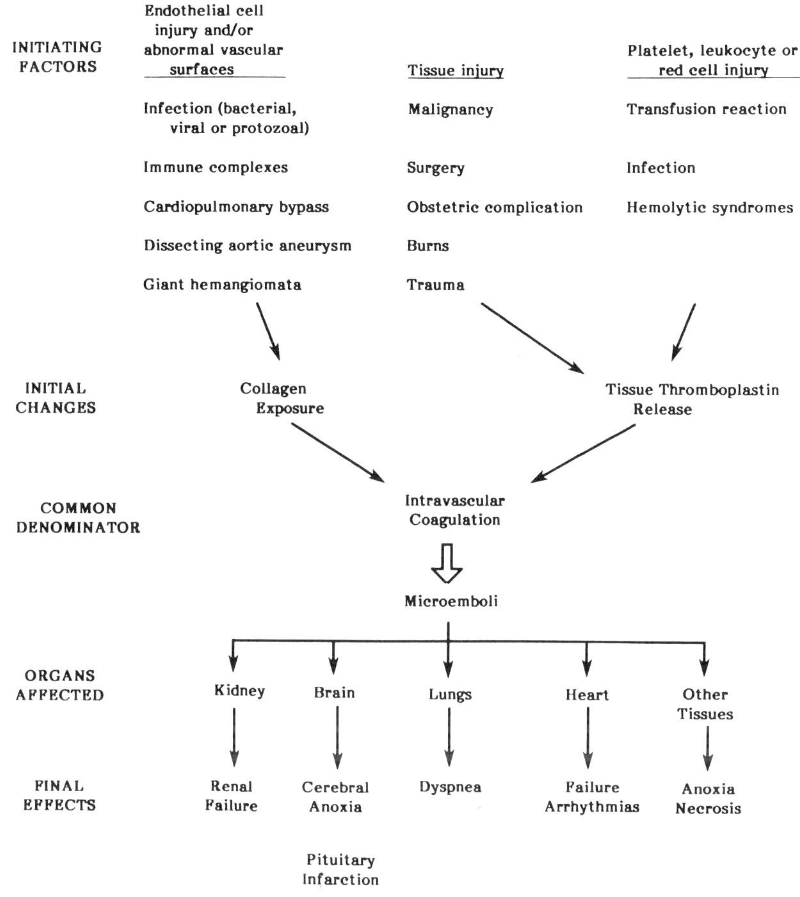

Figure 15-6. Disseminated intravascular coagulation or consumptive coagulopathy.

Partial Thromboplastin Time. The PTT is usually prolonged because of a decrease in factor VIII or for any of the reasons listed for the PT.

Fibrinogen. Most patients with acute DIC have low fibrinogen levels. Fibrinogen levels can be difficult to interpret for several reasons. First, patients with liver disease may have low fibrinogen levels not associated with DIC. Second, fibrinogen is an acute phase reactant that may be elevated as a result of the condition underlying the DIC. In these cases a falling fibrinogen level is helpful.

Platelet Count. Thrombocytopenia is seen in most patients with DIC.

Confirmatory Tests

Fibrin Degradation Products (FDP). With an increasing role of fibrin formation, there is a concomitant increase in fibrinolysis with increasing amounts of FDPs (see Fig. 15–3). There are a number of tests available for detection of FDP.

D-Dimer. Following intravascular coagulation, enzymatic digestion of the formed fibrin results in the formation of crosslinked fibrin derivations, so-called XDP. A simple latex agglutination procedure is used and is reported as positive (>200 ng/ml XDP) or negative (<200 ng/ml).

Fibrin Monomer. Fibrin monomers or dimers are the result of thrombin-cleaved fibrinogen. Tests for these entities provide very sensitive measures of increased intravascular fibrin formation.

Euglobulin Clot Lysis Time. This test measures plasmin and/or plasminogen activators after the inhibitors have been removed. It is performed by reacting a standard clot with the patient's plasma and observing for lysis. Normal lysis time is greater than 3 hours. Specimens with significant fibrinolysis lyse the clots in 1 hour or less.

Other Tests

Antithrombin III (AT III). AT III is a naturally occurring plasma protease inhibitor to factors XII, IX, X, and thrombin. Low AT III levels are seen in DIC. It is not specific for DIC, as low AT III levels can be seen in other conditions such as liver disease or nephrotic syndrome.

Factor Assays. Frequently quantitative assays for the consumable factors (i.e., factors V and VIII) are decreased in DIC.

Thrombin Clotting Time (TCT). The TCT is often increased in DIC because of a decrease in fibrinogen or the presence of FDPs that act as inhibitors.

HEMORRHAGE CAUSED BY ACQUIRED DECREASES IN PROTHROMBIN COMPLEX

Clinical Features

The various factors of the prothrombin complex are normally produced in the liver and are dependent on adequate amounts of vitamin K for their production. If significant liver disease (e.g., cirrhosis) is present or vitamin K is deficient because of malabsorption or dietary lack, the prothrombin complex will be deficient. Likewise, patients receiving chronic anticoagulant therapy have decreased levels of these procoagulants. Finally, in hemorrhagic disease of the newborn, lack of sufficient vitamin K levels can lead to neonatal hemorrhage. This disease is now rarely seen because of the prophylactic administration of vitamin K at or before the time of birth.

Laboratory Studies

Prothrombin Time

The measurement of the one-stage PT is the laboratory test of choice. For whatever reason, if there is a deficiency of the vitamin K dependent factors (i.e., factors II, VII, IX, and X) the PT will be prolonged. In most cases all factors are affected and there is no need to determine individual deficiencies.

INTRAOPERATIVE AND POSTOPERATIVE HEMORRHAGE

Clinical Features

One of the periodic problems on the surgical service is the sudden and unexpected occurrence of a hemostatic defect during or soon after operation. Uncontrollable oozing into the operative site or from serous surfaces usually heralds such an emergency. A number of possible causes are listed in Table 15–12. If a hemostatic defect is truly present, a combined clinical and laboratory investigation should be initiated. This event constitutes a true emergency.

Laboratory Studies

It is important to begin the investigation as soon as possible. The following studies are done immediately: a platelet count or

TABLE 15–12. CAUSES OF OPERATIVE HEMORRHAGE

Multiple transfusions of banked blood

Intravascular coagulation or incompatible transfusion

Unsuspected mild hemophilia

Unsuspected anticoagulant therapy

Platelet deficiency (number or function)

Fibrinolysins (obstetric, extensive surgical procedures especially prostatic surgery)

Shock (from any cause) with anoxia

a blood film for the estimation of platelets, a PT and PTT, and a fibrinogen determination. A clot is drawn for observation of clotting, failure to clot, or clot lysis. In addition, it is observed for retraction and color of serum. These four studies should allow a reasonably quick and accurate diagnosis, and specific therapy should be initiated promptly. Table 15–13 summarizes the findings in some major causes of intraoperative hemorrhage. Clinical judgment allows certain of these possibilities to be discounted or eliminated. The correlation of the laboratory studies with the clinical picture will almost certainly elucidate the cause of the bleeding diathesis.

DEEP VEIN THROMBOSIS

Deep vein thrombosis is a common clinical problem that frequently arises in hospitalized patients, especially when they are confined to bed. The elderly postoperative patient is especially prone to this condition. A number of conditions increase the risk of venous thrombosis (Table 15–14); these risk factors appear to be additive.

Spontaneously arising thrombi most commonly occur in the lower limbs. They form as a small clump of red blood cells in a fibrin network on a venous valve. The underlying endothelium is usually normal. The small nidus of cells and fibrin may be washed away or may be lysed. If stasis persists, the thrombus may grow by successive layering of platelets and fibrin until it occludes the venous channel. Subsequently, there is propagation of the thrombus centrally.

Normally, the intact endothelium resists thrombogenesis. However, with injury and denuding of the endothelial surface, the coagulation process is triggered. Platelets adhere to the

TABLE 15–13. COAGULATION TESTS IN OPERATIVE HEMORRHAGE

Conditions	Platelets	PT	PTT	Fibrinogen	Clot Retraction	Serum
Multiple transfusions	↓ *	↑	↑	Normal	Delayed	Pink
Intravascular coagulation	↓ ↓	↑	↑	↓ ↓ *	Poor	Pink
Incompatible blood transfusion	↓	↑	↑	↓	Poor	Red*
Hemophilia, mild	Normal*	Normal	↑ *	Normal	Normal	Clear
Coumadin therapy	Normal	↑ *	Normal	Normal	Normal	Clear
Platelet deficiency	↓ ↓ *	Normal	Normal	Normal	Poor*	Clear
Excessive fibrinolysins	Normal	↑ or no clot	↑ or no clot	↓ ↓ *	None formed*	Pink
Shock, hemorrhagic†	Normal	Normal	Normal	Normal	Normal	Clear

*Important differential tests.
†Primarily a vascular defect (early); thus, test results are normal.

TABLE 15–14. RISK FACTORS IN VENOUS THROMBOSIS

Primary changes in blood vessels 　　Varicose veins 　　Thrombophlebitis 　　Injury	Primary changes in blood flow 　　Immobility 　　Pregnancy 　　Obesity
Primary changes in blood 　　composition 　　Hemoconcentration 　　Postoperative period 　　Lupus anticoagulant 　　Deficiency of ATIII, protein S, or 　　　　protein C	Multifactorial 　　Previous history of thrombosis 　　Family history 　　Increasing age 　　Estrogen therapy

underlying collagen, the coagulation cascade is activated, and a thrombus forms. Both immediate and remote injury (e.g., major surgical procedures within the abdominal cavity or hip joints) may initiate injury to the venous endothelium.

Blood coagulation is ordinarily kept in check by the normal continuing neutralization of activated coagulation factors. The most important such inhibitor is AT III, also known as heparin cofactor. Activated procoagulants are also cleared by the reticuloendothelial system and the liver. With stasis, however, the normal neutralization and clearance mechanisms are impaired.

A second defensive mechanism (i.e., fibrinolysis) also is continually operative. Even if fibrin is formed, the continuing fibrinolytic process dissolves such clots. This enzyme, called fibrinolysin or plasminogen, is normally present in low concentrations.

Thus, a delicate balance of the coagulation and fibrinolytic processes ordinarily maintains the fluidity of the blood. However, if the scales are tipped by hypercoagulability, increased neutralization of antithrombin, or decreased fibrinolysis, significant problems may result.

Hypercoagulability is a concept implying blood changes that predispose to thrombosis. A number of factors in the normal physiologic response to trauma or illness may predispose to thrombosis in the susceptible patient, i.e., one who has one or more of the risk factors noted in Table 15–14.

A number of laboratory tests (Table 15–15) have been proposed as tests for hypercoagulability. These indirect tests suffer from a number of problems including a considerable overlapping of normal and abnormal results. It is difficult to know, in many cases, whether the abnormality seen is a cause or an effect. Nevertheless, it is apparent that there will be increasing interest in this facet of laboratory medicine, because the more definitive studies (venography, radioactive fibrinogen uptake, and Doppler studies) are so much more difficult to use in the large number of patients at risk.

The accurate diagnosis of deep venous thrombosis (DVT) is difficult at best. Clinical history and physical examination are notoriously inaccurate. Venous angiography and radioactive fibrinogen studies indicate that venous thrombosis is often asymptomatic with pulmonary embolization often being the initial clinical manifestation of this disease. To compound the problem, several conditions (e.g., painful veins, postphlebitis syndrome, calf hematoma, ruptured popliteal cyst, or unaccustomed muscular exercise) may closely mimic DVT.

Laboratory Studies

There are two blood tests that are sensitive to venous thromboembolism in symptomatic patients: the fibrinopeptide A assay and the assay for fibrin/fibrinogen fragment E. Both of these tests are nonspecific and have to be performed by radioimmunoassay, a procedure that is too complicated for routine clinical use. Therefore, there are no good blood tests at present for diagnosing DVT. There are other tests available that are useful in diagnosing DVTs which are discussed on page 252.

TABLE 15–15. CANDIDATE TESTS FOR HYPERCOAGULABLE STATE

Abnormally short PTT
Increased fibrin/fibrinogen degradation products
Increased D-dimer (XDP)
Increased fibrin monomer
Increased fibrinopeptide A
Increased factor VIII_{AG}/factor VIII_c ratio
Increased β-thromboglobulin
Increased platelet factor 4 (PF4)
Decreased antithrombin III (AT III)
Decreased protein C
Decreased protein S

Definitive Procedures

Venography. The intravenous injection of x-ray contrast media is the definitive procedure for the diagnosis of DVT.

Radioactive Fibrinogen Uptake. This rather complex test is dependent on the continuing deposition of fibrin at the site of thrombosis. Thus, it detects only active thrombosis and is of no use if the disease has stabilized. The test appears to correlate quite well with the fibrin monomer or dimer measurement. It is particularly sensitive to distal DVTs (i.e., in the calves).

Doppler Examination. This procedure, when done by well-trained personnel, is sensitive and specific for the diagnosis of DVT, particularly proximal deep vein thromboses (i.e., in the thigh).

Treatment

DVTs are usually treated by anticoagulation. The ideal duration of anticoagulant treatment is not known. Present data suggests continuing therapy between 6 weeks and 6 months for a single proven episode. Heparin should be given for the first 1 to 2 weeks of therapy. The patient may then be switched to oral anticoagulants, i.e., the coumarin drugs. Heparin acts principally by accelerating the reaction between AT III and thrombin. Heparin is given to maintain the PTT about two times the normal control (Table 15–16). Coumadin, the most

TABLE 15–16. LABORATORY MONITORING OF ANTICOAGULANT THERAPY FOR VENOUS THROMBOSIS

	Anticoagulant		
	None	*Heparin*	*Coumarin Drugs*
Activated coagulation time, (secs)	75–120	150–190	Not useful
Prothrombin time (seconds)			
Brain thromboplastin	9–11	Not useful	17–25*
Brain–lung thromboplastin	9–11	Not useful	17–28*
Partial, thromboplastin time (activated seconds)	23–34	50–80	Not useful

Values given are approximate because of significant variability in coagulation system performance.

*International Normalized Ratio (INR) = 1.5–3.0.

common oral anticoagulant, acts by interfering with the gamma-carboxylation of the vitamin K-dependent clotting factors (i.e., factors II, VII, IX, and X). Coumadin is given to maintain the PT about one and a half to two times normal. However, the PT is system dependent. There have been recent attempts to standardize this test for more careful control of the level of anticoagulation.

SUGGESTED READINGS

Aledort L: Current concepts in diagnosis and management of hemophilia. Hosp Pract 17:77, 1982.

Bachman F: Diagnostic approach to mild bleeding disorders. Semin Hematol 17:292, 1980.

Bick RL: Disseminated Intravascular Coagulation and Related Syndromes. Boca Raton, Fla, CRC Press, 1983.

Biggs R, Rizza C (eds): Human Blood Coagulation, Haemostasis and Thrombosis, 3rd ed. Oxford, Blackwell Scientific Pub., 1984.

Bloom A, Thomas D (eds): Haemostasis and Thrombosis. New York, Churchill Livingstone, 1981.

Colman R, et al. (eds): Hemostasis and Thrombosis: Basic Principles and Clinical Practice. Philadelphia, Lippincott, 1982.

Deykin D: Current status of anticoagulant therapy. Am J Med 72:659, 1982.

Glader BE (ed): Perinatal haematology. In Gladder BE (ed): Clinics in Haematology, vol 7, no 1. London, Saunders, 1978.

Hoyer L: The factor VIII complex: Structure and function. Blood 58:1, 1981.

Lowe G: Laboratory evaluation of hypercoagulability. Clin Haematol 10:407, 1981.

Mielke C, Rodvien R: Platelets and disease. Lab Mgmt 16:22, 1978.

Perkins HA: Postoperative coagulation defects. Anesthesiology 27:456, 1966.

Rader M: Coagulation factor disorders. Diagn Med 4:57, 1981.

Sherry S: Fibrinolysis and afibrinogenemia. Anesthesiology 27:465, 1966.

Spector I, Corn M: Laboratory tests of hemostasis: The relation to hemorrhage in liver disease. Arch Intern Med 119:577, 1967.

Thompson A, Harker L: Manual of Hemostasis and Thrombosis. Philadelphia, Davis, 1983.

Triplett D: Anticoagulant therapy: Monitoring techniques. Lab Mgmt 20:31, 1982.

Triplett D (ed): Laboratory Evaluation of Coagulation. Chicago, ASCP Press, 1982.

Zimmerman TS, Ruggeri ZM: Von Willebrand's Disease. In Gladder BE (ed): Clinics in Hematology vol 12, no. 1 London, Saunders, 1983.

16
TRANSFUSION THERAPY

BASIC INFORMATION

Although the clinical laboratory's major role is the provision of diagnostic services, in most hospitals it is also directly concerned with therapy in at least one area, i.e., the provision of blood and blood components for transfusion. Because the procedures to ensure compatibility of these products are primarily immunologic tests and because laboratory personnel are especially well trained in these procedures, it is only natural that this medical service be a part of the laboratory service of most hospitals.

Certain aspects of transfusion therapy, coagulation abnormalities, platelet and white blood cell deficiencies, have already been reviewed. However, certain facets of blood banking apply to many areas of medicine; these topics can be most efficiently covered in a separate section. The emphasis of this chapter varies from other parts of this book in that in this case the diagnosis is assumed to be known and comments are directed at the therapeutic aspects of transfusion.

In addition, those aspects of immunohematology that are of special aid to the clinician are included because most books on clinical pathology do not emphasize the clinical aspects of blood transfusion practice, and therefore this area is not well understood by many medical students. A knowledge of the rudiments of blood banking helps to smooth out the relationships, at times harried, between the blood banker, who wants to ensure the safety of the transfusion, and the clinician, who is concerned with the immediate needs of the patient.

BLOOD TRANSFUSION

With the ready availability of blood and blood products there are tendencies to transfuse for only minimal or even nonexistent indications. However, blood is not an innocuous material by any means, and there are inherent risks associated with each transfusion. The clinician, then, must weigh the relative merits of transfusion against the potential hazards and decide whether to transfuse the patient on the basis of information outlined below.

Blood Component Therapy

The basic indications for transfusion are listed in Table 16–1. The clinical variations are endless, requiring close communication between clinicians and blood bank personnel. It is useful to consider that blood contains various components, i.e., erythrocytes, leukocytes, platelets, and plasma. Each of these components has given functions that can be of therapeutic benefit. The trend in transfusion therapy is to use more specialized blood components instead of whole blood. There are several advantages to this. First, it enables each donor unit to be used for more than one recipient. Second, components can be concentrated so that patients may be treated without circu-

TABLE 16–1. TRANSFUSION CONSIDERATIONS

Indications for Transfusion	Hazards of Transfusion

Restore or maintain:
  oxygen carrying capacity
  blood volume
  coagulation properties,
    including platelets
  leukocyte functions
	Immunologic
	  Hemolytic reactions
	    Immediate
	    Delayed
	  Allergic
	  Febrile

Elimination of antibodies
  (exchange transfusion)
	Sensitization of recipient
	  GVHD
	Nonimmunologic
	  Infection
	    Hepatitis, CMV, EBV, AIDS
	  Hypervolemia
	  Hemosiderosis

GVHD, Graft versus host disease.

TABLE 16–2. BLOOD COMPONENTS AVAILABLE

Product	Content	Indications	Shelf Life	Comments
Whole blood	RBC WBC Plasma	Acute massive blood loss Neonatal exchange transfusion	42 days	
Red blood cells	RBC WBC Some plasma	Anemia	42 days	Minimize volume overload
Leukocyte-poor red blood cells (e.g., washed)	RBC Few WBC Minimal plasma	Anemia Prevent febrile reactions to WBC antibodies	24 hours after washing	Use in patients who have had two or more febrile reactions
Deglycerolized red blood cells	RBC Very few WBC No plasma	Anemia Prevent febrile reactions	24 hours after deglycerolizing	Use to store rare bloods Very expensive
Platelet concentrate	Platelets Few RBC Few WBC Some plasma	Bleeding secondary to low platelet count, or poor platelet function	72 hours	
Leukocyte concentrate	WBC Platelets Few RBC	Serious infections in leukopenic patients	24 hours	Granulocytes and other leukocytes
Fresh frozen plasma	Clotting factors No platelets	Coagulation disorders	6 hours after thawing	Does not contain platelets
Cryoprecipitate	Factor VIII Fibrinogen	Factor VIII deficiency DIC	6 hours after thawing	One bag contains about 100 AHF units and about 150–200 mg of fibrinogen

latory overload. Third, once isolated, that particular component may be stored under optimal conditions for that particular component (Table 16–2 lists the blood components commonly available).

Erythrocytes

Red blood cells are the component of choice for supplementation of oxygen-carrying capacity. If a patient requires blood volume replacement as well, whole blood transfusion may be optimal. One must realize, however, that in most patients loss of up to 20 percent of the blood volume can be safely corrected with crystalloid solutions alone.

In chronic anemia blood should be transfused only to patients who are symptomatic from their anemia or whose anemia is not treatable by other means. Patients with anemias caused by iron deficiency or vitamin B_{12} deficiency should not be transfused unless they are in acute distress from their anemia. The inherent dangers of transfusion (hypervolemia, hepatitis) are avoided, allowing the patient's normal hematopoietic mechanisms to slowly and safely correct the anemia. If transfusion is necessary in these cases or in patients with various hemoglobinopathies and inborn errors of erythrocyte metabolism, the transfusion of packed red blood cells is the preferred method because it replaces only the missing components and avoids the dangers of hypervolemia and potential cardiac failure.

Transfusion policies for surgery deserve special mention. In the past the anticipation of blood loss in elective surgery has led to excessive preoperative orders for blood. Reviews of actual blood usage have indicated more modest requirements. There have been several approaches to this problem. One approach is the establishment of a list of "type and screen" procedures, i.e., procedures that only rarely require transfusions. Patients undergoing these procedures have a blood sample screened the day prior to surgery for unexpected antibodies. If no antibodies are detected, the blood bank will not actually tag units for the patient but will store the patient's sample. In the event blood is required, the operating room personnel notify the blood bank and the crossmatch is then initiated. A companion strategy is the establishment of a maximum surgical blood order schedule (MSBOS) that establishes the appropriate number of units to be crossmatched for various surgical procedures. Table 16–3 gives some guidelines for blood ordering. Both of these approaches reduce the number of unnecessary crossmatches. They also reduce blood wastage caused by outdating. Blood crossmatched for a particular patient is not available to other patients for 1 or 2 days.

Leukocytes

Transfused granulocytes have been shown to function normally and improve the prognosis in a few selected patients. Obtaining leukocyte concentrates is a very involved and complex procedure. Thus, the cost to benefit ratio is very high for granulocyte transfusions. Therefore, the patients must be selected carefully. There are strict guidelines for selection of candidates for granulocyte transfusion. The patient should have a severe neutropenia (i.e., an absolute neutrophil count less than $0.500 \times 10^9/L$); a good prognosis of recovering from the neutropenia; documented septicemia resistant to appropriate antibiotic therapy; and the expectation of a satisfactory quality of life if he or she survives the infection.

TABLE 16–3. GUIDELINES FOR BLOOD ORDERS FOR ELECTIVE SURGICAL PROCEDURES

Surgical Procedure	Blood Order
Amputation (AK or BK)	T&S
Aortic aneurysm resection	8
Breast biopsy	T&S
Carotid endarterectomy	1
Cholecystectomy	T&S
Colectomy (total or AP resection)	2
Dilatation and curettage	T&S
Gastrectomy	3
Hernia, inguinal	0
Hysterectomy	T&S or 1
Laminectomy (for disc repair)	T&S
Laparotomy, exploratory	2
Mastectomy	T&S
Nephrectomy	1 or T&S
Pneumonectomy	4
Porto-caval shunt	4
Splenectomy	3
Thyroidectomy	T&S
Transurethral resection of prostate	T&S
Vagotomy and pyloroplasty	T&S

Number indicates units of packed cells or whole blood to be ordered preoperatively. T&S, type and screen procedure; AK, above the knee; BK, below the knee.

There is no suitable in vitro compatibility test for granulocyte transfusion as there is for red blood cell compatibility. Currently, it appears as if HLA matched granulocytes provide the best product for a particular patient because this method essentially determines the relatedness between donor and recipient. Because leukocyte concentrates contain 25 to 50 ml of red blood cells, the donor and the recipient must be ABO and Rh compatible. One cannot rely on posttransfusion increments in neutrophil count to assess the efficacy of treatment as the neutrophils leave the vascular compartment very rapidly. Instead, effectiveness of treatment must be evaluated clinically, e.g., resolution of fever or improvements in chest x-ray.

Platelets

The decision to use platelet concentrates must be based on several considerations: the clinical condition of the patient, the cause of the thrombocytopenia, the platelet count, and the functional ability of the patient's own platelets. For example, the risk of spontaneous hemorrhage is very small if the platelet count is greater than $20 \times 10^9/L$. In patients with ITP, platelet transfusions are of no benefit. Patients who have received massive transfusions with stored blood may require platelet transfusion because the stored blood they have received contains few functional platelets.

Pooled platelet concentrates do not require major or minor crossmatch prior to transfusion. A platelet concentrate from a single unit of whole blood should raise the platelet count 5 to 6 $\times 10^9/L$ in an average adult and a pool should raise the count more than $30 \times 10^9/L$. The increments are somewhat lower for ABO incompatible platelets as platelets contain ABO antigens on their surface. Patients may also develop platelet antibodies as a result of a previous transfusion or pregnancy and they may have markedly decreased survival of transfused platelets. These patients may benefit from HLA matched platelets obtained by plateletapheresis. Platelets prepared by cytapheresis contain a significant quantity of red blood cells and therefore should be ABO compatible. It is important to obtain pretransfusion platelet counts and posttransfusion counts at 1 and 24 hours. If the increments in the platelet count obtained 1 hour posttransfusion is less than expected, one should suspect the development of platelet antibodies. Other factors that adversely affect the platelet increment are fever, infection, splenomegaly, DIC, and hemorrhage. In these conditions, however, there is usually a good platelet increment at 1 hour.

TABLE 16–4. BIOCHEMICAL PARAMETERS OF BANKED WHOLE BLOOD (CPDA-1)

Parameters	Day					
	0	7	14	21	28	35
Glucose (mg/dl)	400	325	312	280	230	230
Sodium (mmol/L)	173	125	111	102	94	87
Potassium (mmol/L)	4.4	12	17	21	23	25
pH (whole blood)	7.0	6.9	6.8	6.6	6.5	6.5
Hemoglobin (mg/dl)	1.7	8	12	29	29	32

Values for chloride, hematocrit, MCHC and MCV, and fibrinogen showed no clinically significant changes.
Data from Applied Biochemistry Section, Cell Preservation Laboratory, American Red Cross Blood Services.

Plasma

Fresh frozen plasma (FFP) is used in clinical situations where restoration of procoagulants is necessary but should not be used for simple volume expansion. It is useful in patients with bleeding secondary to deficiencies of multiple clotting factors such as liver disease, DIC, or when a specific factor deficiency is suspected but has not yet been established. FFP does not need to be ABO-identical but should be compatible with the recipient's red blood cells. One should remember that the clotting factors have been preserved by freezing and as they are labile at room temperature, the product should be administered as soon as possible after thawing to give maximal benefit to the patient.

Fresh Whole Blood

There are few indications for the use of freshly drawn blood (<24 hours old). In most situations an appropriate blood component, or relatively fresh blood, rather than freshly drawn blood, is entirely adequate for treatment. In doubtful cases the patient's physician should review the entire case with the transfusion service director, so that optimal care is provided. The newer anticoagulant–preservative solutions for blood insure that all blood in the blood bank is suitable for transfusion, and requests for fresh blood (i.e., less than 7 days old) must be justified by clinical (e.g., perinatal transfusions) and laboratory information rather than based on emotion. This may necessitate doing appropriate tests for evaluation of blood coagulation abnormality. Fresh blood is not a panacea for all bleeding problems (Table 16–4). Unless freshly drawn blood is used conservatively and only for proper indications, such blood or its components may not be available for the patient who legitimately requires the product.

Hazards of Transfusion

As noted previously, there are a number of real as well as potential hazards associated with the transfusion of blood or any of its components. These hazards must always be considered, especially when the need for transfusion may be equivocal. Transfusion reactions may be classified as either immunologic or nonimmunologic in nature. Immunologic reactions are the most common and include hemolytic, febrile, and allergic reactions as well as sensitization of the recipient (Table 16–5). Nonimmunologic reactions include infectious diseases, volume overload, and rarely, hemosiderosis.

Immunologic Hazards

Hemolytic Transfusion Reactions

Immediate Reaction. The exact frequency of immediate hemolytic transfusion reactions is not known but has been estimated to occur in 1 out of every 6000 transfusions. It is caused by an antibody in the recipient's plasma reacting with an antigen on the donor's erythrocytes. The vast majority of immediate hemolytic reactions are caused by ABO incompatibility. Most of these reactions are caused by clerical error which could have

TABLE 16–5. INCIDENCE OF IMMUNOLOGIC TRANSFUSION REACTIONS

Reaction	Incidence*
Febrile	1/120
Allergic	1/140
Febrile and allergic	1/500
Hemolytic	
Immediate	1/6000
Delayed	1/80,000
All others	1/3600
Overall incidence	1/60

*One reaction per stated number of transfusions.

been averted by adherence to the strict but necessary rules and regulations associated with blood usage.

The clinical presentation of immediate hemolytic reactions is often dramatic and may include fever, chills, chest pain, back pain, hypotension, and oliguria. In extreme reactions this may progress to shock, acute renal failure, DIC, and even death.

Initial efforts should be directed toward establishing a diagnosis and preventing shock and acute renal failure. The transfusion must be stopped but the IV should be kept open with other fluids. A laboratory investigation should be initiated that includes:

1. Rechecking all the paperwork associated with that particular transfusion. If a discrepancy is found, an immediate search must be undertaken to find if other patient or donor bloods have also been misidentified or incorrectly issued.
2. Comparing the color of pretransfusion and posttransfusion plasma or serum. The appearance of a pink discoloration in the posttransfusion specimen is suggestive of free hemoglobin. In samples drawn later (4 to 10 hours) a deep yellow or brown discoloration is suggestive of increased bilirubin and other hemoglobin breakdown products. These color changes are suggestive of red blood cell hemolysis.
3. Direct antiglobulin (Coombs') test. This test is described in the next section. It is usually positive in immediate hemolytic transfusion reactions because of antibody coating of the incompatible cells.
4. Examination of the first urine specimen voided after the reaction for free hemoglobin.

In most cases negative results in the above investigation will rule out an immediate hemolytic transfusion reaction. In the event of equivocal results or strong clinical suspicion, however, further investigation may be warranted that may include repeating the ABO test, Rh test, antibody screening, and crossmatch on pretransfusion and posttransfusion samples.

Delayed Reactions. There are two types of delayed hemolytic transfusion reactions. One type occurs several weeks after transfusion and is the result of primary alloimmunization, i.e., the recipient forms antibodies to antigens on the donor red blood cells. As the antibody titer rises, hemolysis of the transfused cells is accelerated until they are all destroyed. The second type occurs several days after the transfusion and is caused by an anamnestic response to transfused red blood cell antigens in a previously immunized recipient. Many cases of delayed hemolytic transfusion reactions are clinically silent and are discovered by an unexplained fall in hematocrit coupled by the appearance of a positive direct antiglobulin test and appearance of a new alloantibody.

Allergic Reactions. This type of reaction is probably the least dangerous reaction to transfusions. They are fairly common, occurring in about 1 of every 140 transfusions. These reactions occur when the recipient mounts an antibody response to proteins present in donor plasma. Clinically, they are manifest by urticaria and pruritis. Treatment with antihistamines rapidly alleviates the symptoms. Pretreatment with antihistamines may be of benefit in patients who frequently experience urticaria during transfusion.

The classic example of a severe allergic reaction is the anaphylactic reaction in a patient with IgA deficiency. These patients must receive washed red blood cells or components from special donors who lack IgA.

Febrile Reactions. Febrile reactions are probably the most common reaction to transfusions, occurring in about 1 of every 120 transfusions. These reactions are caused by antibodies in the recipient directed against transfused white blood cells. They usually occur in patients who have had previous pregnancies or transfusions. Clinically they are manifested by chills, fever, nausea, and possibly tachycardia and hypotension. These patients must have a workup initiated for a hemolytic transfusion reaction as one cannot unequivocally distinguish between febrile reactions and hemolytic reactions. If a patient has one febrile reaction there is only 1 chance in 8 that he or she will have one with the next transfusion. Therefore, leukocyte-poor products (e.g., washed red blood cells) should be reserved for patients who have had two or more febrile reactions.

Sensitization of Recipient. As the blood bank usually only matches donor and recipient blood for the ABO, Rh_o (D), and possibly the Kell systems, there is always the possibility of immunizing a patient against one of the many other antigens. In addition, if fresh blood containing intact platelets and white blood cells is transfused, antibodies to these formed elements may also be produced. The changes of immunization or sensitization occurring are noted in Table 16–6.

TABLE 16–6. SENSITIZATION FOLLOWING BLOOD TRANSFUSION OR PREGNANCY

Antigens	Transfusion	Pregnancy
Erythrocyte		
Overall	1:1800	1:43
D	*	1:71†
c	1:5000	1:4100
E	1:4500	1:650
Kell	1:3800	1:720
All others	1:3100	1:1700
Leukocyte antigens	Variable	1:6
Platelet antigens	Variable	?

*Usually avoided by routinely matching for Rh_O (D).
†Without use of hyperimmune anti-D globulin.

Nonimmunologic Transfusion Reactions

Infection. Bacterial, parasitic, and viral diseases have all been transmitted by transfusion. Of these, viral diseases are the most common. The major viruses transmitted via blood products are Epstein-Barr virus, cytomegalovirus and hepatitis viruses. Hepatitis virus is the one most commonly associated with transfusion and therefore the discussion will be limited to it.

Hepatitis. Abnormal liver function tests (LFT) develop in 10 percent of transfused patients compared with 2 percent of non-transfused controls. Overt hepatitis develops in about 3 percent of the 10 percent with abnormal LFTs. Presently non-A, non-B hepatitis accounts for about 85 to 90 percent of post-transfusion hepatitis whereas hepatitis B accounts for most of the rest. The incidence of hepatitis B has decreased in recent years because of the development of sensitive methods for detecting hepatitis B surface antigen (HB_sAg) and the greater

TABLE 16–7. ABO BLOOD GROUP SYSTEM

Group or Phenotype	Genotype	Agglutinogen on Red Blood Cell	Agglutinin in Serum	U.S. Incidence White	U.S. Incidence Black
O	OO	None	Anti-A and anti-B	45	48
A	AA or AO	A	Anti-B	41	27
B	BB or BO	B	Anti-A	10	21
AB	AB	A and B	None	4	4

use of volunteer donors. At present there is no screening test available for non-A, non-B hepatitis. Therefore, the only way to decrease posttransfusion non-A, non-B hepatitis is careful donor screening, elimination of paid donors, and careful follow-up of recipients to detect the disease and discover potentially dangerous donors. (See Chapter 9 for a more complete discussion of hepatitis.)

Volume Overload. Another ever present danger, especially when large amounts of blood or plasma are infused (such as in coagulation disorders), and particularly in patients with poor cardiovascular reserve (such as the elderly), is the decompensation of the cardiovascular system. This is accompanied by venous distension and peripheral or pulmonary edema, or both.

Acquired Immune Deficiency Syndrome. Acquired immune deficiency syndrome (AIDS) is a recently described disease of viral etiology and high mortality. Transmission of AIDS has occasionally been linked to transfusions. The currently available screening test is for antibodies to the HTLV-III virus. Time will tell if this screening test is really effective in eliminating infectious units of blood.

Compatibility Testing

The ABO Blood Group System

Four major blood groups exist in the ABO system; the makeup is determined by the presence or absence on the red blood cell surface of antigen A or B. The A and B genes are both dominant over O, and are co-dominant with each other. In contrast with all other blood group systems, the reciprocal antibody (isoagglutinins) is normally present in the plasma, except in the case of group AB (Table 16–7).

Except for passive transfer of antibodies from the mother, infants do not produce ABO blood group isoagglutinins until they are several months old. Hence, reverse grouping is not ordinarily done in this age group. The red blood cells do, however, react to direct typing serum when the red blood cell type is being determined. Confusion on these points arises in the special case of hemolytic disease of the newborn. In addition to the naturally occurring antibody (isoantibody or isoagglutinin), immune anti-A or anti-B antibody may be produced in response to transfusion of ABO incompatible blood, stimulation of an ABO incompatible pregnancy (ABO hemolytic disease of the newborn), or injection of horse serum or other biologicals.

There are several subgroups of group A (A_1, A_2, and so on), one of which, A_2, is of some importance because A_2 erythrocytes may be antigenic in an A_1 recipient. About 80 percent of all A subjects are A_1.

Other Blood Group Systems

In contrast with the ABO system with naturally occurring serum agglutinins, many other antigens are found on red blood cells but with no corresponding antibodies present in the plasma (Table 16–8). If red blood cells containing these foreign antigens are transfused into a recipient who does not have the antigen, the recipient may become immunized or sensitized. Likewise, an incompatible pregnancy may immunize the mother. The actual development of antibodies depends upon several factors, including the following:

1. Potency of antigen: Rh and K antigens are quite potent.
2. Frequency or absence of antigen in recipients: Recipients at risk may be rare.
3. Age of recipient: Elderly patients are poorer producers of antibodies.

The Routine Crossmatch

Blood for transfusion is crossmatched with the blood of the prospective recipient by the techniques that will permit detection of almost all antibodies that could result in hemolysis of

TABLE 16–8. CLINICALLY SIGNIFICANT ANTIBODIES MOST FREQUENTLY ENCOUNTERED IN BLOOD BANKS

Antibody	Frequency
Anti-Rh_o (D)	Most frequent
Anti-C + D or (G)	
Anti-rh" (E)	
Anti-Kell	
Anti-rh' (c)	↓
Anti-Duffy (Fy^a) or (Fy^b)	
Anti-Kidd (Jk^a) or (Jk^b)	
Anti-hr" (e)	
Anti-S or (s)	Least frequent

donor or recipient erythrocytes. At present one cannot match donor and recipient blood to ensure white blood cell or platelet compatibility, although HLA antigen matching appears to improve both platelet and white blood cell survival.

Several different media and incubation conditions are used to determine red blood cell compatibility. The crossmatch is divided into two parts: (1) the major side (donor cells and recipient serum), as this is the more important (major) part of the match and (2) the minor side (donor serum and recipient cells). If donor blood is checked for unexpected antibodies (as is commonly done), the minor crossmatch is omitted.

The crossmatch mixtures in a saline suspension (saline phase) are immediately centrifuged and are examined for hemolysis or agglutination. ABO incompatibilities will react in this system. Incubation at 37C will reveal some Rh and other incompatibilities. An indirect antihuman globulin (Coombs') test performed on the crossmatch specimens after incubation reveals most beta- and gamma-globulin antibodies. The routine crossmatch requires 45 to 60 minutes to complete.

Antihuman Globulin (Coombs') Test. One of the key laboratory procedures in immunohematology is the antihuman globulin (Coombs') test. The principle of the test is quite simple and the sensitivity is remarkable. Through its use, weakly reacting or incomplete (but clinically important) antibodies can be detected.

Two variants of this test are commonly employed. In the direct Coombs' test, the presumably antibody-coated red blood cells are directly reacted with the antihuman globulin serum. If the cells are coated with antibody, they will clump in the system (Fig. 16–1). In the indirect test the serum suspected of containing antibody is reacted with two or three group O cells containing all the common antigens. If coating occurs, it can be demonstrated by subsequent reaction with antihuman globulin serum (Fig. 16–2).

The Incompatible Crossmatch

Sometimes the blood bank will contact the physician who has ordered blood for a patient and report that the crossmatch is incompatible. In addition to giving the blood bank considerable difficulty in finding compatible blood, the analysis of the incompatibility may provide valuable clinical information. A certain number of these incompatibilities are caused by antibodies formed in patients immunized by previous transfusion or pregnancy (Tables 16–6 and 16–9). At other times the reac-

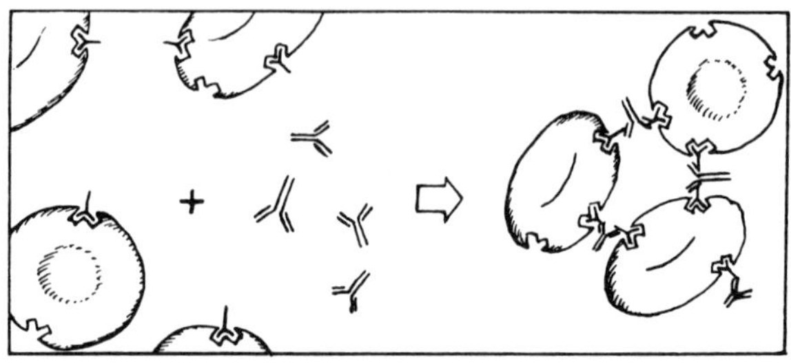

Figure 16-1. Direct antiglobulin test: Is there antibody on the patient's red blood cells?

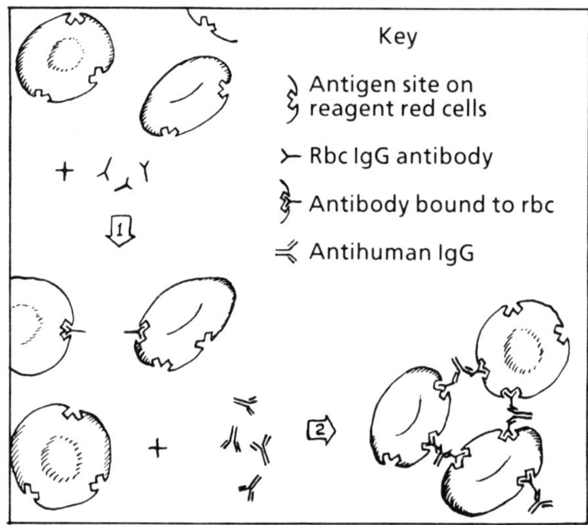

Figure 16-2. Indirect antiglobulin test: Is there antibody in the patient's serum?

TABLE 16–9. INCOMPATIBLE CROSSMATCH

Observed Reaction	Cause	Control Test	% Blood Units Incompatible by Crossmatch	Characteristics
Rouleaux	Dextran, abnormal proteins	+	100	Clumping on typing and major crossmatch, immediate
Polyagglutination or panagglutination	Recent or present viral or bacterial infection	±	Nearly 100	Minor crossmatch, immediate
Cold agglutinins	Viral pneumonia, or unknown	+	Nearly 100	Major crossmatch, immediate; stronger at colder temperatures
Acquired hemolytic anemia	Autoimmunization	+	100	Major crossmatch, AHG phase*
Antibody in recipient				
Anti-Rh$_o$ (D)	Previous transfusion or pregnancy	Negative	85	Major, after incubation, AHG
Anti-rh′ (C)	Previous transfusion or pregnancy	Negative	70	Major, after incubation, AHG
Anti-rh″ (E)	Previous transfusion or pregnancy	Negative	30	Major, after incubation, AHG
Anti-Kell (K)	Previous transfusion or pregnancy	Negative	8	Major, AHG
Anti-hr′ (c)	Previous transfusion or pregnancy	Negative	80	Major, after incubation, AHG
Anti-Duffy (Fy[a])	Previous transfusion or pregnancy	Negative	65	Major, AHG
Anti-Kidd (Jk[a])	Previous transfusion or pregnancy	Negative	75	Major, AHG
Anti-hr″ (e)	Previous transfusion or pregnancy	Negative	98	Major, after incubation, AHG
Anti-S	Previous transfusion or pregnancy	Negative	55	Major, AHG

*AHG indicates antihuman globulin test (i.e., Coombs' test).

tion will be caused by the patient's primary disease, with autoantibodies coating the patient's erythrocytes or abnormal plasma proteins being formed. The incompatibility can appear in any phase of the crossmatch. The experimental conditions under which the strongest reactions occur provide valuable clues for diagnosis and, therefore, the crossmatch should be taken to completion before being discarded. The thermal amplitude of the reactions should also be determined.

Table 16–9 lists some of the more important situations in which the crossmatch indicates incompatibility. Clinical data, including the diagnosis, will usually explain the reason for the apparent incompatibility. Reactions resulting from rouleaux are usually easily handled. The diagnosis is made by microscopic examination of the crossmatched specimens. Panagglutinins and cold agglutinins may be more difficult to cope with.

How does one proceed after discovering the incompatibility? If a true antibody is found, the donor bloods are typed for the corresponding antigen if possible, and those not containing the antigen are crossmatched. Sometimes more than one antibody is found, and finding suitable donors is extremely difficult. Rare donor files or frozen supplies of rare blood may be the only recourse in these situations.

Finally, it may become evident that only an in vivo crossmatch procedure can be done. To accomplish this procedure a small quantity (e.g., 0.5 to 1 ml) of donor blood is radiolabeled with chromium 51. It is infused into the patient and samples are obtained at specified intervals. If the survival at 60 minutes is within normal limits (i.e., >95 percent) the red blood cells are considered compatible. A simpler, though less sensitive, way to perform an in vivo crossmatch is to take a small quantity (10 to 15 ml) of donor red blood cells, slowly infuse them into the patient while carefully observing for any untoward reaction. Control, 15-minute, and 30-minute plasma hemoglobin samples are drawn and observed (or measured) for elevated plasma hemoglobin levels. Control values should be less than 10 mg/dl, and no significant increases should follow the infusion of 50 ml of compatible blood.

Emergency Transfusion

Only rarely do patients require a blood transfusion without prior crossmatch. In the great majority of instances, the blood bank is able to complete the usual 45- to 60-minute crossmatch. True emergencies do arise, however, and the urgent need for immediate transfusion must be met as quickly as possible. Two alternatives exist.

TABLE 16–10. OUT-OF-GROUP TRANSFUSIONS IN EMERGENCY SITUATIONS

Recipient Type	Approximate % of Blood Supply	Packed Cell ABO Type
O pos	38	O pos (or neg)
O neg	7	O neg, (O pos if life threatening)
A pos	35	A pos (or neg), O pos (or neg)
A neg	6	A neg, (A pos, O pos if life threatening)
B pos	8	B pos (or neg), O pos (or neg)
B neg	2	B neg, (B pos, or O pos if life threatening)
AB pos	3	A pos (or neg), O pos (or neg)
AB neg	1	A neg, O neg, (A pos if life threatening)

An emergency crossmatch can be done. The recipient is quickly typed for ABO and Rh_o (D), and a unit of similar blood is set up for crossmatch. If time is available (5 minutes), an immediate-spin crossmatch is read and, if the blood is compatible, it can be released for transfusion with only minimal risks. The crossmatch is completed and reported after the transfusion has been started.

A second alternative is to use low-titer group O blood, the universal donor. This means that the level of reaction of anti-A and anti-B agglutinins is negative at a 1 to 2 dilution. Such blood can be given to an O, A, B, or AB recipient with minimal danger. The blood can also be given as packed cells, most of the plasma with its A and B isoagglutinins having been removed. The anti-A and anti-B agglutinins are diluted by the recipient's plasma to inactive levels. It must be remembered, however, that there is no assurance that incomplete antibodies (e.g., anti-Rh (D), anti-rh' (c), or anti-Kell) are not present; the danger of severe hemolysis due to these antibodies is always present. In all cases, a crossmatch is subsequently performed and reported.

If at all possible, one should try to temporize in these emergency situations by using plasma protein fraction or plasma until a crossmatch is completed. The risks of an incomplete crossmatch are thus avoided. But if blood transfusion is mandatory, the appropriate blood types for emergency transfusion, including out-of-group transfusions, are listed in Table 16–10. One should avoid transfusing Rh positive blood in an Rh negative patient especially in a woman in child-bearing years except in life-threatening situations.

SUGGESTED READINGS

Biggs RP (ed): Treatment of Haemophilia A and B and von Willebrand's Disease. Philadelphia, Davis, 1977.

Blajehman M: Clinical use of blood, blood components, and blood products. Can Med Assoc J 121:33, 1979.

Blood Component Therapy: A Physician's Handbook, 2nd ed. Washington, DC, American Association of Blood Banks, 1975.

Bohnen RF, Ultmann JE, Gorman JG, Farhangi M, Scudder J: The direct Coombs' test: Its clinical significance. Ann Intern Med 68:19, 1968.

Bonal L, Henry J: The type and screen: A safe alternative and supplement in selected surgical procedures. Transfusion 17:163, 1977.

Cash JD (ed): Blood Transfusion and Blood Products. In Clinics in Haematology, vol 5, no. 1. London, Saunders, 1976.

Higby D, Burnett D: Granulocyte transfusions: Current status. Blood 55:2, 1980.

Horowitz C: Blood transfusion therapy. Postgrad Med 69(4):155, 1981.

Huestis DW, Bove JR, Busch S: Practical Blood Transfusion, 3rd ed. Boston, Little Brown, 1981.

Leparc G, Schmidt P: Stop: Transfusion reaction. Diag Med(Sept):49, 1984.

McCullough J (ed): Symposium on blood transfusion. Practice and science. Human Path 14:203, 1983.

Mintz P, et al.: Expected hemotherapy in elective surgery. NY State J Med 76:532, 1976.

Mollison PL: Blood Transfusion in Clinical Medicine, 7th ed. Oxford, Blackwell Scientific, 1984.

Petz LD, Swisher SN: Clinical Practice of Blood Transfusion. New York, Churchill-Livingstone, 1981.

Pineda A: Blood component therapy: Granulocyte and platelet transfusion. Mayo Clin Proc 56:645, 1981.

Schmidt PJ, Grindon AJ: Blood and blood components in the prevention and control of bleeding. JAMA 202:967, 1967.

Tannenbaum S: Blood—Which component and why? Hosp Phys (Aug):41, 1983.

Widmann F (ed): Technical Manual, 9th ed. Arlington, Va, American Association of Blood Banks, 1985.

17
CHANGES IN APPEARANCE

GENERAL COMMENTS

Many reasons for changes in body weight have been discussed in other chapters (see Chapter 6 on edema; Chapter 10 on chronic diarrhea; and Chapter 14 on leukemia). This chapter deals with the endocrine glands and dysfunction of these important structures, which can cause changes in body appearance either by significant gain or loss of weight or by other changes in body configuration. It is fair to say, however, that in the United States the most common cause of weight gain is exogenous obesity, i.e., from overeating and underexercising. This fact should not be forgotten in the evaluation of the overweight individual.

Four endocrine glands (anterior pituitary, thyroid, islets of Langerhans, and adrenal cortex) have major effects on body weight. In the following sections, these glands will be discussed in detail, especially in relation to changes in body appearance. Parathyroid gland function is discussed in Chapter 19, which is devoted to metabolic bone disease.

BASIC INFORMATION

Normal Thyroid Gland Function and Its Assessment

Thyroid hormones are the major regulators of the metabolic rate in the body. There are two thyroid hormones: thyroxine, which is composed of two tyrosine molecules coupled together with four attached iodide ions (T_4), and triiodothyronine, a similar compound except that it contains only three iodide ions (T_3). Both compounds are metabolically active; the T_3 form is

TABLE 17-1. THYROID FUNCTION TESTS

Test	Primary Function Measured
Thyroxine (T_4)	Circulating hormone
Triiodothyronine (T_3)	Circulating more active hormone
Free thyroxine (T_4)	Amount of unbound hormone
Thyroid-stimulating hormone (TSH)	Pituitary stimulation of thyroid
I-131 uptake (6-hour, 24-hour)	Iodide trapping and thyroglobulin storage
Thyroid stimulating immunoglobulins	Thyroid stimulating antibodies, e.g., LATS in Graves' disease
Basal metabolic rate	Total body metabolic rate

several times more active than T_4 microgram for microgram. However, T_4 normally constitutes about 90 percent or more of circulating hormone.

Within the gland there are at least four distinct (and measurable) steps in the biosynthesis of circulating thyroid hormone: (1) iodide trapping by the thyroidal cells; (2) stepwise binding of iodide to tyrosine to form the hormone; (3) storage of the synthesized hormone in the gland acini as thyroglobulin; and (4) release of hormone into the plasma as circulating active hormone.

The hormone circulates bound to a specific carrier protein called thyroid-binding globulin (TBG) with a small fraction (<1 percent) free and in equilibrium with the bound fraction. The free hormone is able to penetrate the cell membrane and is therefore believed to be the physiologically active agent.

Although the clinical history and physical examination still constitute a primary method for the diagnosis of thyroid gland dysfunction, the laboratory is becoming increasingly important in the evaluation of this endocrine gland. There are several specific indications for the use of laboratory procedures: (1) corroboration of clinical diagnosis; (2) screening for mild thyroid disease (e.g., hyperthyroidism masking as nervousness); and (3) monitoring the response to therapy.

Several laboratory tests are used singly and in combination to assess the various aspects of thyroid gland function. The most recently developed is the indirect or direct measurement of free hormone. The choice between the different tests is based upon tentative clinical diagnosis and requires some clinical sophistication, as each test has certain advantages as well as disadvantages (Table 17-1).

Radioactive Iodine Uptake Test

The thyroid gland has the ability to trap and use iodide for the production of thyroid hormone, and the measurement of this function has been widely used as one of the primary assessments of the thyroid function. A variety of tests has been devised; some are simple, whereas others are quite complicated and time-consuming. The choice of procedures should be based on the probable diagnosis. This will become more evident in the following discussion.

The uptake of radioactive iodine at 24 hours is probably the most commonly measured interval because the peak uptake normally occurs before that time and plateaus at about 24 hours. Normally between 5 and 25 percent of the administered radioactive iodine is taken up at 24 hours, but these ranges vary from population to population as well as from laboratory to laboratory, depending on the basal iodine ingestion as well as the technique of measurement. Greater than 25 percent of the iodine will be taken up in hyperthyroidism, whereas less than 5 percent will be trapped in hypothyroidism. The peak uptake may occur much earlier than 24 hours in hyperthyroidism. Measurement of uptake at 6 hours is probably more discriminating than the 24-hour uptake test, especially in hyperthyroidism, and is considered by some to be preferable.

The measurement of the rate of conversion of administered radioactive iodine into circulating radioactive hormone also yields valuable supplementary data in certain patients. The 72-hour conversion ratio is quite helpful, for example, in the differentiation of borderline hyperthyroidism.

In cases of suspected hyperthyroidism with equivocal iodine uptake levels, it is usually possible to distinguish the response of iodine uptake to thyroid hormone. In Graves' hyperthyroidism no change in iodide uptake will be elicited following 8 days of T_3 administration. On the other hand, there will be significant decrease in radioactive iodide uptake in the normal patient.

Measurement of Circulating Thyroid Hormones

Thyroxine and Triiodothyronine. The measurement of thyroid hormone as protein-bound iodine (PBI) has been replaced by more specific tests using radioimmunoassay or radioligand procedures that are both sensitive and specific for T_4 and T_3. These hormones are bound to plasma proteins. About 70 percent of thyroxine is bound to TBG, 15 percent to thyroxine-binding prealbumin (TBPA), and the remainder to albumin. Almost all T_3 is bound to TBG.

TABLE 17–2. THYROID FUNCTION TEST PANEL

Diagnosis	Radioactive Iodine Uptake	Thyroid Scintiscan	Thyroxine (T_4)	Free Thyroxine	TSH
Normal	N*	Uniform	N	N	N
Thyrotoxicosis	↑ ↑	Uniform increase	↑ or N	↑	N
Thyroid adenoma with hyperthyroidism	↑ or N	"Hot nodule"	↑	↑	N
Thyrotoxicosis factitia	↓	Uniform decrease	↑	↑	↓
Euthyroid goiter (iodine lack)	↑	Uniform increase	N	N	↑
Hypothyroidism	↓ or N	Decrease	↓ or low N	↓	↑ or
Adequately treated hyperthyroidism (surgical or irradiation)	↑	Uniform	N	N	↓ N ↑

*N, normal see text for comments.

A hyperthyroid patient usually has elevated T_4 and T_3 levels, whereas a hypothyroid patient has decreased hormone levels. There is good correlation between results obtained by most methods and the clinical condition of the patient.

The normal level of T_4 (95 percent of the normal population) is 4 to 11 μg/dl. Triiodothyronine levels normally vary between 100 and 200 ng/dl. Total thyroxine, bound to thyroid binding globulin, will be artefactually elevated in cases of elevated TBG, e.g., pregnancy and female hormone therapy. Conversely, TBG is decreased during androgen therapy and in nephrotic syndrome, and total T_4 levels are correspondingly lower.

Free Thyroxine. This procedure is based on the fact that TBG binds a large proportion of circulating thyroid hormone. The free or unbound hormone is the metabolically active fraction, and hence its measurement may provide a more valid relationship to the clinical state than some other thyroid function tests. Normally only about 0.03 percent of the total T_4 is free to diffuse into tissues to exert its metabolic effects.

A reliable estimate of free thyroxine is the free thyroxine index (FTI). This value is obtained by multiplying the total T_4 by the T_3 uptake. The T_3 uptake assay gives an estimate of the amount of binding of thyroid hormone to the proteins in the blood. Table 17–2 summarizes the thyroid function test panel in various diseases.

Normal Adrenal Function and Its Measurement

The adrenal cortex is divided into three distinct zones: the zona glomerulosa, the zona fasciculata, and the zona reticularis. Each zone produces its own group of hormones. The zona glomerulosa synthesizes the mineralocorticoids (e.g., aldosterone); the zona fasciculata synthesizes the glucocorticoids (e.g., cortisol); and the zona reticularis synthesizes the sex hormones (e.g., androgens, estrogens, and progesterones). All of the adrenal cortical hormones begin as a cholesterol molecule that is added to via a series of biochemical reactions.

Secretion of cortisol (the major glucocorticoid) by the adrenal cortex is stimulated by adrenocorticotrophic hormone (ACTH), stress, and a diurnal rhythm. ACTH production is regulated by blood cortisol levels, low levels of cortisol stimulating ACTH production, and increased levels decreasing ACTH production. This normal feedback regulation between the adrenal cortex and the pituitary forms the basis for several methods of adrenal cortical functional testing, including the dexamethasone suppression test and the ACTH stimulation tests.

The measurement of these adrenal cortical steroids is based on chemical reactions that occur at reactive groups attached to one or more sites of the basic steroid nucleus. The reactive sites are located by numbering the carbon atoms. The side chains containing carbons 19, 20, and 21 may be absent. For example, the estrogenic steroids contain only 18 carbon atoms. The androgens, on the other hand, have 19 carbons and characteristically a ketone group in the 17-carbon position, i.e., a 17-ketosteroid (17-KS). The glucocorticoids are somewhat more complicated, with regard to both terminology and methodology of measurement. These compounds have 21 carbon atoms. They have a hydroxyl group in the 17-carbon site and therefore have been labeled 17-hydroxycorticosteroids.

The 17-hydroxycorticosteroids are measured in several ways. In one method, the 17-hydroxy group of most important 17-hydroxycorticoids is oxidized to a ketone group. The steroid is changed into a ketosteroid, i.e., it is a ketogenic steroid (17-KGS). The second major method of analysis, the Porter-Silber reaction, measures only those hydroxycorticosteroids having a dihydroxyacetone side chain. The 17-hydroxy compounds not measured by this method include some minor glucocorticoids as well as the progesterone compounds. Cortisol, the major 17-hydroxycorticoid, can now be measured separately by radioimmunoassay as urinary free cortisol.

It is worth mentioning that about one-third of the urine 17-ketosteroids in men are derived from the testes. In women, on the other hand, 17-ketosteroid production is almost entirely adrenal in origin. Thus, this determination is not the method of choice for the biochemical evaluation of adrenal activity, especially in men (Table 17–3).

An absence of or a decrease in the enzymes necessary for the various interconversions between steroids results in several very interesting, although rare, adrenogenital syndromes, the details of which are beyond the scope of this book.

INVESTIGATION OF UNEXPLAINED WEIGHT LOSS

Loss of body weight is associated with a wide variety of diseases, many of which are discussed in other chapters of this

TABLE 17–3. MAJOR STEROIDS AND THEIR MEASUREMENTS

| Class | General Steroids | Major 17-KS | Measurement | |
			Porter-Silber	*17-KGS*
Glucocorticoids	Cortisone	−	+	+
	Cortisol	−	+	+
	Cortilone	−	−	+
	Cortol	−	−	+
Progesterones	Progesterone	*	*	*
	Pregnatriol	−	−	+
Estrogens	Estrone	−	−	−
	Estradiol	−		
Androgens	Etiocholanelone	+	−	−
	Dehydroepiandrosterone	+	−	−
	Androsterone	+	−	−
	Testosterone	−	−	−

*Not excreted in urine.

book. In many of these conditions the accompanying clinical manifestations, such as evidence of malignant disease, chronic infection, or chronic heart disease, will readily explain the concurrent weight loss, and no diagnostic dilemma develops. Some of these conditions are summarized in Table 17–4. In addition, a significant decrease in caloric input or an increase in exercise without an increase in caloric intake will result in loss of weight.

A number of conditions or abnormalities of several endocrine glands may result in apparent unexplained weight loss: diabetes mellitus, hyperthyroidism from whatever cause, adrenal insufficiency, and pituitary insufficiency. These four conditions will be discussed in the following sections.

DIAGNOSIS OF DIABETES MELLITUS

Clinical Features

Diabetes may be present without any manifestation of weight loss, polyuria, polydipsia, or polyphagia. There is a frequent association of diabetes with various degenerative disorders. Table 17–5 lists individuals who have an increased risk of diabetes.

TABLE 17–4. MAJOR DISEASE CONDITIONS THAT MAY BE ASSOCIATED WITH WEIGHT LOSS

Disease	Discussion
Malignancy	Chapter 2 (Chronic disease), Chapter 14 (Leukemia)
Chronic infection	Chapter 20 (Fever)
Heart disease	Chapter 6 (Edema), Chapter 4 (Hypertension)
Chronic liver disease	Chapter 9 (Jaundice)
Chronic renal disease	Chapter 11 (Renal disease)
Sprue	Chapter 10 (Chronic diarrhea)
Diabetes mellitus	Chapter 17
Hyperthyroidism	Chapter 17
Adrenal insufficiency	Chapter 17
Pituitary insufficiency	Chapter 17

The patient with weight loss accompanied by polyuria, polydipsia, and polyphagia rarely causes diagnostic difficulties. On the other hand, the symptoms of the patient in diabetic acidosis and ketosis may clinically resemble those of a variety of disorders, but the diagnosis can be made if the proper laboratory procedures are done.

Laboratory Studies

Screening Procedures

Urine Glucose. The normal renal threshold for glucose is usually about 180 g/dl. Above that amount, enough glucose is filtered to exceed the usual tubular transfer maximum for glucose resorption, and the surplus remains in the urine. The screening of a random urine specimen with glucose oxidase test strips is probably the simplest procedure to screen for diabetes. Clinitest tablet color reactions can be used to confirm the amount of glucose, because they are semiquantitative (Table 17–6), whereas the glucose oxidase test strips are difficult to interpret, especially at low levels of glucose.

If reducing substances are present, a check for ketone bodies (acetone, beta-hydroxbutyric acid, and acetoacetic acid) is usually done to determine whether diabetic acidosis might be present.

Blood Glucose. Because the glucose tolerance test (GTT) is a cumbersome procedure, a simple and effective screening test

TABLE 17–5. RISK FACTORS FOR DIABETES MELLITUS

Individuals with a family history of diabetes

Individuals who are obese

Patients with transitory glycosuria or nondiagnostic hyperglycemia, especially during the course of pregnancy, surgical procedures, trauma, emotional stress, myocardial infarction, cerebrovascular accident, or administration of adrenal steroids

Individuals with unexplained episodes of hypoglycemia

Women who have delivered large babies or who have had pregnancies associated with abortions, premature labor, stillbirths, or neonatal deaths

Patients with unexplained neuropathy, retinpathy, nephropathy, peripheral vascular disease, or coronary artery disease

for diabetes is desirable. The fasting blood sugar (FBS) and the 2-hour postprandial blood glucose level have been used as screening tests for diabetes mellitus. The FBS is normally 70 to 115 mg/dl; patients with levels greater than 140 mg/dl on two separate occasions may be diagnosed as diabetic. Two-hour postprandial blood glucose levels greater than 200 mg/dl are very suggestive of diabetes. In patients with classic symptoms of diabetes mellitus and fasting glucose levels above 140 mg/dl, or nonfasting glucose levels above 200 mg/dl, a formal fasting glucose tolerance test adds little to the understanding of the patient's disease.

Serum and plasma have essentially the same glucose concentrations, whereas simultaneously drawn whole blood glucose levels are said to be about 17 percent lower. Serum or plasma glucose is more conveniently measured, and levels noted in this section are serum or plasma levels, not whole blood levels. When whole blood is allowed to stand at room temperature without a metabolic inhibitor (sodium fluoride), the glucose may decrease at a rate of about 5 percent per hour.

TABLE 17–6. INTERPRETATION OF TESTS FOR GLYCOSURIA

Clinitest Color	Clinitest Reading	Glucose (g/dl)
Deep blue	0	0
Blue-green	Trace	0.25
Green	+1	0.50
Olive green	+2	0.75
Tan	+3	1.0
Orange	+4	2.0

Thus, either the specimen should be refrigerated or better, the serum or plasma should be removed shortly after the blood is drawn.

Definitive Procedures

Oral Glucose Tolerance Test. A glucose tolerance test may be indicated when a diagnosis of diabetes cannot be established with the above laboratory measurements. In those patients in whom the diagnosis of diabetes is obscure, the glucose tolerance test is of value; it also gives the physician an opportunity to identify and possibly to initiate treatment earlier in the course of the disease to reduce or prevent overt symptoms or complications, if this is possible.

The assessment of a patient's reaction to a loading dose of glucose is also useful in the detection and understanding of a number of other metabolic disorders, as, for example, malabsorption states, starvation, hyperinsulinism, or pheochromocytoma.

The oral glucose tolerance test is performed as follows:

1. The patient is maintained on a diet with a normal carbohydrate content (200 to 300 g/day for adults) for at least 3 days before testing.
2. An overnight fast of 12 hours precedes the test.
3. A fasting blood sample is taken before the glucose load is administered.
4. The oral load of glucose is administered over a period of several minutes. The size of the glucose load given is variable; some investigators recommend 1.75 g/kg body weight, whereas the National Diabetes Data Group recommends a 75 g glucose dose for nonpregnant adults.
5. Venous blood samples are taken from adult patients at fasting or zero time, ½, 1, 1½, 2, and 3 hours. Additional specimens may be of value in studying patients with hypoglycemia.

In interpreting the results of this test, it is necessary to be somewhat arbitrary. With the use of the procedure and the doses described, the blood sugar results are usually interpreted in nonpregnant adults as shown in Table 17–7. According to the National Diabetes Data Group (NDDG) there are three ways to make the diagnosis of diabetes mellitus: (1) clinical symptoms of diabetes mellitus (e.g., polyuria, polydipsia, polyphagia, and weight loss) plus elevation of either the fasting glucose level (>140 mg/dl) or elevation of the nonfasting

TABLE 17–7. SERUM GLUCOSE LEVELS IN GLUCOSE TOLERANCE TESTING

Time (hr)	Normal	Diabetic
0.0 (fasting)	70–115*	>140*
0.5	<200	>200
1.0	<200	>200
1.5	<200	>200
2.0	<140	>200
3.0	70–115	>145

*All values given as mg/dl.

glucose level (>200 mg/dl); (2) elevation of the fasting glucose level (>140 mg/dl) on more than one occasion; or (3) a normal fasting glucose level but peak and 2-hour levels both over 200 mg/dl on more than one occasion.

The NDDG recognizes a group of patients with mildly abnormal glucose tolerance tests similar to latent diabetes in the old classification system. These patients have mildly elevated fasting blood sugars (>140 mg/dl) and a single point of the glucose tolerance test curve above 200 mg/dl (either the peak or 2-hour level but not both).

Potassium depletion from thiazide drugs or other causes may result in abnormal test results. Infections or other febrile conditions may also result in abnormal tolerance curves. Vomiting of ingested glucose during the first hour will invalidate the results.

Intravenous Glucose Tolerance Test. This procedure enables the clinican to overcome the variable factor of gastrointestinal absorption in certain cases. For example, glucose absorption may be increased in thyrotoxicosis and in patients with a gastroenterostomy. In sprue and other malabsorption syndromes, glucose absorption may be significantly decreased.

A standard dose of 50 percent glucose in water is given intravenously. Blood samples are drawn before the glucose injection, and at 1/2, 1, 2, and 3 hours after the injection. The criteria for the interpretation of this test are not uniform. Normally the blood glucose level returns to normal by 1 to 1 1/2 hours. The height of the curve has no significance. In diabetes mellitus the blood glucose level may not return to fasting levels by 2 hours and often not even by 3 hours.

DIAGNOSIS OF HYPERTHYROIDISM

Clinical Features

The clinical diagnosis of hyperthyroidism is often straightforward and laboratory studies are only confirmatory. The hyperthyroid patient usually notes a preference for cold temperatures and manifests increased sweating. Weight loss is evident despite a markedly increased appetite. Symptoms of nervousness, tiredness, and possibly palpitations may be present; the physical examination confirms these symptoms. In addition, the thyroid gland may be palpable and even exhibit a bruit. Hyperkinetic movements and tremor may be present. The resting pulse is usually greater than 90 per minute, and atrial fibrillation may be present. Eye signs, such as exophthalmos with lid retraction and lid lag, are helpful in making a diagnosis but are not uniformly present.

There are a significant number of patients in whom diagnosis is uncertain, and distinguishing symptoms from nervousness is not simple. In these cases the laboratory helps to arrive at the correct diagnosis. It may also be desirable to have objective laboratory information even in the obvious clinical case.

There are a number of causes of hyperthyroidism; common causes include diffuse overactivity of the gland (toxic diffuse goiter or Graves' disease) and localized production of thyroid hormone by thyroid nodules (toxic nodular goiter or Plummer's disease). Less common causes include damage to the thyroid, releasing the store of performed hormone in thyroid follicles (subacute thyroiditis or de Quervain's thyroiditis); chronic thyroiditis (or Hashimoto's thyroiditis), ectopic hormone production (struma ovarii), or deliberate ingestion of excess thyroid hormone (thyrotoxicosis factitia).

Laboratory Studies

Screening Procedures

Radioactive Iodine Uptake. The uptake of radioactive iodine in combination with a measurement of the conversion of iodine into circulating hormone is probably the single test most likely to be abnormal. The 6-hour uptake is preferable to a 24-hour uptake because in hyperthyroidism the peak uptake may occur considerably earlier than 24 hours. In hyperthyroidism the 6-hour uptake is greater than 25 percent of the dose. In thyrotoxicosis factitia resulting from the ingestion of thyroid hormone, iodine uptake will be decreased below normal. The determination of the conversion of radioactive iodide to circulating hormone at 48 or 72 hours may add useful additional information. At 48 hours, greater than 0.4 percent of the dose of radioactive iodide per liter of plasma is present as radioactive hormone. At 72 hours, greater than 0.28 percent of the dose indicates hyperthyroidism.

The production of a radioactivity scan for the determination of hot nodules or diffuse radioactive uptake allows the differentiation of thyrotoxicosis caused by diffuse hyperplasia from a toxic nodule.

As the determination of the iodine uptake is both expensive and time-consuming, several alternative laboratory tests may be substituted. However, the agreement of these test results with the clinical diagnosis is not quite as good as the agreement of the iodine uptake with the clinical state.

Thyroxine. The T_4 level is elevated in about 90 percent of patients with thyrotoxicosis (usually in the range of 12 to 20 μg/dl). The small number of thyrotoxic patients with normal T_4 should have T_3 measured because they may have the variant T_3 thyrotoxicosis. It may be that T_3 toxicity precedes the much more common T_4 variety of the disease.

Free Thyroxine. A variety of procedures are at present used to measure either directly or indirectly the amounts of free (and therefore metabolically active) T_4 in hyperthyroidism. This test is about 95 percent accurate. The chief advantage of the procedure is specificity. Therefore, it is the laboratory procedure of choice in complicated situations. Reference ranges vary among laboratories, and the specific procedure reference ranges must be consulted.

Triiodothyronine. In most instances of hyperthyroidism, total and free levels of both T_4 and T_3 are elevated. In about 5 percent of cases, however, only the total T_3 level is raised, whereas the total T_4 level is within the reference interval (T_3-toxicosis). In these cases a total T_3 level is necessary for the diagnosis.

Definitive Procedures

Thyrotropin Releasing Hormone (TRH) Stimulation Test. This test has been used as a confirmatory test for hyperthyroidism. Failure of the thyroid-stimulating hormone (TSH) level to rise after an intravenous injection of TRH is compatible with primary hyperthyroidism, i.e., high levels of thyroid hormone inhibit the release of TSH even under strong stimulation from the administered TRH.

Thyroid Suppression Test. In cases of borderline hyperthyroidism, the administration of exogenous hormone (5 μg of T_3 four times per day for 8 days) will reduce the 24-hour radioactive iodine uptake to less than 10 percent or less than one-half of the baseline value in the euthyroid patient. If no suppression occurs the results are taken as strong evidence of hyperthyroidism. If suppression occurs it rules out hyperthyroidism. The rationale of the test is that TSH production is normally suppressed by increased levels of thyroid hormone. In hyperthyroidism, the thyroid is no longer controlled by TSH, and it becomes autonomous in its production of increased quantities of hormone.

Thyroid Stimulatory Immunoglobulins (Long-Acting Thyroid Stimulator [LATS]). These are circulating immunoglobulins that appear to be antibodies directed against the TSH receptor sites or a closely related membrane antigen in the thyroid. These immunoglobulins act as thyroid stimulators and play an important role in the pathogenesis of the hyperthyroidism of Graves' disease. These substances can now be measured in some laboratories. Increased levels correlate with those patients who are difficult to manage clinically and may also indicate those patients who are prone to relapse when therapy is stopped.

DIAGNOSIS OF ADRENAL INSUFFICIENCY

Clinical Features

Adrenal insufficiency is characterized by unexplained weakness and increased fatiguability as well as loss of weight and anorexia. Hypotension with accompanying dizziness and syncope are also usually present. Vitiligo as well as a characteristic skin pigmentation may also be present.

Primary adrenal insufficiency, sometimes known as Addison's disease, may follow adrenal destruction from a variety of conditions such as autoimmune adrenalitis, tuberculous or histoplasmic destruction of the adrenal cortices, leukemic or other tumor infiltration of these glands, or rarely amyloidosis. The clinical manifestations of these diseases are also present. Secondary adrenal insufficiency is caused by a lack of pituitary ACTH production.

Laboratory Studies

Screening Procedures

A number of laboratory determinations may point to possible adrenal insufficiency, but as they are nonspecific, in effect, they do not constitute screening procedures. Table 17–8 lists laboratory abnormalities that may be present in adrenal insufficiency.

Urinary Steroids. The urinary excretion of corticosteroids, 17-hydroxysteroids, or 17-ketogenic steroids (or even 17-ketosteroids) is often decreased, although low normal levels of excretion are also seen on occasion. Therefore, normal levels of steroid excretion do not rule out the possibility of adrenal insufficiency. The insufficiency may only be latent and manifest only when the patient is under stress.

Plasma Cortisol Levels. As with urinary steroid excretion, plasma cortisol levels may be normal (5 to 20 μg/ml), therefore normal concentrations do not rule out the possibility of adrenal failure. Diurnal variation may also be evident.

ACTH Stimulation (Single Dose). The ability of the adrenal cortex to respond to ACTH stimulation allows for the differentiation of primary from secondary adrenal insufficiency. A synthetic ACTH that does not cause allergic reactions, cosyntropin, is now available.

After drawing a baseline plasma cortisol, 0.25 mg of cosyntropin is given intramuscularly. At 1 hour a second plasma cortisol level is drawn. Normally the cortisol level rises to more than 15 μg/dl over the baseline level. A failure to rise indicates primary adrenal insufficiency. Patients with secondary adrenal insufficiency theoretically should have a normal

TABLE 17–8. LABORATORY ABNORMALITIES IN ADRENAL INSUFFICIENCY

Anemia, normochromic, normocytic	Hypochloremia
Neutropenia	Hyperkalemia
Lymphocytosis, relative	Na/K ratio <30:1
Eosinophilia	Decreased basal metabolic rate

response. Some patients with pituitary insufficiency may have a subnormal response. These patients may be diagnosed by the formal ACTH stimulation test (discussion follows).

Metyrapone Test (Single Dose). This test has been used to assess pituitary ACTH reserve. Cortisol is the physiologic inhibitor of ACTH secretion by the well-known feedback mechanism. A heightened blood level of cortisol decreases ACTH secretion, whereas a diminished blood cortisol level promotes the pituitary secretion of ACTH. The drug metyrapone inhibits 11-β-hydroxylation in the adrenal cortex, thereby interfering with the normal production of cortisol. The fall in cortisol levels causes a primary discharge of ACTH, which stimulates the adrenal cortex, resulting in increased amounts of 11-deoxycortisol (compound S) proximal to the block. Compound S has little or no inhibitory effect on ACTH output and has relatively weak glucocorticoid biological activity.

To carry out the test, metyrapone (30 mg/kg) is given at midnight with a snack. A blood sample for 11-deoxycortisol (compound S) and ACTH is drawn at 8:00 AM. Normally, the serum compound S level rises to greater than 7 μg/dl and ACTH rises to greater than 100 pg/ml. In patients with secondary adrenal insufficiency the response is poor.

Definitive Procedures

ACTH Stimulation Test. The response of the adrenal cortex to ACTH infusion (0.25 mg of cosyntropin in 500 ml of 5 percent dextrose in normal saline given over 8 hours for 2 days) is measured by noting a rise in urinary or plasma cortisol levels (Table 17–9). This method distinguishes primary ($<$10 μg/dl rise in serum) from secondary (increases $>$15 μg/dl) adrenal insufficiency.

DIAGNOSIS OF PITUITARY INSUFFICIENCY

Whenever there is evidence of endocrine gland failure, either partial or complete, there is the question of whether this failure is caused by insufficiency of the particular endocrine gland itself (primary failure) or whether it is a result of failure of the pituitary (master) gland to supply the tropic (stimulating) hormone in sufficient quantities (secondary failure). Further complicating the issue is the fact that the hypothalamus controls pituitary secretion of several hormones, therefore hypothalmic dysfunction may also result in endocrine gland abnormalities.

TABLE 17–9. ADRENAL RESPONSE TO ACTH INFUSION*

	Control	Day 1	Day 2	Day 3
Normal	7	30	35	35
Adrenal insufficiency, primary	5	5	6	5
Pituitary insufficiency	5	7	10	15

*All values reported in milligrams 17-KGS per 24 hours.

At times the clinical history and manifestations of pituitary failure are clear-cut and the diagnosis is easily made. Often, however, the picture is not evident, possibly suggestive only after laboratory investigation of individual endocrine glands. One such endocrine deficiency, Schmidt's syndrome, which has features of both hypothyroidism and adrenal insufficiency, may resemble pituitary failure but more probably is a combined thyroid–adrenal insufficiency.

The anterior pituitary produces the following hormones: growth hormone (GH); prolactin; adrenocorticotrophic hormone (ACTH); melanocyte stimulating hormone (MSH); thyroid stimulating hormone (TSH); and the pituitary gonadotropins i.e., follicle stimulating hormone (FSH) and lutenizing hormone (LH). The posterior pituitary produces antiduretic hormone (ADH) and oxytocin. It is beyond the scope of this book to discuss all the pituitary hormones in detail but selected hormones are discussed. TSH and ACTH were previously discussed in the sections on the thyroid and the adrenal, respectively.

Growth Hormones

Clinical Features

GH deficiency is probably the most frequent pituitary hormone deficiency, either in overall pituitary failure or as an isolated defect leading to growth retardation in childhood. GH assay has been used as an overall screen for pituitary insufficiency, but not all cases of pituitary insufficiency have an associated GH deficiency.

Laboratory Studies

Screening Procedures

Growth Hormone Assay. The most widely used screening test for GH deficiency is the serum GH assay. Serum GH is usually measured by radioimmunoassay. The level may be elevated by sleep, exercise, or various foods. Therefore, the blood specimen should be collected in the morning, after an overnight fast with the patient still in bed. The result is only helpful if the level is high, which rules out GH deficiency. Low levels may be due to GH deficiency or may simply be normally low.

Definitive Procedures

Growth Hormone Stimulation Tests. There are a variety of stimulation tests for GH assessment. The classic procedures are the insulin tolerance test and arginine infusion. An arbitrary absolute value of serum GH defined differently by different investigators must be exceeded for a response to be classified as normal. Generally, peak poststimulus GH values of less than 9 ng/ml are considered subnormal; values from 9 to 10 ng/ml are considered indeterminate; and values greater than 10 ng/ml are considered normal.

Pituitary Gonadotropins

Pituitary production of LH and FSH is controlled by specific releasing factors from the hypothalamus. Production of these factors is under feedback control by the hormones or other active substances from the gonads.

FSH and LH are usually measured by radioimmunoassay. The reference ranges vary from laboratory to laboratory and reference ranges differ for men and women. For women, the values must be interpreted with consideration of the age and menstrual status of the patient. It is beyond the scope of this book to discuss the LH and FSH levels in various diseases. In general, however, patients with lesions in the hypothalamus or pituitary have low gonadotropin levels and low sex hormone levels, whereas patients with lesions in the gonads have low sex hormone levels with elevated gonadotropin levels.

Antiduretic Hormone

As mentioned above, the posterior pituitary produces ADH, or vasopressin. This hormone plays a major role in control of water resorption by the distal convoluted and collecting tubules of the kidneys. In patients with polydipsia and polyuria, but without glycosuria or azotemia, there may be impaired production of ADH or psychogenic polydipsia (compulsive water drinking). The functional state of the neurohypophyseal–

renal system can be evaluated by several tests, including intravenous hypertonic saline and vasopressin under constant water-loading conditions. The water deprivation test (discussion follows) is probably the most convenient and helpful procedure.

Water Deprivation Test

Comparison of the renal concentrating capacity after dehydration and after vasopressin administration is a simple and reliable way of diagnosing diabetes insipitus and of differentiating vasopressin deficiency from other causes of polyuria.

The following timed measurements are required. The patient may have breakfast but without coffee or tea. Thereafter no fluids or foods are allowed until after the completion of the test. At the beginning, after 5 hours, and at 8 hours, carefully weigh the patient, collect a 1-hour urine specimen and draw a blood sample. If the body weight decreases by more than 3 percent serious complications might occur.

Give five units of aqueous vasopressin (Pitressin) subcutaneously after the second (5-hour) samples are collected. Send the urine and blood specimens to the laboratory for osmolality determinations. Remember to correctly label each specimen as to the time of collection.

In normal individuals, the osmolality of the serum specimens never exceeds 295 mOsm/L and the osmolality of the second (5-hour) urine specimen is greater than 500 mOsm/L (Table 17–10).

TABLE 17–10. WATER DEPRIVATION TEST*

	Control		Water Deprivation (5 hr)		After Pitressin (8 hr)	
	Urine	*Serum*	*Urine*	*Serum*	*Urine*	*Serum*
Normal	—	<295	>500	<295	—	<295
Pituitary diabetes insipidus	<300	—	<300	>300	>400	—
Nephrogenic diabetes insipidus	<300	—	<300	>300	No change	—
Compulsive water drinkers	—	—	—	<295	—	<295

*All values given as mOsm/L.

INVESTIGATION OF UNEXPLAINED WEIGHT GAIN

The majority of patients who gain weight do so because of an intake of foodstuffs in excess of need. Probably the next most common cause of weight gain includes the various types of edema, as discussed in Chapter 6.

There are, in addition, several abnormalities of the endocrine glands that result in increased body weight or unusual distribution of fatty tissue in the body. These endocrine conditions include hypothyroidism and Cushing's syndrome attributable to pituitary or adrenal hyperfunction.

Other uncommon or even rare endocrine abnormalities include adiposogenital dystrophy, pseudohyperparathyroidism, acromegaly, and thalamic disease. Our discussions are limited to the more common disorders.

DIAGNOSIS OF HYPOTHYROIDISM

Clinical Features

The hallmark of severe hypothyroidism, myxedema, is well known. The condition includes a dull, disinterested facial expression with puffiness around the eyes, and dry, cold, coarse, thick, and sallow skin with brittle nails, and dry and thinning hair. A thick tongue and slow, deep voice are also characteristics. Menstrual abnormalities are common. But rarely are all these features fully developed; thus, a high degree of clinical suspicion backed up by sensitive laboratory procedures is essential for making the diagnosis.

Primary hypothyroidism (failure of the thyroid gland) is far more common than pituitary (secondary) or hypothalmic (tertiary) hypothyroidism. Most cases of primary hypothyroidism are caused by chronic thyroiditis.

Laboratory Studies

Screening Procedures

As expected with any chronic disease, a variety of laboratory changes may be evident. Many of these changes are quite nonspecific and are of little aid in making the diagnosis. Nonspecific laboratory changes that may be seen in hypothyroidism are: anemia, normocytic or (uncommonly) macrocytic;

hypercholesterolemia; decreased plasma and blood volume; and decreased basal metabolic rate.

Thyroxine. The measurement of serum T_4 is probably the single most reliable thyroid function test in hypothyroidism. Thyroxine levels below 3.5 µg/dl indicate hypothyroidism. Levels at or below 1.0 µg/dl are usually associated with frank myxedema. The free T_4 index will give essentially the same information but will take into account the amount of protein binding (discussion follows).

Definitive Procedures

Thyroid Stimulating Hormone. The availability of an accurate and sensitive procedure to measure TSH has made the diagnosis of hypothyroidism much more definitive than in the past.

TSH levels are low in hypothyroidism because of pituitary or hypothalamic insufficiency, whereas the TSH concentrations are elevated in hypothyroidism because of primary thyroid gland problems. Patients with pituitary insufficiency almost invariably have evidence of other endocrine gland insufficiency. The TRH test is useful in distinguishing between hypothyroidism caused by pituitary or hypothalamic insufficiency (discussion follows).

Occasionally a patient with early thyroidal hypothyroidism will have elevated TSH levels with only normal T_4 levels. In this case the TSH seems to be the more sensitive test for thyroid insufficiency.

Thyrotropin Releasing Hormone Test. The TRH test is helpful in distinguishing between hypothyroidism caused by pituitary or hypothalamic insufficiency. In pituitary disease the serum TSH should not rise after the TRH administration, whereas in hypothalamic disease there is a rise in serum TSH after TRH injection.

Antithyroid Autoantibodies. In a number of thyroid diseases associated with hypothyroidism, autoantibodies to thyroglobulin can be demonstrated. Many different techniques are in use, and the diagnostic specificity must be equated with the relative sensitivity of each procedure. As a general rule, as the sensitivity of the procedure increases, the number of false-positive results also rises. The most commonly used method is the tanned cell hemagglutination test. Table 17–11 shows the prevalence of antithyroid antibodies in various diseases.

TABLE 17–11. PREVALENCE OF ANTITHYROID ANTIBODIES IN VARIOUS DISEASES

Clinical State	Prevalence of Antithyroglobulin Antibody (%)
Hashimoto's disease	75–95
Idiopathic myxedema	75
Graves' disease	40
Nontoxic goiter	20–30
Thyroid cancer	40
Normal	10
Normal >70 yrs old	20

DIAGNOSIS OF CUSHING'S SYNDROME

Clinical Features

Although Cushing's syndrome (except for the iatrogenic form) is a relatively rare disorder, it has many features that it shares with more common disorders. These manifestations include obesity, hypertension, glucose intolerance, osteoporosis, menstrual abnormalities, and hirsutism. Because the syndrome is often curable, it behooves the physician to consider the diagnosis in patients manifesting any of the signs and symptoms noted above.

In addition to those symptoms, there are skin changes, including unusual fragility with poor healing properties and striae of a characteristic purple hue. Rather than gross obesity, an unusual distribution of body fat is seen, i.e., cervical and supracervical fat pad, so-called moon facies, and a relative increase of truncal rather than extremity fat.

Laboratory Studies

Screening Procedures

There are nonspecific changes in the blood count, including some increase in hemoglobin levels, and relative polymorphonuclear leukocytosis with lymphopenia and eosinopenia. An eosinophil count about $0.1 \times 10^9/L$ is considered strong evidence against the diagnosis of Cushing's syndrome. Although overt diabetes is not common, impaired glucose tolerance is commonly found. Hypokalemic alkalosis is found in severe cases.

Plasma Cortisol. In recent years, the measurement of plasma cortisol concentrations has become a convenient procedure for the evaluation of adrenal cortical hyperfunction. Cortisol measured at 8:00 AM and 6:00 PM may reveal the failure of normal diurnal variation in Cushing's syndrome as well as elevated levels of plasma cortisol. Normally the 6:00 PM levels are about half the morning levels. However, the sometimes erratic fluctuations of cortisol secretion caused by diurnal as well as day-to-day variation make the measurement of cortisol by itself not very helpful unless it is markedly elevated.

Urinary Corticosteroids. Approximately 1 percent of plasma cortisol is excreted in the kidney in its original or unconjugated state; the remainder appears in the urine as conjugated metabolites. Urinary free cortisol can be quantitated by radioimmunoassay with a satisfactory degree of specificity. Urinary free cortisol in 24-hour collections is elevated in about 95 percent of patients with Cushing's syndrome.

The 24-hour output of 17-ketogenic steroids (17-KGS) or 17-hydroxycorticosteroids (17-OHCS) will be elevated in most cases of Cushing's syndrome. The measurement of urinary creatinine levels to determine the completeness of collection procedures is stressed.

Dexamethasone Suppression Test (Single Dose). The secretion of pituitary ACTH is maximal in the early morning and minimal in midafternoon. Dexamethasone inhibits the maximal output if given late in the evening. For this procedure a control

---

TABLE 17–12. CONDITIONS ASSOCIATED WITH CUSHING'S SYNDROME

Bilateral adrenal hyperplasia due to excess ACTH production
  1. Pituitary hyperfunction
  2. ACTH-like substances produced by nonendocrine tumors (lung, thymus, pancreas, bronchial adenoma)
  3. ACTH treatment (iatrogenic)
Adrenal adenoma
Adrenal carcinoma
Nodular or adenomatous hyperplasia of the adrenals
Corticosteroid therapy (iatrogenic)

cortisol level is drawn at 8:00 AM on day 1. At 11:00 PM of day 1, dexamethasone, 1 mg, is given orally and, on the following morning (day 2), a second plasma cortisol specimen is drawn.

Healthy persons and patients with obesity caused by conditions other than Cushing's syndrome have cortisol levels on day 2 under 5 μg/dl or less. Individual laboratories may have somewhat different normal and abnormal values.

Definitive Procedures

A number of different conditions can cause Cushing's syndrome, and additional laboratory studies, which can help to further delineate these conditions, are noted in Table 17–12.

Urinary 17–Ketosteroids. In contrast with most studies of adrenal hyperfunction, adrenal adenomas characteristically are associated with decreased 17-ketosteroid production. The other conditions noted above usually are associated with increased 17-ketosteroid production, which is especially pronounced in adrenal carcinomas and ACTH-like substances that are produced by tumors of nonendocrine origin.

Metyrapone Test. As noted previously, metyrapone selectively inhibits 11-β-hydroxylation in the adrenal cortical biosynthesis of cortisol. This results in decreased cortisol production with a subsequent increase in pituitary ACTH production. Of the hyperfunctional conditions noted above, only bilateral hyperplasia and nodular hyperplasia respond to metyrapone by a further significant increase in steroid production. Adrenal adenomas may show a slight increase, whereas carcinomas are totally unresponsive.

To carry out this procedure after collecting a 24-hour control urine specimen, administer metyaprone, 750 mg orally every 4 hours for six doses. Also collect all urine voided during this second 24-hour period. The 17-ketogenic steroids or 17–hydroxycorticosteroids are measured on both specimens and interpreted as outlined in Table 17–13.

Dexamethasone Suppression Test. Dexamethasone, a synthetic steroid, normally suppresses ACTH production by the pituitary gland. By use of a low-dose and high-dose procedure, adrenal cortical reaction to normal or excessive ACTH production or possibly nonsusceptibility to ACTH may be inferred.

After a control urine specimen is collected, 0.5 mg of dexamethasone is given orally every 6 hours for a total of eight doses. On the second day of dexamethasone administration, a

TABLE 17–13. SUMMARY OF DIFFERENTIAL TESTS IN CUSHING'S SYNDROME*

	Normal	Hyperplasia	Adenoma	Nodular Hyperplasia	Carcinoma
Control urine 17-KGS	N	↑	↑	↑	↑
Metyrapone test	$2-5 \times N$	$1\frac{1}{2} \times N$	No change	$1\frac{1}{2} \times N$	No change
Dexamethasone suppression (2 mg/day)	↓	No change	No change	No change	No change
Dexamethasone suppression (8 mg/day)	↓	↓	No change	No change	No change
ACTH stimulation	$3-5 \times N$	$3-5 \times N$	$3-5 \times N$	$3-5 \times N$	No change

*All data given as urinary 17-KGS levels; N, normal.

24-hour urine specimen is again collected. The dose of dexamethasone is then increased to 2.0 mg orally every 6 hours for eight doses, and another 24-hour urine specimen is collected on the second day of the larger dosage schedule. Ketogenic steroids or 17-hydroxycorticosteroids are measured on all three specimens. On the lower dosage schedule, the urine steroid excretion normally falls whereas, in adrenal hyperplasia as well as the various adrenal tumors, no significant change is noted. The increased dosage will suppress the hyperplastic adrenal steroid production by at least 50 percent but will fail to affect steroid production caused by adrenal tumors, either benign or malignant.

ACTH Stimulation Test. A final functional test that helps to differentiate adrenal carcinomas is the determination of the effect of ACTH on steroid excretion. In this procedure, autonomous adenocarcinoma fails to react to ACTH (0.25 mg of cosyntropin in 500 ml of 5 percent dextrose in saline intravenously over 8 hours), but normal glands as well as benign tumors of the adrenals react by increasing 17-ketogenic steroid excretion three- to fivefold.

SUGGESTED READINGS

Alsever R, Gotlin R: Handbook of Endocrine Tests, 2nd ed. Chicago, Year Book Medical Publ., 1978.

Bray GA, Jordan HA, Sims EAH: Evaluation of the obese patient. 1. An algorithm. JAMA 235:1487, 1976.

Bray GA, Jordan HA, Sims EAH: Evaluation of the obese patient. 2. Clinical findings. JAMA 235:2008, 1976.

Crapo L: Cushing's syndrome: A review of diagnostic tests. Metabolism 28:955, 1979.

Edwards C: Vasopressin and oxytocin in health and disease. Clin Endocrinol Metab 6:223, 1977.

Gold E: Cushing's syndrome: A tripartite entity. Hosp Pract 14:67, 1979.

Hershmon J: Endocrine Pathophysiology: A Patient-oriented Approach. Philadelphia, Lea and Febiger, 1982.

Howanitz PJ, Howanitz JH (eds): Issues in Laboratory Endocrinology. Clinics in Laboratory Medicine. Philadelpia, Saunders, 1984.

Knowles HC: Evaluation of a positive urinary sugar test. JAMA 234:961, 1975.

McHardy-Young, et al.: Single-dose dexamethasone suppression test for Cushing's syndrome. Br Med J 2:740, 1967.

Musa BU, Dowling JT: Rapid intravenous administration of corticotropin as a test of adrenocortical insufficiency. JAMA 201:663, 1967.

National Diabetes Data Group: Classification and diagnosis of diabetes mellitus and other categories of glucose intolerance. Diabetes 28:1039, 1979.

Netter FH: Endocrine System and Selected Metabolic Disease. Summit, NJ, Ciba Pharm., 1965.

Rosenberg IN: Evaluation of thyroid function. N Engl J Med 286:924, 1972.

Spiger M, et al.: Single-dose metyrapone test. Arch Intern Med 135:698, 1975.

Streck W, Lockwood D (eds): Endocrine Diagnosis: Clinical and Laboratory Approach. Boston, Little, Brown, 1983.

Williams R (ed): Textbook of Endocrinology, 6th ed. Philadelphia, Saunders, 1981.

18

JOINT AND MUSCLE PROBLEMS

BASIC INFORMATION

Criteria for the Diagnosis of Diseases Associated with Arthritis

There are several major and numerous minor causes of arthritis or rheumatism that must be considered in the patient with a single or multiple painful joints or muscles. The conditions can be conveniently divided into degenerative and inflammatory varieties. At times even this gross division is difficult to make in the individual patient, especially if he or she has an acute exacerbation of the chronic degenerative diseases; however, the two major classes are nevertheless quite useful.

By far the most common cause of arthritis is degenerative joint disease, or osteoarthritis. This type of joint pain is a result of the ceaseless minor trauma to joints occurring over many years. It usually occurs in the elderly patient in those joints, such as the knees, hips, or hands, that take the brunt of the trauma. The degenerative changes are hastened in the obese patient and in those joints previously injured by fracture or other trauma. The characteristic Heberden's nodes are a diagnostic aid, but their absence does not militate against this cause of arthritis.

A special type of degenerative joint disease, the ruptured intervertebral disc, has a characteristic clinical history of previous strain or trauma. Symptoms of dorsolumbar pain and clinical evidence of sensory deficits and muscle wasting are found frequently.

Traumatic arthritis usually follows known, but at other times forgotten, damage to the joints. The rare but interesting arthritis following neural degeneration, such as Charcot joints of tertiary syphilis or diabetes mellitus, is, in reality, a type of traumatic arthritis that follows loss of sensory perception in these joints. The x-ray changes are usually diagnostic.

The clinical picture in gout is variable except in one point, the initial episode quite often occurs in the great toe. Thereafter other joints may be involved. The hot, extremely tender, and extraordinarily painful joint in the gouty patient is characteristic, although all gradations of the clinical picture can and do occur.

The clinical manifestations of rheumatoid arthritis, rheumatic fever, and systemic lupus erythematosus (SLE) are quite variable. Because of the potentially ominous complications and sequelae of these diseases, there has been a need for the sharpening of diagnostic criteria.

The American Rheumatism Association (ARA) has developed 11 criteria for the diagnosis of rheumatoid arthritis (Table 18–1). Of the 11 criteria, seven are needed for the diagnosis of classical rheumatoid arthritis (RA), five for the diagnosis of definite RA, and three for the diagnosis of probable RA. The reader is referred to a more complete treatise for any further discussion of the individual criteria. The close cooperation of the attending physician, radiologist, clinical pathologist, and

TABLE 18–1. ARA CRITERIA FOR THE DIAGNOSIS OF RHEUMATOID ARTHRITIS

Morning stiffness

Joint pain on motion or tenderness

Swelling of a joint

Swelling of a second joint

Symmetric joint swelling

Subcutaneous nodules

Typical x-ray changes

Positive rheumatoid factor test

Poor mucin clot from synovial fluid

Characteristic histologic changes in the synovium

Characteristic histologic changes in the subcutaneous nodules

Seven criteria are required for the diagnosis of classic rheumatoid arthritis, five are required for the diagnosis of definite rheumatoid arthritis, and three criteria are necessary for the diagnosis of probable rheumatoid arthritis.

TABLE 18–2. AHA CRITERIA FOR THE DIAGNOSIS OF RHEUMATIC FEVER

Major criteria
  Carditis (murmur, enlargement, pericarditis, failure)
  Polyarthritis
  Chorea
  Subcutaneous nodules
  Erythema marginatum
Minor criteria
  Fever
  Arthralgia
  Prolonged PR interval on ECG
  Increased sedimentation rate, white count, or presence of C-reactive protein
  Previous rheumatic fever or inactive rheumatic heart disease

Two major or one major and two minor criteria indicate a high probability of rheumatic fever. Evidence of preceding streptococcal infection, e.g., elevated ASO titer or positive throat culture for group A streptococcus, is also required.

surgeon is especially well illustrated by the criteria listed in Table 18–1 for the diagnosis of rheumatoid arthritis. Some of these criteria are purely clinical manifestations, whereas others are laboratory examinations that help to establish or reject this diagnosis.

Many rheumatologists strongly believe that this entity should be labeled rheumatoid disease rather than rheumatoid arthritis, as serous surfaces in addition to the joint spaces may also be involved. The occurrence of pleural or pericardial effusions indicate a relationship between this entity and the other collagen diseases such as SLE. Although most cases are primarily arthritic in nature, the physician should not be surprised when nonarthritic manifestations occur.

Because of the difficulty in diagnosing rheumatic fever as well as its frequent overdiagnosis, the American Heart Association (AHA) published a listing of major and minor criteria to guide in the establishment of this diagnosis (Table 18–2). At least two major or one major and two minor criteria indicate a high probability of rheumatic fever provided that there is supporting evidence of a recent streptococcal infection. As rheumatic fever has certain features in common with rheumatoid disease (e.g., polyarthritis, arthralgia, and subcutaneous nodules), the criteria for the diagnosis of rheumatic fever are given in this table.

Although rheumatic fever is a major consideration in the young patient with arthritis or arthralgia, SLE is a more important consideration in the middle-aged patient. The criteria for the diagnosis of SLE are listed in Table 18–3.

For the diagnosis of SLE at least four criteria must be satisfied. It can be seen that the manifestations of this disease are variable and usually nonspecific; again, they include both clinical and laboratory features. Such listings as those given above help to sharpen the criteria for the diagnosis of these diseases that are extremely variable in their manifestations and have serious prognostic significance.

With the widespread use of antibiotics, the occurrence of septic arthritis has become a rarity. However, the possibililty of a suppurative process must be considered in any case of a painful, swollen, and tender joint accompanied by systemic signs of sepsis such as chills and fever. A resemblance to other causes of arthritis is evident, and at times only examination of the synovial fluid will yield the diagnosis.

Other less common causes of painful joints include sarcoid, Reiter's syndrome, leukemia, and lymphoma. Because the joint manifestations may at times precede identifiable disease, these diagnoses are occasionally quite difficult. As the diagnosis may be missed and the condition mistakenly diag-

TABLE 18–3. ARA REVISED CRITERIA FOR THE CLASSIFICATION OF SLE

Criteria	Sensitivity	Specificity
Malar rash	57	96
Discoid rash	18	99
Photosensitivity	43	96
Oral ulcers	27	96
Arthritis	86	37
Serositis—pleuritis or pericarditis	56	86
Renal disorder—proteinuria greater than 0.5 g/day or cellular casts	51	94
Neurologic disorder—seizures or psychosia	20	98
Hematologic disorder—hemolytic anemia, leukopenia, lymphopenia, or thrombocytopenia	59	89
Immunologic disorder—positive SLE prep, anti-DNA or anti-SM, or false-positive serologic test for syphilis	85	93
Antinuclear antibody	99	49
Overall	96	96

The diagnosis of SLE requires 4 or more of the 11 criteria be present.

nosed as one of the more common causes of arthritis, periodic review of the case is necessary.

CLINICAL INVESTIGATION

Laboratory Studies

Several approaches are available for the study of joint diseases, including synovial fluid analysis, x-ray examinations, and certain blood chemical determinations. In the laboratory, blood constituents or aspirated synovial fluid can be examined. Because of the ready accessibility of blood, it is the more widely studied of the two fluids.

Synovial Fluid Analysis. The examination of synovial fluid aspirated from symptomatic joints is a simple but very useful procedure. Several aspects are considered, including the gross appearance, the viscosity of the fluid, its ability to form a mucin clot, and finally, a microscopic examination including a cell count and a search for cartilaginous fibrils, urate crystals, and bacteria. Culture of the fluid is at times extremely useful. Table 18–4 summarizes the characteristic changes seen in various arthritic conditions.

If large numbers of white blood cells or bacteria are found in the examination of the synovial fluid, septic arthritis is a most likely diagnosis. A portion of the aspirated fluid should be, kept in a sterile container for appropriate microbiological procedures. Several different organisms are associated with septic arthritis, and each requires different culture media for isolation and identification. A Gram stain of the synovial fluid sediment will usually indicate the appropriate culture media for isolation, as shown in Table 18–5.

The failure to see organisms in fluids with markedly elevated numbers of white blood cells may result from a sampling difficulty (very few organisms present), staining difficulties (acid-fast bacilli or PPLO fail to stain with Gram stain), or asepsis (caused by a burned-out infection or noninfectious inflammatory arthritis). For these reasons culture on all four media listed in Table 18–5 is appropriate in all cases where no reasonable alternative explanation is found.

X-ray Studies

If synovial fluid examination fails to reveal the diagnosis or if the examination is not performed, which procedures can be

TABLE 18–4. CHARACTERISTIC SYNOVIAL FLUID ANALYSIS IN ARTHRITIC CONDITIONS

	Appearance	Viscosity	Hyaluronic Acid (Mucin Clot Test)	White Cell Count ($\times$ 10^9/L)	Neutrophils (%)	Other
Healthy	Clear, straw	High	Good	<0.2	<10	—
Degenerative joint disease	Clear, straw	Variable	Good	<0.7	~15	Cartilage fibrils present
Gouty arthritis	Yellow, cloudy	Low	Poor	~20	~70	Negatively birefringent urate crystals present
Pseudogout	Slightly cloudy	Fair to low	Fair to poor	~15	~70	Positively birefringent CPPD crystals present*
Rheumatoid disease	Yellow, green, cloudy	Low	Poor	~20	~70	RA cells may be present, low complement

(*cont.*)

TABLE 18–4. CHARACTERISTIC SYNOVIAL FLUID ANALYSIS IN ARTHRITIC CONDITIONS (cont.)

	Appearance	Viscosity	Hyaluronic Acid (Mucin Clot Test)	White Cell Count ($\times 10^9$/L)	Neutrophils (%)	Other
Rheumatic fever	Yellow, slightly cloudy	Low	Good	~14	~50	
Systemic lupus erythematosus	Straw, slightly cloudy	High	Good	~2	~30	LE cells may be present, low complement
Septic arthritis	Purulent, bloody	Low	Poor	~90	~90	Gram stain and culture positive in about one-half of cases
Traumatic arthritis, acute	Bloody or turbid	High	Good	~1	~25	Fat globules may be present

*Negatively birefringent (urate) crystals are yellow when parallel to the compensator axis and blue when perpendicular. Positively birefringent (CPPD) crystals are blue when parallel to the compensator axis and yellow when perpendicular.

done to delineate the cause of the patient's arthritis or arthralgia? The roentgenographic examination of the involved joint or joints can yield diagnostic information, especially in degenerative joint diseases or gout, and therefore this examination is recommended; in fact, it is mandatory. The reader is referred to the radiologic literature for discussions of these examinations.

Laboratory Studies in Gout

Uric Acid. Following degenerative joint disease, gout is probably the most common disease associated with arthritis. It would seem appropriate, therefore, to test for this disease, if possible.

Uric acid is the major product of purine metabolism and is formed from xanthine by the action of xanthine oxidase. Gout is a disorder of purine metabolism or renal excretion of uric acid. An elevation of serum uric acid levels will usually be seen in gout, although at times the values may be within the normal range during inactive stages of the disease. Methodologic differences have resulted in variations in normal, or reference, ranges. Therefore, each laboratory should publish its own normal ranges. Men normally have uric acid levels about 1.5 mg/dl greater than women.

In interpreting elevated levels of uric acid, one must keep in mind the artifactual elevations that occur in a significant number of patients receiving thiazide diuretics.

Laboratory Studies in Rheumatic Fever

Throat Culture. Two procedures are generally available for the confirmation of streptococcal infections. The first study, the throat culture, is positive only during the stage of acute pharyngitis and usually is negative when the sequelae of rheumatic

TABLE 18–5. MICROBIOLOGICAL EXAMINATION OF JOINT FLUID

Gram Stain	Possible Organism	Appropriate Isolation Media
Gram-positive cocci	*Staphylococcus* *Streptococcus* *Pneumococcus*	Blood agar
Gram-negative cocci	*Neisseria*	Chocolate agar
No organisms seen	*Mycobacterium* PPLO	Lowenstein's or other TB media PPLO media

fever or acute glomerulonephritis occur. A positive culture is dependent on the obtaining of an adequate sample and also on the use of appropriate culture techniques including proper media and reduced oxygen incubation. Physicians contemplating the use of this test as an office procedure (a commendable idea) must use acceptable bacteriologic techniques when processing these cultures. Without adequate control of this procedure, up to half of the streptococcal infections may be missed. The reader is referred to Chapter 24 for a complete discussion on how to obtain bacteriologic specimens as well as accepted methods of plating and culturing.

Antistreptolysin Titer. The second laboratory procedure of value in the diagnosis of rheumatic fever is the measurement of the antistreptolysin-O (ASO) titer. Streptolysin O is an enzyme-like toxin produced by most group A streptococci that is capable of hemolyzing red blood cells. Measuring the ASO titer is of aid in the diagnosis of rheumatic fever as well as other sequelae of streptococcal infections such as acute glomerulonephritis. In these diseases, increased titers of ASO are the usual (80 percent) finding. It is also of value in the differential diagnosis of diseases that simulate rheumatic fever, but in such cases the ASO titer is not increased.

Essentially, serial dilutions of the patient's serum are reacted with streptolysin-O reagent, a hemolytic agent. If antistreptolysin is present in the patient's serum, the streptolysin will be inactivated and no hemolysis of the indicator erythrocytes will occur. The converse will occur if no antistreptolysin is present. For laboratory convenience, to obtain dilutions in concentrations of clinical applicability, a rather unusual set of dilutions is used in this test. The reciprocals of these dilutions are the units in which test results are reported (Todd units).

It is also of some importance to obtain serial ASO titers and to seek changes of two tubes or more when testing at biweekly intervals. A rising titer points to a recent (within the past month or 6 weeks) streptococcal infection, whereas a falling titer indicates recovery. An ASO titer above 200 in a single specimen is evidence of a recent group A streptococcal infection.

Anti-DNAse Titer. This enzyme produced by the hemolytic streptococcus can also be measured following a presumed streptococcal infection. It has fewer false positives than the ASO titer because the overlap of the normal and abnormal titers is less extensive than with the ASO titer. The test is valuable in those patients who may not produce antibodies to streptolysin-O, or in diagnosing more remote infections, as the anti-DNAse titer remains elevated longer than the ASO titer.

A rise in titer of two or more dilution units between acute and convalescent serum is considered evidence of a recent streptococcal infection. An anti-DNAse titer above 200 on a single specimen is considered evidence of a recent streptococcal infection.

Laboratory Studies in Collagen Vascular Diseases

Several procedures are available to measure immunoglobulins or other abnormal globulins. Some of these globulins have some of the characteristics of autoantibodies (e.g., antinuclear antibodies) and are inconsistently elevated in rheumatoid disease as well as other collagen-type disorders.

Although the demonstrations of the SLE phenomenon (intracytoplasmic phagocytosis of denatured nucleoprotein) is comparatively well standardized in many laboratories, the demonstration of rheumatoid fever and antinuclear antibody is not. A variety of methods are available, and they vary considerably in sensitivity, specificity, and reproducibility. It is, therefore, necessary to be aware of these factors when interpreting a particular test result.

Rheumatoid Factor. In patients with rheumatoid disease there is concurrent appearance of a rheumatoid factor in the serum. This factor, an IgM gamma-globulin with anti-gamma-globulin activity, can be demonstrated by a number of techniques, none of which is, as yet, entirely specific. Hence, there are a variety of diseases in which increased quantities of gamma-globulins are present and in some cases rheumatoid factor is present, although rheumatoid disease is not present in these patients. As a rule increased sensitivity of any particular test is necessarily associated with an increased incidence of false-positive reactions.

The rheumatoid factor is usually demonstrated by use of a latex fixation procedure. In the latex fixation test, latex particles coated with normal IgG (immune gamma-globulin) are reacted with serum. If it contains the rheumatoid factor, the particles clump or agglutinate. Several commercial preparations are available. As mentioned previously there are significant numbers of false-positive and false-negative results when one tests for the rheumatoid factor. These facts must be borne in mind when interpreting the results of a single test in a patient.

TABLE 18-6. LABORATORY TESTS IN ARTHRITIC CONDITIONS*

Clinical Condition	Rheumatoid Factor	LE Test	Antinuclear Antibody	Anti-DNA (Double-Stranded)
Normal individuals	2–3	0	<5	1–2
Arthritic conditions				
Rheumatoid disease	80	15	25–30	15
Degenerative joint disease	6	0	<5	
Gout	10	0	<5	
Systemic lupus erythematosus	20–30	70–80	>95	70–80
Scleroderma	30	15	60–70	30
Dermatomyositis	15	12–15	<10	15
Mixed collagen-vascular disease	—	20	100	25

*All figures are given as percentage of patients with positive results.

SLE Cell Test. In the LE cell test a serum IgG reacts with nuclei from in vitro damaged cells to form a hematoxylin body. In the presence of complement, phagocytosis of the hematoxylin body by a neutrophil results in an SLE cell, clearly demonstrated by Wright stain. The demonstration of a positive SLE cell phenomenon requires the finding of several (five or more) typical LE cells on each preparation. The intracytoplasmic inclusion must be large and round and exhibit smooth, homogeneous, purplish staining. Table 18–6 lists the incidence of a positive LE test in various arthritic conditions. Occasionally free protein material, or extracellular material (ECM), or rosette formation is found in LE preparations. Because of the relative nonspecificity of this procedure it is being replaced by newer immunologic procedures such as the antinuclear antibody.

Antinuclear Antibody. The demonstration of antinuclear antibodies (ANA) has proved to be a sensitive indicator of a wide variety of collagen-vascular diseases. The indirect immunofluorescence ANA assay is the standard screening test for collagen vascular disease with positive results in greater than 95 percent of patients with SLE. The sensitivity of the test depends on the source of cell nuclei for the procedure, i.e., different nuclear sources do not have equal sensitivity.

The titer of the result and the pattern of nuclear fluorescence are important. A high ANA titer (i.e., 1:160 or greater) strongly suggests SLE, whereas noncollagen diseases usually have titers below 1:160. A peripheral (rim) staining pattern

TABLE 18–7. ANTINUCLEAR ANTIBODY STAINING PATTERNS

Nuclear Staining Pattern	SLE	RA	Scleroderma	Mixed Collagen-Vascular Disease
Homogeneous	+ +	+	+	
Nucleolar	+	0	+ +	
Speckled	+	+	+	+ +
Peripheral	+ +	+	0	

SLE, systemic lupus erythematosus; RA, rheumatoid arthritis.

suggests SLE, whereas a nucleolar pattern suggests scleroderma (Table 18–7).

A wide variety of specific ANAs have been demonstrated, reactive against either nuclear or cytoplasmic constituents with varying degrees of tissue and cellular constituent activity. The most popular of these assays detects antibodies to double-stranded DNA. This test may be somewhat more specific for SLE than the screening ANA test. Other specific autoantibodies may be associated with specific diseases (Table 18–8). These assays are generally available only in large reference laboratories. Table 18–6 summarizes the results of these various tests in a variety of arthritic conditions.

Complement. A number of the components of the complement system are measured, in particular total hemolytic complement and the C3 and C4 components. Complement components are decreased in a number of immunologic diseases, and during the active phases these proteins would be expected to be decreased or even undetectable. C3 is a somewhat more sensitive indicator of complement consumption. With response to therapy, C3 and C4 return toward normal levels.

MUSCLE WEAKNESS AND ATROPHY

CLINICAL INVESTIGATION

The differential diagnosis of neuromuscular disorders and muscle wasting is dependent on a careful family history and

TABLE 18–8. DISEASE ASSOCIATED WITH SPECIFIC AUTOANTIBODIES

Autoantibody	Associated Disease
DNA, Double stranded	SLE
SM (Smith)	SLE
RNP	Mixed connective tissue disease
Scl-78	Scleroderma
Nucleolar	Scleroderma
Centromere	CREST syndrome*

*Calcinosis, Reynaud's phenomenon, esophageal dysfunction, sclerodactyly, and telangiectasia in a patient with systemic scleroderma. The syndrome carries a more favorable prognosis.

physical examination coupled with appropriate laboratory studies including biopsy, if necessary.

Clinical Features

The family history is quite important, as many diseases of muscle are known to occur in family groups. The age of onset, progression, as well as the distribution of affected muscle groups provide invaluable diagnostic information. Associated features such as skin changes (e.g., dermatomyositis), muscle tenderness (e.g., trichinosis), and fasciculations (e.g., amyotophic lateral sclerosis) are also helpful. Rapid fatigue points to myasthenia gravis. Observation of patient movements such as arising from the floor or while walking may reveal the characteristic movements associated with muscular dystrophy.

Laboratory Studies

Many enzymes, including the transaminases (AST, ALT), lactic dehydrogenase, aldolase, and creatine phosphokinase, are especially abundant in skeletal as well as cardiac muscle. When muscle tissue is damaged or diseased, these enzymes are released into the interstitial and intravascular compartment. Muscle wasting and atrophy secondary to neural lesions do not produce elevated enzyme levels.

Creatine Phosphokinase

Creatine phosphokinase (CK) is abundant in muscle tissue and has become a most reliable and sensitive indicator of acute muscle damage. Serum CK is prominently elevated in several muscular dystrophic syndromes (e.g., Duchenne's disease) as well as in myositis from any cause. In dermatomyositis and polymositis all muscle enzymes are elevated. Creatine kinase may be elevated in the acute stages of myocardial infarction, although this rarely presents a problem in interpretation; when in doubt, CK isoenzymes should be obtained. Skeletal muscle contains almost 90 percent of the MM isoenzyme and only 10 percent of the MB isoenzyme. Thus, when skeletal muscle is damaged almost all of the elevation is due to the MM isoenzyme.

Aldolase

This enzyme has proved to be useful in the differential diagnosis of muscular disease. It is especially abundant in muscle, although lesser amounts are widely distributed in the body. As erythrocytes contain considerable amounts of aldolase, hemolysis must be carefully avoided when blood is collected for this assay. Progressive muscular dystrophy in its active stages regularly produces greatly elevated serum levels of aldolase. Aldolase levels are highest in the Duchenne's disease, especially early in the disease when the patient is still in relatively satisfactory clinical condition. The enzyme concentrations gradually decline and finally reach low levels when the patient becomes bedridden. Serum aldolase is elevated in hepatitis, but it is not as useful in the diagnosis of liver disease as are the transaminases.

Electromyography

This modality provides valuable information for the differentiation of the various disorders associated with muscle weakness. Discussion of this test is beyond the scope of this book.

Muscle Biopsy

The most valuable study in muscle weakness is the muscle biopsy. Care must be taken in selecting the site for biopsy, choosing an affected muscle. Careful handling and preparation of the biopsy specimen is imperative to obtain the maximal benefit from this procedure.

Other Laboratory Studies

The laboratory evaluation of adrenal cortical dysfunction, thyroid gland hyperfunction, or plasma potassium abnormalities are indicated in appropriate cases. One can use the cholinergic drug neostigmine as an agent to diagnose myasthenia gravis. An intramuscular injection of this drug promptly relieves the muscular weakness in these patients.

SUGGESTED READINGS

American Heart Association: Jones criteria (revised) for guidance in diagnosis of rheumatic fever. Circulation 32:664, 1965.

Dubois EL: LE cell test and antinuclear antibodies. JAMA 200:1053, 1967.

Fries JF, Mitchell DM: Joint pain or arthritis. JAMA 235:199, 1976.

Greenwald C, et al.: Laboratory tests for antinuclear antibody (ANA) in rheumatic diseases. Lab Med 9:19, 1978.

Hollander JL, Jessar RA, McCarty DJ Jr: Synovianalysis: An aid in arthritis diagnosis. Bull Rheum Dis 12:263, 1961.

Horwitz C: Laboratory diagnosis of rheumatic diseases. Postgrad Med 67:193, 1980.

Kalmin N, et al.: Relative values of laboratory assays in systemic lupus erythematosus. Am J Clin Pathol 75:846, 1981.

McCarty D: Arthritis and Allied Conditions. Philadelphia, Lea & Febiger, 1985.

McCarty DJ Jr, Gatter RA: Pseudogout syndrome (articular chondrocalcinosis). Bull Rheum Dis 14:331, 1964.

Molden D: ANA profiles in systemic rheumatic disease. Diag Med (June):12, 1985.

Nofman D, et al.: Profiles of antinuclear antibodies in systemic rheumatic diseases. Ann Intern Med 83:464, 1975.

Ropes M, et al.: 1958 revision of diagnostic criteria for rheumatoid arthritis. Bull Rheum Dis 9:175, 1958.

Stevens MB, Abbey H, Shulman LE: The clinical significance of extracellular material (ECM) in LE cell preparations. N Engl J Med 268:976, 1963.

Taborn J, Walker S: Rheumatoid factor: A review. Lab Med 10:392, 1979.

Tan E: Antinuclear antibodies in diagnosis and management. Hosp Pract 18:79, 1983.

Tan E, et al.: The 1982 revised criteria for the classification of systemic lupus erythematosus. Arthritis Rheum 25:1271, 1982.

19

METABOLIC BONE DISORDERS

BASIC INFORMATION

Bone is composed of an organic matrix in close association with a solid mineral phase. The organic matrix (osteoid) consists of 90 to 95 percent collagen, small amounts of proteoglycans, and some noncollagenous proteins. The mineral phase is composed primarily of calcium and phosphorus salts, and small amounts of other minerals.

Bone grows and is continually reformed or remodeled in a systematic and orderly manner. Pathologic processes in bone are usually associated with either a decrease or increase in the normal growth activity. No matter what the cause, either endogenous or exogenous, the process of change continues. An understanding of the normal processes is therefore important to the understanding of the abnormal conditions. It should be emphasized that remodeling of bone is a lifelong process in which the ratio of bone formation to bone resorption varies with age. For example, in children there is a high rate of bone formation as well as resorption, resulting in a high turnover rate of bone. In young adults, the bone is remarkably stable with a low turnover rate, and the bones are quite compact. Later in life there is normally a gradual increase in the rate of resorption, particularly in the endosteal zones, without compensating bone formation. Therefore, the bones of older individuals become less compact and more fragile.

Bone growth and remodeling are regulated and affected by many hormones as well as dietary factors all acting in harmony and resulting in a normal skeletal system. It is readily evident that any abnormal increase or decrease in amounts of critical hormones or nutrients may have a profound effect on bone metabolism, especially during certain critical periods of life but especially in the childhood growth period. The final common pathway of many of these factors is the regulation of the osteoclasts and osteoblasts. Simply stated, the osteoblasts are concerned chiefly with the formation of new bone (bone growth), whereas the osteoclasts continually lyse already formed bone (bone remodeling). The major effects of these various hormones on bone are summarized in the following sections.

A deficiency of ovarian hormones in a young but growing person results in the slowdown of endochondral and membranous bone ossification and in the appearance of ossification centers, resulting in delicate and fragile bones. In the postmenopausal adult there is, on the other hand, a slowly progressive osteoporosis of the axial skeleton. Abnormally increased amounts of estrogen in the developing individual inhibit endochondral growth of long bones and increase the rate of growth plate closure, leading to abnormally small stature.

A deficiency of testicular hormones in young persons leads to prolonged but slowed growth of bone with delayed epiphyseal closure, which results in a person with a short trunk and long extremities. In adults a male hormone deficiency may lead to osteoporosis of the axial skeleton. Testosterone in small doses stimulates, but in large doses suppresses, linear growth but always accelerates skeletal maturation.

Glucocorticoids from the adrenal glands decrease the proliferation of cartilage in the growth zone and in other locations. Increased levels result in axial skeletal osteoporosis, probably because of the mechanism of gluconeogenesis or suppression of osteoblasts.

In growing persons, growth hormone causes increased proliferation but delayed maturation of cartilage, thus enhancing the size of the bones in young people. It also affects membranous bone formation to a lesser degree. In adults the effect is also generalized but as the growth plates have closed, the effects are on residual cartilage at the articular surfaces and adjacent to the periosteum. This leads to skeletal distortions because only certain portions of bone are affected by the hormone.

In infants, a decrease in thyroid hormones appears to decrease the proliferative zone at the growth plate and also to decrease conversion of cartilage to bone (endochondral bone formation). Thus, cretins are actually dwarfs. An increase in thyroid hormone matures cartilage but does not stimulate growth.

Parathyroid hormone (PTH) stimulates osteoclastic activity while inhibiting osteoblastic activity, thus leading to osteoporosis if excessive quantities of hormone are secreted. The effect of PTH on the osteoclasts results in increased bone resorption of calcium and phosphate. Serum alkaline phosphatase activity increases because of the increased osteoclastic activity. PTH, or parathormone as it is sometimes called, also augments renal tubular reabsorption of calcium while decreasing renal tubular reabsorption of phosphorus. Another effect of parathormone is increased renal biosynthesis of 1,25-dihydrocholecalciferol (1,25-DHCC) which results in increased calcium absorption from the intestinal tract. This effect, however, is also dependent on the presence of vitamin D. The net effect of PTH is elevation of serum calcium levels and depression of serum phosphorus levels.

Calcitonin is a hormone secreted by the thyroid gland. Although its physiologic role is still not clear, this hormone appears to play a role in the remodeling of bone. Although its measurement in relationship to bone diseases is not yet helpful, calcitonin is found in increased concentrations in the serum of patients with familial medullary carcinoma of the thyroid.

In addition to these hormones, a number of vitamins have important effects on bone growth. Some of the effects of these nutritional elements are noted in the following sections.

A deficiency of vitamin D and its various congeners results in a decrease in calcium and phosphate concentrations in serum, thus delaying the primary calcification of the growth plate as well as all subsequent processes of remodeling that require calcium and phosphorus. Osteoid is deposited in the bone matrix but does not calcify, leading to osteomalacia in the adult. In growing children, rickets is the resulting abnormality. This disease may be accentuated if, in addition to vitamin D deficiency, there is also a deficiency of calcium and phosphorus in the diet. Lack of these elements will, of course, also retard normal bone growth.

Vitamin A deficiency causes a decrease in cartilaginous growth and decreased osteoclastic activity. As osteoblastic activity is unaffected, there is excessive focal periosteal bone formation, for example, at the base of the skull. An excess of this vitamin stimulates osteoclasts, especially in flat bones. The basic effect of a decrease in vitamin C is abnormal and decreased bony matrix formation with suppression of osteoblastic activity. Osteoporosis is the final result.

METABOLIC BONE DISEASE

CLINICAL INVESTIGATION

Metabolic bone disorders can be conveniently divided into two major categories, i.e., osteoporosis and osteomalacia. Osteoporosis is, by definition, a decreased total amount of normally mineralized bone. Essentially there is an imbalance between osteoblastic and osteoclastic activities, resulting in a decrease in quantity rather than quality of bone. Histologically, osteoporosis is characterized by a decrease in the number and size of the trabeculae of cancellous bone with normal width of the osteoid seams. Osteomalacia is, by definition, soft bone and essentially results from failure to mineralize the osteoid matrix. Therefore, this is a disturbance of quality rather than quantity of bone. Histologically, osteomalacia is characterized by poorly mineralized bone with wide osteoid seams.

TABLE 19–1. CAUSES OF OSTEOPOROSIS

Generalized	Localized
Primary	Atrophic osteoporosis
Senile or postmenopausal	Disuse, e.g., postfracture
Endocrine disease	Osteomyelitis
Hypogonadism	Sudeck's atrophy caused by prolonged active hyperemia
Hyperadrenocorticism	
Hyperthyroidism	Osteitis fibrosis cystica (brown tumor), the localized lytic lesion of hyperthyroidism
Hyperparathyroidism	
Diabetes mellitus	
Gastrointestinal disease	
Subtotal gastrectomy	
Intestinal malabsorption	
Biliary disease	
Bone marrow disorders	
Multiple myeloma	
Connective tissue disorders	
Osteogenesis imperfecta	
Other	
Immobilization	

Clinical Features

As the essential feature of osteoporosis is a reduction of bone mass, the disorder can result from a diminished rate of new bone formation, an increased rate of bone resorption, or a combination of the two. Although any of these mechanisms may be the primary problem, it is important to identify the cause so that appropriate therapy can be initiated. From the previous discussion it is evident that osteoporosis can be secondary to a wide variety of clinical conditions. In addition, this condition can be generalized or at times only localized to a specific area, i.e., a single bone or limb. Table 19–1 lists the major causes of osteoporosis.

Except in the case of the localized lytic lesions associated with hyperparathyroidism, laboratory examinations are usually unrewarding in the study of localized or focal osteoporosis. The clinical history and physical examination will usually provide an explanation of these localized changes. However, bone biopsies are useful at times.

In generalized osteoporosis, laboratory investigations may be complicated and prolonged, and the results may often be entirely normal. Several of the endocrinologic etiologies are discussed elsewhere (see Chap. 17) and will not be considered further in this chapter. Atrophic osteoporosis of disuse and senile or postmenopausal osteoporosis are frequently diagnosed on clinical grounds, although these diagnoses are strengthened by excluding the endocrinologic causes of reduction in bone mass.

Osteomalacia refers to deficient mineralization of bone resulting from various disturbances in calcium and phosphorus

TABLE 19–2. CAUSES OF OSTEOMALACIA

Disorders in the vitamin D system
  Decreased bioavailability
    Nutritional deficiency
    Intestinal malabsorption, e.g., postgastrectomy, sprue, hepatobiliary disease, pancreatic disease
  Abnormal metabolism, e.g., liver disease, chronic renal failure, anticonvulsant therapy

Disorders of phosphate homeostasis
  Decreased intestinal absorption, e.g., ingestion of nonabsorbable antacids
  Increased renal loss, e.g., de Toni-Franconi syndromes

Calcium deficiency, e.g., dietary insufficiency

Other, e.g., hypophosphatasia, aluminum toxicity

metabolism. The term rickets has been used synonymously with osteomalacia but it is generally restricted to persons in whom the epiphyseal plates have not yet closed. The many causes of osteomalacia are listed in Table 19–2.

It is important to realize that in a given patient a combination of osteoporosis and osteomalacia is possible. Being able to identify these mixtures in a patient is important, as this knowledge can help to identify the underlying cause and therefore result in proper therapy. Although there may be clinical clues pointing to a preponderance of one or the other of these processes, the principal method of diagnosis is the x-ray evaluation of the skeleton specifically for these lesions. Often one may be faced with an x-ray picture of generalized bone rarefaction but no significant evidence pointing to osteomalacia or osteoporosis. It is in these cases that well-chosen and well-performed laboratory determinations are important in arriving at a diagnosis.

Laboratory Studies

Screening Procedures

Serum Calcium, Phosphorus, and ALP. The simultaneous measurement of serum calcium, phosphorus, and ALP is mandatory in patients presenting with generalized or focal rarefaction of the bones. With the exception of hyperparathyroidism, most types of osteoporosis have normal levels of these analytes. In contrast, the several kinds of osteomalacia may show significant changes in the concentrations of these substances in the blood. Table 19–3 notes some of these variations.

The normal range of calcium must be determined for each laboratory, because it is dependent on the method of analysis. It is also quite important to remember that when one interprets calcium levels about half of the ion is normally bound to albumin. If serum proteins are decreased for any reason, the referent or normal levels in these patients are also decreased. Ionized calcium is not affected by serum protein changes and thus is a more helpful measurement in the difficult case.

Hypophosphatemia is found in about 80 percent of patients with hyperparathyroidism and is even more common in rickets and malabsorption.

Both calcium and phosphorus measurements require the utmost care in the drawing and processing of blood specimens. Venous stasis, hemolysis, and delays in processing can result in artifactual changes and should be avoided.

TABLE 19-3. LABORATORY STUDIES IN BONE DISEASES

Disease	Serum Calcium	Serum Phosphorus	ALP	PTH
Osteoporosis (senile)	N	N	N	N
Primary hyperparathyroidism	↑	↓	N or ↑	↑
Renal osteodystrophy with secondary hyperparathyroidism	↓ or N	↑	↑	↑
Vitamin D and calcium deficiency	↓ or N	↓	↑	↑
Malabsorption	↓ or N	↓	↑	↑
Bone marrow tumor	N or ↑	N or ↑	N or ↑	↑, N, ↓
Hypoparathyroidism	↓	↑	N	↓

N, Normal; ↑, increased; ↓, decreased.

Repeated analyses (up to five or six over a period of several weeks) may be necessary in patients with borderline hypercalcemia or hypophosphatemia before a final decision is made. This is a critical area of clinical and laboratory medicine, as a major operative procedure (neck and superior mediastinal exploration) may be carried out depending on the laboratory data. The availability of accurate assays for PTH has improved this situation.

Serum ALP activity parallels the osteoblastic activity in bone. In all diseases in question, this enzyme activity may be significantly elevated. Although the specific function of ALP in bone formation is unknown, the association of ALP with osteoblasts and bone formation is well established. The rapid rate of bone growth in children parallels the higher serum ALP levels seen in children. If there is interference with bone growth (as in hypothyroidism or cystic fibrosis), serum ALP decreases to normal adult levels. Serum ALP concentration is also greatly elevated in vitamin D deficiency, rickets, and Paget's disease.

TABLE 19-4. REPORTING METHODS FOR ALKALINE PHOSPHATASE

Units	Conversion Factor	Reference Interval
Bodansky (units/dl)	5.37	5.6–22.4
King-Armstrong (units/dl)	7.1	4.2–16.9
Bessey-Lowry-Brock (units/dl)	16.67	1.8–7.2
International (IU/L)	1.00	30–120

Elevated levels can also be seen in hyperparathyroidism, healing fractures, and tumors that have metastasized to bone. Obstruction of the hepatobiliary system is likewise associated with elevated ALP levels. Very low levels of this enzyme are observed in scurvy. Reference values are listed in Table 19–4; this table also illustrates the reasons for the proposed change to international units.

PRIMARY HYPERPARATHYROIDISM

Primary hyperparathyroidism is a generalized disorder of calcium, phosphate, and bone metabolism that results from an increased secretion of PTH. Elevated PTH levels lead to hypercalcemia and hypophosphatemia. There may be recurrent nephrolithiasis, peptic ulcers, mental changes, and excessive bone resorption. With routine multiphasic screening of blood calcium, the diagnosis is made with increasing frequency and earlier in the course of the disease.

Laboratory Studies

Screening Procedures

Serum Calcium, Phosphorus, and ALP. Serum calcium is elevated and phosphorus is decreased in primary hyperparathyroidism. ALP is elevated in patients with bone involvement (about 25 percent of cases) and normal in patients without bone involvement.

Definitive Procedures

PTH Assay. The recent development and widespread availability of the reliable and accurate measurement of PTH has done much to untangle the problems of the differential diagnosis of hypercalcemia. The test is especially useful in sorting out patients with mild to moderate elevations of serum calcium. The rather complex interrelationships between PTH and serum calcium levels are illustrated in Figure 19–1. It is possible, by measuring calcium and PTH in a single serum sample, to correctly categorize 80 to 90 percent of patients with hypercalcemia. Thus, this is the preferred test to perform initially in patients with hypercalcemia.

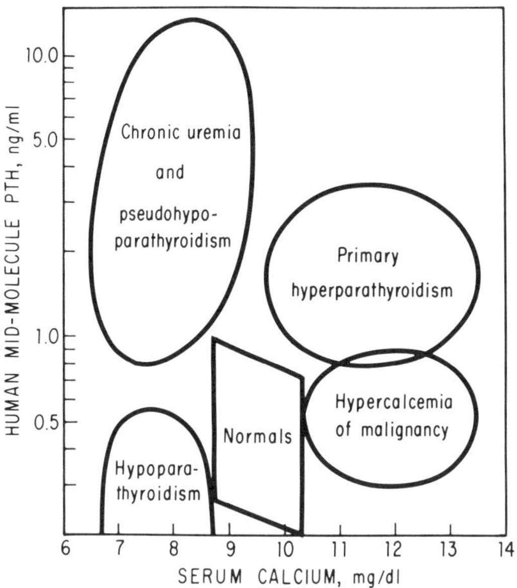

Figure 19–1. Parathyroid hormone and serum calcium interrelationships. *(Modified from University of North Carolina Memorial Hospital report form.)*

Other laboratory procedures that may be useful in evaluating hypercalcemic patients are listed below.

Other Tests

Serum Chloride. Serum chloride levels are often 104 mmol/L or greater in primary hyperparathyroidism. This contrasts with the hypercalcemia of malignancy, in which chloride concentrations tend to be normal.

Urinary Calcium. If dietary calcium intake is controlled, urinary calcium excretion rarely exceeds 250 mg/day in normal individuals. In primary hyperparathyroidism calcium excretion is almost always less than 400 mg/day, whereas many other conditions associated with hypercalcemia (e.g., malignancy or sarcoidosis) frequently exceed this level.

Renal Phosphorus Excretion. PTH increases phosphorus excretion by decreasing the renal tubular resorption of this element. The measurement of the phosphorus clearance or the percent tubular reabsorption of phosphorus (TRP) takes advantage of this hormonal effect. The advantage of TRP is that strict urine

TABLE 19-5. RENAL PHOSPHORUS EXCRETION TESTS

	Phosphorus Clearance (ml/min)	Tubular Reabsorption of Phosphorus (%)
Normal	6.3–15.5	80–90
Hyperparathyroidism	> 12	50–80
Hypoparathyroidism	< 8	90–100

volume timing measurements are not necessary because the measurement of creatinine compensates for this. Appropriate substitution into the following formulas yields the values in question.

$$\text{Phosphorus clearance (ml/min)} = \frac{\sqrt{V} \times Up}{Sp}$$

$$\frac{\text{Percent tubular reabsorption}}{\text{of phosphorus}} = 1 - \frac{Up \times Sc}{Uc \times Sp} \times 100$$

where V is the milliliters of urine per minutes; Up is urine phosphorus in milligrams per deciliter; Sp is serum phosphorus in milligrams per deciliter; Uc is urine creatinine in milligrams per deciliter; and Sc is serum creatinine in milligrams per deciliter.

Renal phosphorus excretion values are given in Table 19–5. Unfortunately, this test has relatively poor specificity in mild cases of parathyroid disease, and other more definitive studies may be required in more difficult cases.

Steroid Suppression of Parathyroid Function. In the steroid suppression test, one attempts to lower serum calcium levels by the administration of prednisone (60 mg/day) for 10 days. Elevated levels of calcium resulting from hyperparathyroidism rarely are lowered, whereas most cases of hypercalcemia caused by malignancy, sarcoidosis, vitamin D intoxication, or myeloma do result in a lowered serum calcium.

Ionized Calcium. Patients having equivocal elevations of serum calcium (confirmed by multiple determinations) may have significant elevations of the ionized fraction if they have hyperparathyroidism.

Nephrogenous Cyclic AMP. Measurement of nephrogenous cyclic AMP (cAMP) may be used as a biologic test of PTH function. About 50 percent of the cAMP excreted in the urine is derived from the renal tubular cell. Its production and release into the urine is almost entirely under the control of PTH. This component of urinary cAMP can be accurately estimated and is termed nephrogenous cAMP. Nephrogenous cAMP is calculated as follows:

$$\text{Nephrogenous cAMP} = \frac{(\text{UcA} \times \text{V}) - (\text{PcA} \times \text{Ccr})}{\text{Ccr}} \times 100$$

where Ccr is creatinine clearance, UcA is the urinary concentration of cAMP, PcA is the plasma concentration of cAMP, and V is the urine flow rate.

It is reported to be elevated in about 80 percent of patients with hyperparathyroidism.

SECONDARY HYPERPARATHYROIDISM

The pathogenesis of bone disease in chronic renal failure is very complex. Decreased renal excretion of phosphate as a consequence of impaired glomerular filtration is important. Diminished responsiveness to vitamin D and decreased renal biosynthesis of 1,25-DHCC are also important. The hyperphosphatemia leads to hypocalcemia. Hypocalcemia leads to increased PTH secretion, i.e., secondary hyperparathyroidism. However the effectiveness of PTH is compromised by the functional deficiency of vitamin D and the inability of the renal tubules to respond with a phosphate diuresis. All of these factors combine to cause diffuse bone disease including osteoporosis, osteomalacia, osteosclerosis, osteitis fibrosa cystica, and metastatic calcification. This disease complex is sometimes called renal osteodystrophy. Figure 19–1 shows the relationship between serum PTH and calcium in secondary hyperparathyroidism.

HYPOPARATHYROIDISM

Clinical Features

The history of previous thyroid surgery or thyroid irradiation for hyperthyroidism always should alert the clinician to the possibility of secondary hypoparathyroidism. In contrast, primary hypoparathyroidism is a rare disease.

The clinical manifestations are primarily a result of acute

hypocalcemia and begin with circumoral and peripheral numbness and tingling, followed by muscle spasms that may progress to laryngeal stridor and convulsions. Chronic hypoparathyroidism is manifested by mental retardation, personality changes, blurring of vision caused by cataracts, and alopecia with or without moniliasis.

Laboratory Studies

Serum Calcium, Phosphorus, and ALP

The measurement of calcium, phosphorus, and ALP levels will usually provide adequate evidence for the diagnosis of this disease. Serum calcium is low, phosphate is elevated, and ALP is normal.

Parathormone

Levels of this hormone are low, or the hormone may be absent. Figure 19–1 shows the relationship between serum PTH and calcium in hypoparathyroidism.

Therapeutic Trials

The therapeutic response to calcium infusion in cases of hypocalcemic tetany as well as response to PTH therapy usually corroborates this diagnosis. Long-term therapy, however, includes a high-calcium diet and vitamin D in large doses. Accurate measurement of serum vitamin D and calcium levels is necessary in following the therapy of these patients.

PSEUDOHYPOPARATHYROIDISM

Clinical Features

The syndrome called pseudohypoparathyroidism results from a genetic defect in which the renal tubules fail to react to endogenous (or exogenous) PTH and there is no inhibition of renal tubular reabsorption of phosphate. As a result urine phosphate is low, serum phosphate is elevated, and, reciprocally, serum calcium is low. This biochemical picture, of course, resembles primary hypoparathyroidism. There are additional genetic defects, including short stature, round face, and short metacarpal bones, which should alert the clinician to this disorder.

Laboratory Studies

Serum Calcium, Phosphorus, and ALP

The concentration of these substances is similar to that seen in hypoparathyroidism, i.e., calcium is low, phosphorus is elevated, and ALP is normal.

Parathormone

Figure 19–1 shows the relationship between serum PTH and calcium in pseudohypoparathyroidism. In contrast to hypoparathyroidism, PTH levels are increased. Thus, this examination serves to differentiate these two conditions.

CONGENITAL DISORDERS OF CALCIUM AND PHOSPHORUS METABOLISM

These inborn errors associated with bone rarefaction are not discussed in depth but must be mentioned. Familial vitamin D-resistant osteomalacia is characterized by increased urine phosphate, decreased serum phosphate, normal serum calcium, decreased urine calcium, and decreased intestinal absorption of calcium.

Fanconi's syndrome is characterized by renal glucosuria, increased urinary excretion of many amino acids, and decreased tubular reabsorption of the phosphate ion. Other findings may be similar to those of hyperchloremic renal acidosis. In children there may be cystine deposits in the conjunctivae, liver, and spleen, as well as in lymph nodes and bone marrow.

Hypophosphatasia is characterized by a reduced activity of ALP in serum and in many tissues including the intestinal tract, kidney, and bone. Phosphoryl ethanolamine and phosphoryl choline, two abnormal substances, are excreted in the urine.

FOCAL BONE LESIONS

Focal bone lesions are most often a result of tumors in bone, either primary or metastatic. At present, the possibility of focal lesions caused by osteomyelitis is quite remote, but it should

TABLE 19-6. IMPORTANT FOCAL BONE LESIONS

Bone Lesions	Other Clinical Features
Benign lesions	
Osteomyelitis	Focal infection
Subperiosteal hemorrhage	Vitamin C deficiency
Infarction	Hemoglobinopathy, steroid therapy
Marrow erythroid hyperplasia	Thalassemia, sickle cell anemia
Hyperplasia	
Pseudotumor of hemophilia	Factor VIII or IX deficiency
Malignant lesions	
Primary	
Myeloma	Anemia, old age, protein abnormalities
Lymphoma	Lymphadenopathy, splenomegaly
Ewing's sarcoma	Bone pain
Osteogenic sarcoma	Bone pain, mass
Chondrosarcoma	Bone pain, mass
	Metastatic tumors
Carcinoma of breast	Primary tumor
Carcinoma of prostate	Primary tumor, elevated acid phosphatase
Carcinoma of thyroid	Primary tumor

always be considered if the patient has accompanying fever and localized bone pain.

A wide variety of bone tumors should be considered when focal bone lesions (Table 19–6) are found. The clinical manifestations may be occult or may merely be localized pain and tenderness. Bone pain is notoriously difficult to relieve.

Acid Phosphatase

Elevation of serum acid phosphatase is regularly seen in metastatic carcinoma of the prostate gland. A variety of acid phosphatase isoenzymes have been demonstrated in various tissues, however, including the liver, bone, kidney, erythrocytes, and platelets. It has been shown that the prostate isoenzyme fraction is sensitive to l-tartrate inhibition. This fact is used to determine the prostatic acid phosphatase level. Elevations of serum prostatic acid phosphatase are seen in prostatic cancer once the tumor has invaded beyond the prostatic capsule or metastasized. Total acid phosphatase may be elevated in various bone disorders (e.g., Paget's disease, Gaucher's disease or fractures), excessive platelet destruction (e.g., ITP), or various liver diseases (e.g., hepatitis or obstructive jaundice).

SUGGESTED READINGS

Avioli L (ed): The Osteoporotic Syndrome: Detection, Prevention and Treatment. New York, Grune and Stratton, 1983.

Burk M: Calcium and phosphorus studies: Interpretation of results and strategies for further testing, Postgrad Med 68:69, 1980.

Fowler WM: Muscle weakness and atropy: Clinical and laboratory evaluation. Calif Med 108:25, 1968.

Frame B, Parfitt A: Osteomalacia: Current concepts. Ann Intern Med 89:966, 1978.

Habener J: Recent advances in parathyroid hormone research. Clin Biochem 14:223, 1981.

Juan D: Differential diagnosis of hypercalcemia: A mechanistic approach. Postgrad Med 66:72, 1979.

Korenman SC, Granner DK, Scherman BM: Practical Diagnosis: Endocrine Disease. Boston, Houghton Mifflin, 1979.

Netter FH: Endocrine System and Selected Metabolic Disease. Summit, NJ, Ciba Pharm, 1965.

Nusynowitz M, Frome B, Kolk F: The spectrum of hypoparathyroid states: A classification based on physiologic principles, Medicine 55:105, 1976.

Raisz L, Kream B: Regulation of bone formation. N Engl J Med 309:29, 1983.

Wong E, Freier E: The differential diagnosis of hypercalcemia: An algorithim for more effective use of laboratory tests. JAMA 247:75, 1982.

20

UNEXPLAINED FEVER

GENERAL COMMENTS

One of the most common clinical manifestations of disease is fever; therefore, this finding is very nonspecific. Usually the presence of fever is easily explained, as, for example, in the patient who is suffering from infection or any process that results in necrosis of tissue. The common denominator in these processes is inflammation. From the very first day in a course in pathology the student is charged to remember the four cardinal signs of inflammation: heat, pain, swelling, and redness or, "calor, dolor, tumor et rubor" as the ancient Roman Celsius said. Although heat in this context is thought of as a localized phenomenon, more extensive inflammatory or infectious processes will result in an elevation of the body temperature or, in fact, in fever.

This chapter is concerned primarily with a discussion of the investigation of unexplained fever. Unexplained fevers are often associated with malaise, fatigue, weight loss, and sometimes chills. They are defined as having been present for more than 3 weeks and still unexplained after 1 week of study in the hospital. The approach to unexplained fever—or, as it is more often called, fever of undetermined origin (FUO)—is often haphazard and hit or miss. Unexplained fever is usually associated with a chronic inflammatory reaction. We present a logical and systematic way to investigate these interesting but, at times, very frustrating problems. These cases require all the diagnostic acumen of the physician and the full use of the diagnostic troika of clinical history, physical examination, and laboratory investigation. It is estimated that about 40 percent of patients with unexplained fever have an infection, 20 percent have a malignancy, 20 percent have a connective tissue disorder, about 10 percent have other diagnoses (e.g., drug fever), and about 10 percent of cases remain undiagnosed.

BASIC INFORMATION

Body temperature is closely regulated by a number of mechanisms that control the production and dissipation of body heat. These complex physiologic mechanisms are regulated by the hypothalamus, which responds to temperature receptors in the skin as well as receptors in or near the hypothalamus itself. Small changes in the temperature of the blood are sufficient to evoke a hypothalamic response.

Fever is defined as an oral temperature greater than 38.3C (101F). In the febrile patient, the thermostat setting in the hypothalamus is raised and maintains a higher body temperature. The rise in the setting of the hypothalamus apparently results from the outpouring of a pyrogen derived from injured leukocytes that stimulates the thermoregulatory centers of the brain. In addition to the polymorphonuclear granulocytes, monocytes also release endogenous pyrogens. Thus, we have an explanation for fever in acute inflammatory reactions (chiefly granulocytic pyrogen) as well as in chronic inflammation (monocytic pyrogen). Phagocytosis of bacteria and foreign materials apparently stimulates the production of this pyrogen. In addition, however, pyrogens are released in sterile granulocytic exudates such as in myocardial infarction, thus explaining the occurrence of low-grade fever in these instances.

Fever Types

There are several types of fevers that become evident when periodic temperatures are charted. Body temperatures must be measured several times a day to visualize these patterns. The elevations of temperature apparently are correlated with the release of endogenous pyrogen from granulocytes. Four general types of temperature records are frequently seen.

Intermittent or Septic Fever

This type of fever is characterized by daily elevations of temperature with interspersed periods of normal or even subnormal temperature. This fever is typical of acute bacterial infections such as pneumonia, acute cystitis, or acute pharyngitis.

Remittent Fever

With remittent fever the temperature falls each day but does not return to normal. Although this is a common type of fever curve, it is not characteristic of any particular disease.

Sustained or Continued Fever

This type of fever characteristically has an elevation of temperature that is maintained for several days or even weeks, but there are only minimal variations between individual determinations. Subacute bacterial endocarditis, miliary tuberculosis, typhoid fever, malignancy, or central nervous system lesions are associated with this type of fever.

Relapsing Fever

This temperature curve shows short febrile periods occurring between one or several days of normal temperature. The microorganism *Borrelia* is the classic associated disease; another example is the Pel-Ebstein fever seen in Hodgkin's disease.

A relapsing fever is associated with several types of malaria, such as quartan (every fourth day provided the first attack is counted as day one) in *Plasmodium malariae* and tertian (every third day) in *P. vivax* or *P. falciparum* malaria.

It may be valuable to obtain temperature charts in patients with vague illnesses, with temperatures recorded every 4 to 6 hours. The procedure should be discontinued as soon as practical to avoid unnecessary work for the nursing service.

CLINICAL INVESTIGATION

Clinical Features

Although this book is not primarily concerned with physical diagnosis, certain aspects of the clinical examination are mentioned because they are directly related to the laboratory investigation of unexplained fever.

The clinical history, especially with regard to present as well as past occupations, living quarters, and previous travels of the patient, may be of great help in determining the cause of fever. Likewise, a history of previous infection and the possible occurrence of a carrier status may provide valuable clues to the correct diagnosis of the present illness.

The physical examination of the patient should be complete and thorough. In addition, it cannot be stressed too strongly that the examination should be repeated frequently. It is in this way that growing tumor masses or abscesses, changing murmurs, or early jaundice are discovered, although they may have been imperceptible or not previously evident.

The examination of the skin may reveal the manifestations of systemic lupus erythemotosis (SLE), purpuric spots (e.g., in septicemia or subacute bacterial endocarditis), or scratches from animals (e.g., in cat-scratch fever). Early jaundice is best appreciated in natural rather than incandescent light and is usually first discernible in the sclerae.

The auscultation of the chest may reveal the rales or crackles of early pneumonia, or heart murmurs, sometimes changing, as in bacterial endocarditis.

The examination of the abdomen may reveal splenomegaly, which may be associated with a variety of causes of fever, including bacterial endocarditis, protozoal infections such as malaria, or blood dyscrasias. Perirenal masses or tenderness may be associated with a perirenal abscess or renal tumor.

The findings of enlarged or otherwise abnormal lymph nodes on biopsy may reveal granulomata, leukemia, or lymphoma (including Hodgkin's disease) or possibly a focus of chronic nonspecific inflammation and resultant fibrosis. Pain or swelling of joints should alert the physician to consider rheumatoid disease, SLE, or other collagen-vascular diseases.

Other causes of unexplained fever such as regional ileitis, cirrhosis, pelvic abscess, or occult tumor may give no physical signs or symptoms whatsoever. Sometimes x-ray or laboratory examination may be of help, whereas at other times only the passage of time results in discovery of the underlying cause.

These explanations are not intended to be exhaustive but only illustrative of the value of thorough and repeated examinations in such patients.

Laboratory Studies

Screening Procedures

Leukocyte Count, Including the Differential Count. As a general rule most conditions causing a febrile reaction also have an associated leukocytosis, i.e., an elevated total white blood cell count. It is important to remember that there are several different types of leukocytosis, the terms of which are sometimes used incorrectly. Table 20–1 defines some of the common leukocyte reaction patterns.

The most common abnormality of the white blood cell

TABLE 20-1. COMMON LEUKOCYTE REACTIONS DEFINED

Reaction	Definition
Leukocytosis	Elevation of the total white cell count above 12×10^9/L
Neutrophilia, relative	Elevation of the granulocyte percentage above 75%
Neutrophilia, absolute	Elevation of the total granulocyte count above 9.0×10^9/L
Lymphocytosis, relative	Elevation of the lymphocyte percentage above 47%
Lymphocytosis, absolute	Elevation of the total lymphocyte count above 3.2×10^9/L
Eosinophilia	Elevation of the eosinophil percentage above 7% or the total eosinophil count above 0.5×10^9/L
Monocytosis	Elevation of the monocyte percentage above 10% or the total monocyte count above 0.85×10^9/L
Leukopenia	Depression of the total white cell count below 4.0×10^9/L
Neutropenia, relative	Depression of the granulocyte percentage below 40%
Neutropenia, absolute	Depression of the total granulocyte count below 1.75×10^9/L

TABLE 20-2. DIAGNOSTIC LEUKOCYTE PATTERNS

Reaction	Possible Diagnoses
Neutrophilic leukocytosis, relative	Associated with lymphopenia (as in Hodgkin's disease and lymphosarcoma)
Neutrophilic leukocytosis (neutrophilia), absolute	Pyogenic infections, massive tissue necrosis, steroid therapy
Lymphocytosis, relative or absolute	Caused by granulocytopenia, viral diseases, infectious mononucleosis, pertussis, infectious lymphocytosis
Eosinophilia	Visceral phase of parasitic infestation, allergic disease, periarteritis
Monocytosis	Tuberculosis, malaria, trypanosomiasis, subacute bacterial endocarditis*
Granulocytopenia or neutropenia	Toxic drugs and chemicals, irradiation, typhoid fever, early phases of viral diseases, SLE, aleukemic phase of leukemia, malaria

*The finding of phagocytic histiocytes (monocytes) in ear lobe capillary blood is suggestive of subacute bacterial endocarditis.

count is neutrophilia. This reaction is characteristic of pyogenic infections including abscesses and extensive tissue necrosis. The total white blood cell counts generally are between 15 and $30 \times 10^9/L$ with greater than 80 percent neutrophils. In addition to these changes, a left shift (increased numbers of immature forms) is usually present, and occasionally this change may even precede the granulocytosis. The finding of this change is predicated on a strict interpretation of the morphologic differences between segmented and band neutrophilic granulocytes. Finally, the finding of toxic granulation of the neutrophils and the formation of Döhle bodies is indicative of the more severe infections.

Other types of white blood cell changes are also found, however, and may give valuable clues to the cause of the patient's complaints. Table 20–2 lists some of the possible diagnoses suggested by various leukocyte reaction patterns.

Erythrocyte Sedimentation Rate (ESR). This is a sensitive but very nonspecific test. It is increased in a variety of diseases, i.e., any active inflammatory disease such as rheumatoid arthritis, chronic infection, collagen vascular disease, and neoplastic disease. This test can be used to demonstrate or confirm the presence of occult organic disease in patients with a fever of unknown origin.

Urinalysis. The microscopic examination of the urine sediment (and urine culture, if indicated) may provide clues to the cause of the patient's fever. One is especially interested in the discovery of white blood cells, red blood cells, and bacteria, as their presence may indicate disease within the urinary tract (Table 20–3).

TABLE 20–3. MICROSCOPIC URINALYSIS IN UNEXPLAINED FEVER

White Blood Cells	Red Blood Cells	Bacteria*	Diagnostic Considerations
Many, with glitter cells	0 to trace	+	Acute pyelonephritis
Many, with clumping	0 to trace	+ +	Acute cystitis
Many	Trace to + +	0	Urinary tract tuberculosis
Few	Trace to + +	0	Renal or bladder tumor, Subacute bacterial endocarditis

*Evident on routine microscopic examination.

On the basis of such findings in the febrile patient, further studies may be suggested. For example, if unexplained erythrocytes are found in the sediment, intravenous pyelography and culture of a 24-hour urine specimen for tuberculosis are indicated. Likewise, blood cultures should be taken if there is any possibility that bacterial endocarditis may be causing the patient's illness.

Blood Culture. Blood cultures are probably done as frequently as leukocyte counts on patients who are markedly febrile or who have unexplained fever. This is wise because when bacteria are cultured from the blood they almost invariably are the cause of the infection (Table 20–4). Also, with the determination of the antibiotic sensitivity of the microorganism, the infection can be effectively treated.

Most investigators agree that obtaining more than three blood cultures within a 24-hour period does not result in an increase in positive results. In cases of proven septicemia, the cumulative rates of organism recovery from three blood cultures are 99 percent or greater. Obtaining the culture immediately before a temperature spike is ideal because this is the time of the highest concentration of circulating organisms. Because a temperature spike usually cannot be predicted, however, it is generally recommended that routine blood cultures be obtained from different venipuncture sites at least 1 hour apart. At least 10 ml of blood should be obtained from adults for each venipuncture. It is generally accepted that two blood culture bottles be inoculated from each venipuncture: an aerobic vented bottle and an anaerobic closed bottle.

Definitive Procedures

Serologic Tests. Early in the work-up of a patient with a fever of undetermined origin it is advisable to collect the first of paired serum specimens, the acute-phase specimen. If the disease continues to be undiagnosed, the second specimen, the convalescent-phase specimen, can be collected about 3 weeks later. Both specimens are examined simultaneously for a change in antibody titer. For the disease in question, a fourfold rise in the titer is considered to be diagnostic. Blood for these studies should be collected in a clean and uncontaminated manner without anticoagulants or preservatives. The serum is separated carefully and stored until the second specimen is collected. Then both are examined at the same time.

In most hospitals the paired specimens are shipped to a special virus diagnostic laboratory, which is often operated by

TABLE 20-4. DISEASES ASSOCIATED WITH BACTEREMIA AND SEPTICEMIA

Organism	Disease or Condition
Staphyloccus aureus	Various
Streptococcus viridans	Subacute bacterial endocarditis
Escherichia coli and other gram-negative organisms	Bacteremic shock secondary to genitourinary, biliary, or gastrointestinal tract disease or manipulation
Streptococcus pneumoniae	Pneumonia
Neisseria meningitidis	Meningitis
Neisseria gonorrhea	Urethritis, arthritis
Salmonella typhi	Typhoid fever
Brucella	Acute brucellosis
Staphylococcus epidermidis	Intravascular line bacteremia

the city or state health department. As a host of serologic tests are available, some system of choosing the possible or probable viral or rickettsial infections present is necessary. This problem is usually handled by the submission of a data form with the specimen. The information required includes clinical manifestations (e.g., respiratory tract, gastrointestinal tract, or central nervous system involvement); previous vaccinations and immunizations; contact (e.g., birds, animals); and other pertinent information. It is the responsibility of the physician ordering the test to supply this information so maximal benefit will be obtained from the laboratory examination.

Febrile Agglutinins. Febrile agglutinins are easily performed and are available in most hospital laboratories. In this procedure whole bacterial cell antigens are used, and the tests detect or rule out antibodies to *Salmonella*, *Brucella*, and *Francisella*. Although paired specimens are preferred, single specimens can also be done. Repetition after several days or more may show a rise in titer of one of the agglutinins being measured, and the diagnosis will be established. A rising titer is considerably better evidence of disease than a single elevated titer. It is important to realize, however, that negative febrile agglutinin test results or low titers do not rule out the diagnosis of any of these diseases.

Salmonella Antibodies. The large number of *Salmonella* (typhoid and paratyphoid) species share a somatic antigen, and hence antibodies directed against *Salmonella* O indicate that a *Salmo-*

nella infection of some kind has occurred. *Salmonella* O titers of 1:80 are suspicious, whereas titers of 1:160 or greater usually indicate infection. The antiflagellar titer, anti-*Salmonella* H, usually rises later and persists longer than anti-O titers. Titers of 1:40 are suspicious, and those of 1:80 or greater indicate infection. Both anti-O and anti-H titers rise following typhoid immunization. Finally, there is a more specific antibody directed against virulent (Vi) typhoid bacilli. Although the titers usually are less than with O or H antigen, this serologic test is probably more specific for typhoid infection.

These studies are usually much more useful for epidemiologic investigations than for individual case studies, therefore they are generally not available in most hospital laboratories.

Tuleremia Antibody. The agglutinin directed against *Francisella tularensis* becomes diagnostically elevated (>1:80) during the second week of illness and may rise to extremely high levels such as 1:2560. The agglutinin titer may persist for many years even though the disease is not active. There may be cross-reaction between *Brucella* and *Francisella*. Repeat titers may help in this situation, the specific disease titers are usually higher.

Rickettsial Antibodies (Weil-Felix Test). Certain strains of the *Proteus* species share a common antigenic structure with a number of rickettsiae. These *Proteus* antigens will cross react with rickettsial antibodies causing agglutination. Because the various rickettsial diseases display characteristic patterns of agglutination with different combinations of *Proteus* strains, differential diagnosis is possible. The Weil-Felix test becomes positive after about 1 week of illness, peaking at about 2 weeks. Table 20–5 shows the array of reactions between the *Proteus* strains and the rickettsial diseases. Titers above 1:40 are suspicious of infection, whereas titers above 1:160 are compatible with active infection. Here again a rising titer is of considerable diagnostic importance.

TABLE 20–5. SEROLOGIC REACTIONS IN RICKETTSIAL DISEASES

Proteus	Typhus Epidemic and Murine	Scrub Typhus	Rocky Mountain Spotted Fever
OX-19	+ +	0	+ +
OX-K	0	+ +	0
OX-2	+	0	+

There are a significant number of false-positive and false-negative results with the Weil-Felix test, therefore better tests for diagnosing Rocky Mountain spotted fever have been developed. These include complement fixation tests, immunofluorescence tests, and latex agglutination tests. These tests are more specific and sensitive than the Weil-Felix test. Again these studies are more useful for epidemiologic investigations than for routine care.

Fungal Serologic Tests. These tests play an important role in the diagnosis of mycotic infections, although they often provide only tentative evidence of infection. They are technically difficult tests and consequently are usually done only in reference laboratories. There are serologic tests available for aspergillosis, blastomycosis, candidiasis, coccidioidomycosis, cryptococcosis, histoplasmosis, and sporotrichosis. The main advantage of these tests is that they provide evidence of infection (albeit tentative) in a much shorter time than is required for fungal cultures to become positive.

Other Serologic Tests. There are other serologic tests that can be performed to evaluate unexplained fever. ASO, anti-DNAse and antihyaluronidase titers are helpful in diagnosing rheumatic fever. Rheumatoid factor and ANA titers are useful in diagnosing collagen vascular diseases. The heterophil antibody (Monospot test) and Epstein-Barr virus antibody titer are useful in diagnosing infectious mononucleosis. An elevated carcinoembryonic antigen (CEA) level, although certainly not specific, may suggest a diagnosis of malignancy.

Liver Function Tests

Measurement of bilirubin, hepatic enzymes, and especially ALP has, at times, been quite useful in the evaluation of patients with unexplained fever. Liver scans with radioactive isotopes may help to identify mass lesions within the liver, which may then be biopsied.

Bone Marrow Examination

Examination of the bone marrow is one of the more specialized studies undertaken after the initial group noted above. The physician is primarily searching for evidence of several disease groups: granulomatous disease, primarily tuberculosis or histoplasmosis; malignant diseases such as leukemia, lymphoma, or metastatic tumor; or reticuloendothelial disorders as widely divergent as malaria, kala azar, or the various reticuloendothe-

TABLE 20–6. INTRADERMAL SKIN TESTS

Type	Reagent	Disease	Response
Bacterial	Tuberculin	Tuberculosis	Delayed
Mycotic	Blastomycin	Blastomycosis	Delayed
	Coccidioidin	Coccidioidomycosis	Delayed
	Histoplasmin	Histoplasmosis	Delayed
Viral	Cat scratch	Cat-scratch fever	Delayed
	Frei	Lymphogranuloma venereum	Delayed
Parasitic	Trichinin	Trichinosis	Immediate
	Casoni	Echinococcosis	Immediate
Other	Kveim	Sarcoid	Delayed

lioses. It is also said that the possibility of culturing organisms from the marrow is greater than from the peripheral blood, and this fact may at times warrant a marrow aspiration.

Many diseases discussed previously can be found on examination of the marrow if the marrow is properly biopsied as well as aspirated (see Chap. 24). The marrow biopsy is processed to make tissue sections, and histologic lesions characteristic of the above diseases, if present, are easily seen. Metastatic tumor to marrow is most easily diagnosed by using this sectioning technique. Special staining for acid-fast bacilli or fungus is also easily done with this technique.

Biopsy and Thin Needle Aspiration

The use of the biopsy (muscle, skin, liver, or nerve) in unexplained fever is extremely valuable, but usually only when there is evidence of some localization of the disease. For example, if enlarged lymph nodes are discovered, they should be examined. Focal lesions of all sorts should be biopsied or aspirated because they may reveal the cause of the patient's fever. Generalized organ enlargement, such as hepatomegaly, is also an indication for needle biopsy.

The biopsy should be done only after consultation between the patient's physician and the surgeon performing the biopsy. All too often the biopsy is taken from the wrong area only because it is more convenient or to achieve a better cosmetic result. In the process the diagnosis may be missed. Of course, an adequate portion of tissue should be obtained, and then handled gently and processed quickly. If cultures are indicated they should be initiated before the specimen is contaminated. Muscle biopsies are especially easy to ruin by poor technique.

Intradermal Tests

A wide variety of skin tests are available to the clinician; these are of variable merit and specificity, depending on many factors. Some of the important skin tests are listed in Table 20–6. The reader is referred to the manufacturers' directions for more detailed information.

Because positive reactions indicate either present or past infection, the results must be interpreted in that light. This is of special importance in diseases in which there is a relatively high incidence of positive reactors, such as to histoplasmin, tuberculin, or trichinin, especially in certain geographic areas.

Therapeutic Trial

When the gamut of diagnostic procedures has been run and no positive diagnosis has been obtained, the question of a therapeutic trial with an antibiotic arises. After due consideration it may be decided to use a narrow-range antimicrobial agent in adequate dosage for a reasonable period of time. If the fever disappears, it may well be due to the therapy, although the possibility of a natural regression of the disease should not be forgotten. Also, if the therapy is successful, the physician will never be able to identify with complete certainty the cause of the illness.

On the other hand, if the therapeutic trial is unsuccessful, the emergence of resistant organisms may become manifest (if the disease was caused by a bacterium) and further diagnostic and therapeutic efforts may become more difficult.

SUGGESTED READINGS

Austrian R: The role of the microbiological laboratory in the management of bacterial infections. Med Clin N Am 50:1419, 1966.

Hall B, Dowling HF: Negative blood cultures in bacterial endocarditis: A decade's experience. Med Clin N Am 50:159, 1966.

Herrmann EC Jr: Experience in providing a viral diagnostic laboratory compatible with medical practice. Mayo Clin Proc 42:112, 1967.

Jacoby G, Swarz M: Fever of undetermined origin. N Engl J Med 289:1407, 1974.

Larson E, et al.: Fever of undetermined origin: Diagnosis and follow-up of 105 cases, 1970–1982. Medicine 61:269, 1982.

Petersdorf RG, Beeson PB: Fever of unexplained origin: Report on 100 cases. Medicine 40:1, 1961.

Vickery DM, Quinnell RK: Fever of unknown origin: An algorithmic approach. JAMA 238:2183, 1977.

Wolff S, et al.: Unusual etiologies of fever and their evaluation. Ann Rev Med 26:277, 1975.

Wood WB, Jr: Leukocytes and fever. Hosp Pract 1:36, 1967.

Zuerlein T, Smith P: The diagnostic utility of the febrile agglutinin tests. JAMA 254:1211, 1985.

21
PREGNANCY

PREGNANCY TESTING

In addition to many of the maladies already discussed in other chapters, the pregnant woman is susceptible to several diseases (or potential diseases) that are unique to the pregnant state. Laboratory examinations play a key role in these diagnoses. In addition, the laboratory confirmation of pregnancy has become a common and important laboratory procedure, especially in the diagnosis of ectopic pregnancies or in the management of tumors of placental tissue.

As they grow and mature, placental villi produce a hormone called chorionic gonadotropin. This substance, produced in largest quantities during the first trimester of pregnancy, is excreted in the urine (Fig. 21–1). Human chorionic gonadotropin (hCG) is a glycoprotein consisting of two subunits, an alpha subunit and a beta subunit. The alpha subunit is very similar to the alpha subunit of three other human glycoproteins, LH, FSH, and TSH. However, the beta subunits of the four hormones differ significantly. Convenient immunologic procedures for the determination of hCG are available and are sensitive as well as specific. They are even more specific when they assay for the beta subunit of hCG. In fact, these test parameters make the immunologic pregnancy test one of the most satisfactory in the laboratory. They have replaced the earlier bioassay techniques for pregnancy testing.

There are a number of commercial kit assays available today. There are two major methods for immunoassays, tube tests and slide methods. The tube tests (e.g., hemagglutination inhibition) are sensitive at approximately 0.2 IU/ml and take 1 to 2 hours to perform. The slide tests (e.g., latex particle agglutination imhibition) are slightly less sensitive (0.5 to 1.5 IU/ml)

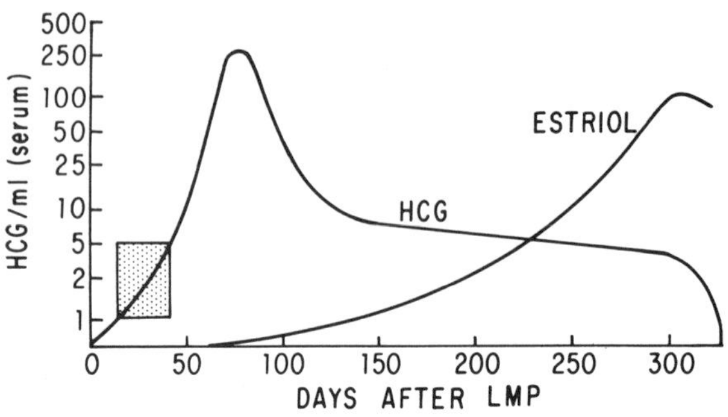

Figure 21–1. Characteristic levels of human chorionic gonadotropin excretion in a normal pregnancy. The production of estriol rises to about 24 mg/24 hours at term and thus appears to be a sensitive indicator of fetal and placental viability.

but take only minutes to perform. Radioimmunoassays are also available; they are very sensitive (0.03 to 0.5 lU/ml but take 5 to 24 hours to perform.

Because the various pregnancy tests have different sensitivities, the time at which a given pregnancy test becomes positive varies. A radioimmunoassay will reliably detect pregnancy 1 to 2 weeks after conception. A beta hCG tube test will reliably detect pregnancy 2 to 3 weeks after conception. A slide test will reliably detect pregnancy 2½ to 3½ weeks after conception.

The hCG levels in ectopic pregnancy are usually quite low (0.15 to 0.8 IU/ml). Studies have shown that even the most sensitive tube tests detect only about one-half of ectopic pregnancies. One can see that very sensitive tests (e.g., radioimmunoassays) are often needed to detect ectopic pregnancies.

The measurement of hCG, including quantitation, is a valuable adjunct in the evaluation of threatened abortion in the first trimester. If less than 3000 IU/24 hours is excreted, the fetus is almost invariably dead, and definitive treatment can be planned. Later in pregnancy the levels of hCG are normally lower (mean of 5000 IU/24 hours) (Fig. 21–1). During the later stages of pregnancy the estriol levels have been correlated with placental function and fetal viability. This procedure is discussed in the next sections.

The quantitation of hCG is also valuable in the care of patients with possible or proven tumors of the placental villi. Both benign (hydatidiform mole) and malignant (choriocarcinoma) variants are seen. As a rule, these tumors excrete large quantities of hCG, but levels comparable with normal pregnancy levels are also known to occur. In contrast with a normal pregnancy in which this hormone secretion drops markedly at the beginning of the second trimester, these tumors continue to produce increased amounts of hormone. After the diagnosis of mole or choriocarcinoma has been made, serial gonadotropin assays are an excellent means of monitoring the response to surgical therapy or chemotherapy. If the treatment is successful, hCG excretion gradually falls to undetectable levels.

Finally, in certain malignant testicular tumors of germinal tissue in men (teratoma, embryonal carcinoma, and seminoma), hCG excretion may be detectable. This information is helpful from a diagnostic, therapeutic, and prognostic point of view.

LABORATORY TESTING IN PREGNANCY

There are certain conditions or diseases to which the pregnant woman or the developing fetus is particularly prone. Although most of these disorders may be evident on clinical examination, they are sometimes diagnosed only when the condition has become far advanced or after irreparable harm has come to the developing fetus. The rationale of the prenatal laboratory evaluation lies in the effort to discover these problems long before they may be clinically evident. By prompt preventive and definitive treatment a viable and healthy infant will be delivered.

Table 21–1 presents the common complications of pregnancy that may be discovered by appropriate laboratory examination. Because the list is short and most of the procedures are simple, it has become accepted practice for many of these procedures to be done at the time of the first visit to the physician. As toxemias usually are seen late in pregnancy, the urinalysis or, more specifically, the check for proteinuria is repeated frequently until after delivery. (The reader is also referred to Chapter 2 for a more complete discussion of screening procedures.)

Anemias of Pregnancy

Although all types of anemia can occur or become more evident during pregnancy, three types have generally been prominently associated with the pregnant state. These three are iron-deficiency anemia (the most common variety), hemoglo-

TABLE 21–1. LABORATORY TESTING IN PREGNANCY

Potential Complications	Laboratory Examination
Maternal	
Anemia, iron deficiency or megaloblastic	Hemoglobin or hematocrit, blood film
Urinary tract infection	Urinalysis microscopic and culture, if indicated
Toxemia	Urinalysis for proteinuria (repeated at each prenatal visit)
Diabetes mellitus	Urinalysis for glycosuria
Carcinoma of cervix	Papanicolaou smear
Tuberculosis, heart disease	Chest x-ray
Fetal	
Hemolytic disease of the newborn	Rh typing and unexpected antibody screening, amniocentesis (repeated at 28 and 35 weeks of gestation)
Congenital syphilis	Serologic test for syphilis
Neural tube defect	Alpha fetoprotein in maternal serum and amniotic fluid
Rubella	Rubella virus antibodies
Threatened fetal death	Urinary estriol
Immature lungs	Amniotic fluid analysis

binopathies (especially sickle cell disease and thalassemia), and megaloblastic anemia of pregnancy. The last variety, although extremely interesting to the hematologist and obstetrician, is actually quite unusual.

Before proceeding further it is proper to define anemia in pregnancy. During pregnancy there are significant changes in the maternal blood so that a new set of reference values must be used as a standard against which to judge hematologic measurements. What changes normally occur? There is a fall in the hematoglobin level during the pregnancy, because the increase in plasma volume (up to 45 percent) is relatively greater than the increase in erythrocyte mass (up to 25 percent). This leads to the physiologic anemia of pregnancy. In addition, a slowly rising white blood cell count is noted. About one-quarter of pregnant women may show an evident left shift of the differential white count. All of these changing hematologic values are summarized in Table 21–2.

If the hemoglobin level is significantly below the normal levels in pregnancy the physician must determine the cause of

TABLE 21-2. HEMATOLOGIC CHANGES IN PREGNANCY*

	Healthy Woman	Third Trimester
Hemoblobin (g/L)	12.0–16.0	9.0–13.0
Hematocrit (L/L)	0.38–0.47	0.30–0.40
White blood cell count (x 10^9/L)	3.7–12.0	5.0–14.0
Leukocyte alkaline phosphate (score)	50–125	250–280

*All values given as mid-95 percentile estimates.

this abnormality. The investigation is very similar to that described in the chapter on anemia (see Chap. 13). In fact it is usually much less complicated, as the three types of anemia noted previously constitute the great majority of all anemias found in pregnancy.

The examination of a well-prepared and well-stained blood film will almost always point to the exact diagnosis. The measurement of serum iron and iron-binding capacity, serum ferritin, hemoglobin electrophoresis and fetal or A_2 hemoglobin quantitation, and sickle cell preparations help corroborate the diagnosis. Again, for more complete discussions of the laboratory investigations in these anemias the reader is referred to Chapter 13.

An extremely interesting, although rare, anemia is the megaloblastic anemia of pregnancy (also called the pernicious anemia of pregnancy). This type of anemia is usually seen only in the third trimester. It is apparently caused by the competition between mother and fetus for folic acid. The developing fetus appears to be the more efficient competitor, and only the mother becomes folate deficient. This anemia reverts following delivery so that any confirmatory laboratory studies (e.g., serum folate levels or bone marrow examination) should be carried out prior to delivery. The marrow morphology is similar to that seen in pernicious anemia, although the changes are usually less marked. Howell-Jelly bodies are rare, megaloblastosis is less prominent, and the anemia is not as severe as in pernicious anemia.

Urinary Tract Infections in Pregnancy

The urinary tract stasis and dilation, possible instrumentation or catheterization, and the trauma of childbirth all increase the susceptibility of the woman to urinary tract infection during or following pregnancy. The discussions on urinary tract infection in Chapters 4 and 11 are also pertinent to this problem. It is sufficient in this context to mention that an initial urinary tract infection is often associated with pregnancy.

The periodic microscopic examination of the urine sediment for white blood cells and bacteria as well as screening procedures to detect significant bacteriuria (e.g., colony forming units) is almost mandatory for the proper care of the pregnant patient. Appropriate follow-up studies are outlined in Chapter 11, which examines renal disease in more detail.

Toxemia of Pregnancy

Although improved prenatal care has significantly decreased the incidence of toxemia, this feared complication is still seen and should not be forgotten. Along with periodic measurements of blood pressure and weight, the check for proteinuria is a valuable screening procedure for this complication, because proteinuria and renal impairment are prominent features of this disease.

If the toxic state proceeds to preeclampsia and frank eclampsia (convulsions), a wide variety of chemical determinations, especially as related to renal and hepatic function, may become abnormal. Most importantly, serum creatinine and uric acid levels rise, although blood urea nitrogen may fall because of hepatic failure. Serum bilirubin and transaminase levels, reflecting hepatic involvement, tend to become elevated.

Placental Function

In recent years the measurement of placental function and its relationship to fetal viability have been extensively studied. A number of basic facts have become evident, and the application of these data has been instrumental in reducing perinatal mortality and morbidity.

After the second month of pregnancy the fetoplacental unit becomes the major source of estrogen production in the pregnant woman. These estrogens (90 percent are sodium estriol glucosiduronate) are excreted in the urine and are thought to be proportional to the amount and type of trophoblastic tissue in the placenta as well as the blood flow through the placenta. Mean excretion in the last 6 weeks is about 16 mg/day, with a range of about 20 to 24 mg/day.

Impending fetal death has been associated with decreased urinary estrogen excretion in pregnancies complicated by maternal diabetes, toxemia, or hypertension. In all these patients urinary estriol levels are less than 12 mg/day during the last weeks of the pregnancy. Levels below 4 mg/day almost invariably indicate fetal death.

The serial determination of estriol levels has been shown to be valuable in the management of these patients at risk, providing objective criteria for possible intervention when the fetus is in jeopardy. Sudden falls in estriol levels, for example, from above 12 mg to 4 or 6 mg, indicate serious fetal difficulties and prompt delivery must be considered. There are problems associated with urine estriol measurements including the difficulties of 24-hour urine collections as well as false-positive and false-negative results. Therefore, many clinicians use other procedures to monitor fetal well-being, e.g., the nonstress test.

Assessing Fetal Lung Maturity

The lungs are among the last of the fetal organs to mature. Thus, mature lungs usually indicate that the fetus is ready for birth. Fetal lung maturity is evaluated by measuring the amount of surfactant in the amniotic fluid. Surfactant is a substance that decreases the work of breathing by lowering the surface tension in the alveoli, reducing resistance to expansion during inspiration and avoiding alveolar collapse during expiration. A deficiency in surfactant leads to the development of respiratory distress syndrome (RDS) in neonates. One can see that evaluation of fetal lung maturity is indispensible for the obstetrician when he or she must decide whether to delay a delivery or allow it to proceed.

Surfactant is composed of a variety of chemicals. Approximately 75 percent of the surfactant consists of phosphatidyl choline (lecithin); about 10 percent consists of phosphatidyl glycerol; and the remainder consists of various phospholipids and sphingomyelin.

There are a number of different assays for surfactant. They can be divided into functional assays and biochemical assays. The functional assays do not measure phospholipids directly, but instead test for the biophysical properties of surfactant present in amniotic fluid. Functional assays include: surface tension lowering ability, capillary flow rate changes, optical density, microviscosity measurements, and foam stability. The foam stability test is the only functional assay that is popular at this time. The biochemical assays measure the concentration of various components of surfactant. Biochemical assays include: lecithin/sphingomyelin (L/S) ratio; lung profile (measures the relative amounts of the components of surfactant); or desaturated phosphatidyl-choline analysis. The most popular biochemical assay is the L/S ratio.

Foam Stability Index (FSI)

Most biologic compounds can form relatively stable foams when air is introduced to an aqueous solution. Adding ethanol to these mixtures acts as an antifoaming agent in most biologic compounds. Surfactant can produce such low surface tensions that it produces stable foams even in the presence of ethanol. Based on these findings a semiquantitative "shake test" has been developed. In this test a series of ethanol–amniotic fluid mixtures are made such that the percentage of ethanol varies in each tube. The tubes are agitated and then evaluated for the presence or absence of stable bubbles. The highest ethanol fraction that supports the presence of stable bubbles is defined as the FSI. An FSI value of 47 or greater suggests that the fetal lungs contain enough surfactant so that RDS will not occur.

Lecithin/Sphingomyelin Ratio

In this procedure the lecithin and the sphingomyelin are extracted from the amniotic fluid with organic solvents, and purified by precipitation with cold acetone. The extract is then separated using thin layer chromatography and visualized by charring with sulfonic acid. In the first 35 weeks of pregnancy, the levels of lecithin increase only gradually relative to sphingomyelin. At approximately 35 weeks the levels of lecithin increase dramatically relative to sphingomyelin. An L/S ratio equal to or greater than 2.0 suggests that the fetal lungs are mature enough that RDS will not occur.

Hemolytic Disease of the Newborn

In hemolytic disease of the newborn (HDN), the red blood cells of the fetus are coated with maternal IgG antibody and are destroyed in the infant's reticuloendothelial system. Several blood group systems have been associated with HDN, for example, the Rh system [anti-Rh$_o$ (D), anti-Rh' (C), or anti-Rh'' (E)], the ABO system (anti-A, anti-B, or anti-A,B), and other groups that form IgG antibodies (e.g., anti-Kell).

Because HDN is treatable, and now also preventable, it is imperative to determine if and to what the extent the fetus is affected by the antibodies being produced in the mother. Only in this way can proper obstetric management be planned and exchange transfusions and laboratory studies be anticipated.

At present there are no laboratory procedures that can predict ABO hemolytic disease during the prenatal period. However, this variant is usually much milder than Rh HDN.

Prenatal Blood Studies

The objective of prenatal blood studies is to identify women at risk for having babies affected with HDN. To this end, the following studies should be done early in pregnancy: (1) ABO grouping; (2) Rh testing, including tests for D^u in patients who are apparently D negative; and (3) screening for unexpected antibodies (indirect Coombs' test). Mothers with a negative antibody screen should have a repeat test at 28 weeks. If this is negative, no further prenatal studies are required. All positive antibody screening tests require identification of the antibody. Increasing levels of antibody are associated with HDN. The best way to evaluate the degree of intrauterine hemolysis is to examine the amniotic fluid for a bilirubinlike pigment. The fluid is obtained by amniocentesis and is then analyzed spectrophotometrically.

Amniocentesis

If one or more irregular antibodies associated with hemolytic disease are detected, it is then important to examine amnionic fluid obtained by needle aspiration. The amnionic fluid is examined for the presence of an abnormal 450 nm absorption peak in the spectral absorption curve caused by bilirubin. This has proved to be a reliable and practical guide to the obstetric management of mothers carrying fetuses affected with hemolytic disease.

The test specimen is obtained by aspiration of a small amount of amnionic fluid. The procedure is done by using only local anesthetic and is well suited to office or outpatient service. The deeply yellow stained fluid aspirated from a uterus containing a severely affected fetus is usually obtained too late to be of benefit. If aspirations are done early, however, and the diagnostic 450 nm peak is found, indicating as yet mild disease, intrauterine transfusion and early delivery will increase the chance of fetal salvage.

Blood Studies at the Time of Delivery

In cases of suspected HDN the following tests should be performed on cord blood: (1) ABO group; (2) Rh group and D^u if apparently Rh-negative; and (3) direct antiglobulin test. If the direct antiglobulin test is positive an eluate should be made to

TABLE 21–3. CHOICE OF BLOOD FOR EXCHANGE TRANSFUSION IN HEMOLYTIC DISEASE OF THE NEWBORN*

Rh$_o$ Hemolytic Disease		Transfusion		ABO Hemolytic Disease		Transfusion	
Mother's Type	Baby's Type	First Choice	Second Choice	Mother's Type	Baby's Type	First Choice	Second Choice
O–	Any	O–		O+	A+	O+	
					O+		
					A–	O–	
					B–	O–	
A–	O+	O–		A+	B+	O+	
	A+	A–	O–		AB+	A+	O+
	B+	O–			B–	O–	
	AB+	A–	O–		AB–	A–	O–
	B–	O–					
	AB–	A–	O–				
B–	O+	O–		B+	A+	O+	
	A+	O–			AB+	B+	O+
	B+	B–	O–		A–	O–	
	AB+	B–	O–		AB–	B–	O–
	A–	O–					
	AB–	B–	O–				
AB–	A+	A–	O–	AB+			
	B+	B–	O–				
	AB+	AB–	A–,O–		ABO HDN not possible		
	A–	A–	O–				
	B–	B–	O–				
	AB–	AB–	O–				

*Plus and minus signs refer to presence or absence of Rh$_O$(D) antigen.

identify the antibody. The concurrent measurement of hemoglobin levels and bilirubin (either total or unconjugated) and the examination of a well-prepared blood film will provide a final check for hemolytic disease. If hemolytic disease is a possibility, daily bilirubin levels are measured to determine the severity of the disease. Remember, prior to delivery, fetal bilirubin is cleared by the placenta into the maternal circulation. If bilirubin levels approach the dangerous level (20 mg/dl), exchange transfusion is indicated. The choice of blood for exchange is noted in Table 21–3.

Use of Rh$_o$ Immune Globulin

Hyperimmune globulin has proved to be remarkably effective in the prevention of immunization to the Rh$_o$ antigen. Only certain mothers, however, are eligible for its use. When an Rh$_o$ (D) negative woman delivers an Rh$_o$ (D) positive infant, she is a candidate for Rh$_o$ (D) immune globulin, provided that the following conditions are met:

1. The mother is Rh$_o$ (D) negative and D^u negative.
2. The mother has no anti-Rh$_o$ (D) antibodies in her serum.
3. The infant is Rh$_o$ (D) positive or D^u positive.

The immune globulin is injected intramuscularly within 72 hours of delivery although it is said to be effective even up to 5 days after delivery.

If there has been a fetal–maternal hemorrhage exceeding 30 ml of blood, a larger dose of globulin is required. The amount of hemorrhage can be estimated using a Kleihauer-Betke stain on a maternal blood film. Using this procedure the clinician estimates the number of fetal red blood cells per maternal red blood cells. An estimate of the maternal blood volume allows one to calculate the total volume of fetal blood lost into the maternal circulation, and the appropriate amount of immune globulin is determined. Turbidometric test procedures are also available.

There are several other circumstances in which immune globulin is indicated in Rh-negative women. These include: amniocentesis, abortion, ruptured ectopic pregnancy, or third trimester vaginal bleeding. It also appears that a small proportion of Rh-negative women with an Rh-positive fetus become immunized during pregnancy. This has lead to trials of injecting immune globulin during the third trimester of pregnancy at around 28 weeks. It appears as if combined prenatal and postnatal treatment may be more effective than postnatal treatment alone in preventing immunization.

Neural Tube Defects

Neural tube defects are among the most common fatal congenital malformations. The cause of these disorders is not known. Many open neural tube defects can be detected by elevated alpha-fetoprotein (AFP) levels in maternal blood and amniotic fluid. AFP is an alpha-1-glycoprotein produced in the fetal liver and excreted into the amniotic fluid via fetal urine. From there it reaches maternal blood. Many antenatal screening programs for open neural tube defects have been set up.

Screening Procedures

Maternal Serum. Elevated maternal serum AFP levels are seen in about 85 percent of open neural tube defects. Normal levels for maternal AFP differ for each week of gestation and ideally should be determined for each laboratory. Most screening programs recommend determining maternal AFP levels between 16 and 18 weeks' gestation. Elevated maternal serum AFP levels should be confirmed by a repeat test in 1 week.

Definitive Procedures

Amniotic Fluid AFP. After maternal serum AFP is found to be elevated, the level of AFP in the amniotic fluid should be determined. Elevated amniotic fluid AFP is about 95 percent sensitive for open neural tube defects. As with maternal serum AFP levels, amniotic fluid AFP levels are gestational age-related. False-positive results may be due to contamination by fetal blood, therefore a test for fetal red blood cells or hemoglobin is recommended when the amniotic fluid AFP is elevated.

Ultrasound. Obstetric ultrasound examination can be very useful in diagnosing anencephaly or other neural tube defects. It is also useful to accurately date the fetus so the correct reference range for AFP can be used. Further discussion of this test is beyond the scope of this book.

SUGGESTED READINGS

AMA Council on Scientific Affairs: Maternal serum alpha-fetoprotein monitoring. JAMA 247:1478, 1982.

American College of Obstetrics and Gynecology: Prevention of Rh$_o$(D) isoimmunization. Tech Bull 79 (Aug), 1984.

Bates H: Estriol assays in monitoring fetal/placental function. Lab Mgmt 21:17, 1982.

Brown L, Duck-Chong C: Methods of evaluating fetal lung maturity. In Batsakis J, Savory J (eds): Critical Reviews in Clinical Laboratory Sciences. Boca Raton, Fla, CRC Press, 16:85, 1982.

Freer D, Statland B: Measurement of amniotic fluid surfactant. Clin Chem 27:1629, 1981.

Haddow J: Screening for spinal defects. Hosp Pract 17:128, 1982.

Plauché W, et al.: Phosphatidyl glycerol and fetal lung maturity. Am J Obstet Gynecol 144:167, 1982.

Polesky H: Diagnosis, prevention and therapy in hemolytic disease of the newborn. In Myhre B (ed): Clinics in Laboratory Medicine, vol 2. Philadelphia, Saunders, 1982, p 107.

Widmann F (ed): Technical Manual. Arlington, Va, American Association of Blood Banks, 1985.

22

HEADACHE, COMA, AND OTHER CENTRAL NERVOUS SYSTEM DISORDERS

BASIC INFORMATION

Pathogenesis of Headaches

There are many causes of headache; therefore, head pain is a symptom of a wide variety of disorders. Headaches may originate from changes in the structure, biochemistry, physiology, or even psychology of the patient. The many mechanisms can be conveniently divided into several groups or classes, which are of aid both in the diagnosis and in the treatment of the patient.

The most obvious cause, an intracerebral lesion, should always be considered first, especially when headache is a new symptom. The following sections complete the differential diagnosis of headaches.

A large and important group is the vascular headache, which includes migraine and related disorders. Unilateral headache with associated scotomata, anorexia, or even nausea and vomiting characterizes this type. Cranial arterial distension is presumed to cause the associated head pain.

Headache associated with muscle tenseness is probably the most common type of headache. Nervous tension with associated skeletal muscle contraction results in sensations of tightness, pressure, or constriction in the head, most commonly in the posterior portions. Congestion and edema of the nasal and paranasal mucous membranes, such as in allergic rhinitis or chronic sinusitis, are common causes of headache. Other diseases of the ocular, aural, or dental structures may also produce headache.

Traction headache is usually caused by traction on vascular structures by an intracranial mass such as a tumor, hematoma, or abscess. This type of headache is closely related to those of an intracranial inflammation. The causes of inflammation are multiple, but the two major types are infections with meningitis and meningeal reactions secondary to subarachnoid hemorrhage.

A veritable host of systemic diseases can produce headaches that are primarily vascular in type. Systemic infection, hypoxia, postconcussion or postconvulsive states, hypoglycemia, and some cases of essential hypertension are frequently associated with headache.

Finally, headache accompanies psychosomatic or neurotic illnesses such as delusional, hypochondriacal, or conversion reactions. Posttraumatic headaches may be of this type, although other mechanisms such as muscle contraction, vascular constriction, or focal injuries may be causal.

Spinal Fluid Examination

Spinal fluid is a transudate of the plasma formed by the choroid plexuses of the lateral, third, and fourth ventricles. The fluid bathes and supports the brain and spinal cord. The fluid is reabsorbed into the venous system via the arachnoid villi, which lie over the superior aspect of the cerebral hemispheres.

Because of the circulation of the spinal fluid around and about all the structures of the central nervous system, this substance provides a convenient fluid to examine in disorders of the central nervous system. Spinal fluid can be easily obtained by aspiration from the lower lumbar spinal canal. Examination of the spinal fluid is particularly useful in the laboratory investigation of cerebrovascular diseases, meningitis, central nervous system tumors, and neurosyphilis.

There are, however, certain inherent dangers in the performance of lumbar puncture. The chief contraindication is increased intracranial pressure with or without papilledema. A lumbar puncture should never be attempted in these cases unless preparations for immediate surgical intervention are also made. Cerebellar tumors may fail to show signs of increased intracranial pressure, and when lumbar aspiration of spinal fluid is made, the cerebellar tonsils may herniate through the foramen magnum and result in dire and sometimes fatal consequences. In the case of spinal cord tumors potential complications also make lumbar puncture a dangerous procedure. The techniques for routine lumbar puncture are outlined in Chapter 24.

Normally almost all of the leukocytes found in the spinal

fluid are lymphocytes. Total counts may range up to 10/mm³ but usually are less than 4/mm³. Infection is usually associated with moderate (e.g., 100/mm³) to marked (e.g., 2000/mm³) elevations of the cell count (pleocytosis). The differential count is predominantly lymphocytic in viral, tuberculous, fungal, or luetic disease. Tumors, unruptured abscesses, multiple sclerosis, tabes, and rabies are also associated with predominant lymphocytosis. Polymorphonuclear leukocytes in counts above several hundred are indicative of pyogenic meningitis (e.g., pneumococcus, *Haemophilus influenzae*), but may also be seen in early viral encephalitis and tuberculous meningitis. As expected, ruptured abscesses also show a predominance of neutrophils.

The differentiation of lymphocytes from neutrophils, although usually causing no problem, may be difficult especially when the counts are only mildly elevated. Considerable shrinkage of the neutrophils may occur, making identification difficult or even impossible. Smears stained with several different stains (e.g., Wright, Gram, or Wayson) will help to overcome this difficulty.

POSSIBLE MENINGITIS

Clinical Features

The syndrome of headache, stiff neck, and fever is immediately recognized as evidence of possible meningitis. The syndrome is usually acute in onset and may progress rapidly to stupor and coma. Bacterial meningitis is most likely, but certain viruses and fungi may also present with a similar clinical picture. Table 22–1 lists the various microbiologic causes of meningitis.

TABLE 22–1. MICROBIOLOGICAL CAUSES OF MENINGITIS

Age Group	Common Causes
Infants and children	*Haemophilus influenzae, Neisseria meningitidis, Streptococcus pneumoniae*
Adolescents	*S. pneumoniae, Mycobacterium tuberculosis, N. meningitidis*
Adults	*M. tuberculosis, S. pneumoniae*, fungus, especially cryptococcus

TABLE 22–2. CEREBRAL SPINAL FLUID IN VARIOUS DISEASES

Disease	Cells (per mm³)	Glucose*	Protein	Other
Normal	0 pmns, 0–4 monos	60%	<50 mg/dl	—
Bacterial	500—10,000 pmns	<20%	↑	+ Gram stain + Culture
TB	20–500 monos	20–40%	↑ ↑	+ Acid fast stain in 10% + Culture
Viral	20–1000 monos	N– ↑	Mild– ↑	+ Culture (rarely)
Fungal	25–500 monos	20–40%	↑	+ India ink in cryptococcosis + Culture
Carcinomatosis	5–500 monos	20–40%	↑	+ Cytology
Traumatic tap	1 to 3 × 10⁶ RBCs 1 WBC/750 RBCs	N– ↑	↑ by 1 mg/dl for each 700 RBC	Fluid clears with successive tubes Clear supernatant
Subarachnoid hemorrhage	500–3 × 10⁶ RBCs 1 WBC/750 RBCs	N– ↑	↑ by 1 mg/dl for each 700 RBC	Fluid does not clear in successive tubes Xanthochromic supernatant

*As percentage of peripheral blood levels.

Laboratory Studies

Cerebrospinal Fluid (CSF) Examination

The lumbar puncture will show an increase in spinal fluid pressure. Gross examination of the fluid shows a cloudy or turbid, slightly yellow fluid. A smear of the spinal fluid sediment obtained by centrifugation is stained with Gram or Wright stain. This smear is thoroughly examined for organisms, because rapid (albeit tentative) identification is essential before appropriate therapy is initiated.

Protein levels are increased because of the greater number of white blood cells. Glucose levels are usually decreased in bacterial meningitis caused by accelerated glycolysis by white blood cells and bacteria. These chemical studies are only secondary in importance to the smear examination and probably are not necessary in many cases. The measurement of chloride levels is rarely helpful except in cases of tuberculous meningitis, in which instance chloride levels are quite low. Thus, a routine request for chloride determinations on spinal fluids is not justified. Table 22–2 shows the characteristic CSF findings in meningitis.

Counterimmunoelectrophoresis (CIE) is a technique that has been widely used for the rapid diagnosis of bacterial meningitis. The technique involves the use of commercial antisera against the most common infectious agents (*H. influenzae, Neisseria meningitidis, Steptococcus pneumoniae,* and streptococcus group B) to detect specific bacterial antigens in the CSF. The major technical difficulty has been variation in patency of commercial antisera. CIE is currently being replaced by latex agglutination methods.

The culture of the spinal fluid is necessary for definitive diagnosis of the organism as well as for the determination of antibiotic susceptibility of the organism. Special culture media are required for meningococcus (chocolate agar) as well as tubercle bacilli (Lowenstein's or equivalent), and the laboratory should be made aware of the clinical impressions so that appropriate media are inoculated.

DISTURBANCES IN CONSCIOUSNESS/COMA

Clinical Features

Disturbances in consciousness may follow a wide variety of conditions or intoxications, which in general can be grouped into several large categories. These reactions may occur acutely and be initially accompanied by delerium, which later progresses to deepening stupor and coma, termed acute brain syndrome. A short-lived variety, syncope or simple faint, presents no special diagnostic problem and will be mentioned no further.

The most common cause of coma is a cerebrovascular accident secondary either to cerebral atherosclerosis or after trauma. The clinical manifestations and localizing as well as general neurologic changes are well known and require no further mention in this context.

A large number of cases of coma result from intoxications from endogenous (e.g., diabetic ketoacidosis, uremia, or liver disease) or exogenous causes (e.g., acute alcoholism, barbiturate or opiate overdosage, or other drug effects).

Coma also occurs in diabetic patients. In these cases there may be difficulties in the differentiation of diabetic ketoacidosis from insulin shock. Diabetic coma is relatively slow (days) in onset and follows the discontinuation or an inadequacy of insulin dosage. Or it may be precipitated by intercurrent infection in a usually well-controlled diabetic. The skin is dry and the patient appears dehydrated. Respirations are deep and labored (Kussmaul). The blood pressure is low, and the pulse is weak and rapid.

Insulin shock, on the other hand, rapidly follows insulin overdosage. The skin is moist, and there is no evidence of dehydration. Convulsions may occur because of the hypoglycemia. Respiration is normal.

Infections with meningitis or encephalitis may be primarily manifested by coma. Tuberculous meningitis, rabies, viral encephalitis, trypanosomiasis, and malaria are well-known examples of this cause of loss of consciousness. Fever usually is a prominent feature of these infections. These diseases were discussed earlier.

Brain tumors, either primary or metastatic, or brain abscess may have associated stupor and coma. Neurologic examination should help to differentiate this condition from the other conditions noted.

Laboratory Studies

Screening Procedures

CSF Examination. Except for the contraindications to lumbar puncture noted above, obtaining a specimen of spinal fluid for appropriate examination is almost mandatory in the study of the patient with coma.

The gross examination of the spinal fluid often yields a diagnosis. For example, nonclearing blood-tinged, or grossly bloody fluid indicates some type of vascular accident. Xanthochromic (yellow-orange) fluid is found in patients who have suffered an intracerebral hemorrhage at least several days prior to lumbar puncture. As stated previously, a cloudy or turbid fluid points to infection, and further definitive microbiological studies are necessary. If a traumatic tap has occurred there will be an artifactual evaluation of the CSF protein level. Each increment of 700 red blood cells per cubic millimeter results in about a 1 mg/dl increment in the protein concentration (Table 22–2).

Brain tumors usually result in mildly elevated spinal fluid protein levels as opposed to the moderate or great evaluations that follow infections processes.

Glucose. Blood glucose levels can be very useful in diagnosing diabetic ketoacidosis and insulin shock. Tests for urine glucose and acetone will also effectively screen for the presence of diabetic acidosis.

In the case of differentiating diabetic coma from insulin shock, the blood glucose level is quite elevated in diabetic coma, whereas it is subnormal in insulin shock. A therapeutic trial of intravenous glucose (50 percent solution) may yield an immediate diagnosis, hypoglycemia, if the patient quickly responds to this treatment. The additional glucose in ketoacidosis is not harmful if appropriate therapy is begun promptly.

Creatinine. The serum creatinine level is a good screen for renal insufficiency with uremia. Normal or only mildly elevated levels essentially rule out uremia as the cause of coma.

Serum Electrolytes, Calcium. These determinations may give a clue as to the etiology of coma.

Blood Ammonia. In many cases of hepatic coma the blood ammonia levels are raised to 5 times normal. Blood ammonia is not elevated in all patients with hepatic coma, therefore, a normal ammonia level does not rule out the diagnosis.

Definitive Procedures

Drug or Other Intoxications. No simple procedures are available to screen for drug or other intoxications. The clinical history and physical examination will often point to the intoxicant (e.g., ethanol, barbiturate). In these cases specific procedures can be done to corroborate the diagnosis. Consultation with the toxicologist is most valuable in these cases. (Also refer to Chapter 23, which deals with drug reactions.)

Endogenous Intoxication. The laboratory investigation of diabetic ketoacidosis and its treatment involves serial blood glucose determinations and the measurements of pH, bicarbonate, and potassium levels.

In both the definitive diagnosis of renal insufficiency with uremia and the monitoring of therapy (e.g., peritoneal or extracorporeal dialysis), the laboratory is called on to perform multiple procedures such as pH, carbon dioxide content, potassium, sodium, urea, and creatinine on blood or urine. Most of these procedures are discussed in the chapters on renal function (see Chap. 11) or acid-base disorders (see Chap. 12).

Roentgenologic Studies. Computerized tomography (CT) scanning has revolutionized the diagnostic workup of patients with possible central nervous system lesions. It is indispensible in diagnosing CNS hemorrhage, tumor, or abscess. Arteriography is of help in the diagnosis of focal (and surgically correctable) atherosclerotic disease.

DEMENTIA

The goal in the workup of a patient with dementia is to identify a treatable cause of the dementia. Treatable causes include brain tumor, normal pressure hydrocephalus, subdural hematoma, vitamin B_{12} deficiency, liver disease, syphilis, fungal meningitis, drug intoxication, uremia, myxedema, Cushing's disease, hypercalcemia, carcinoma of the lung, and subacute bacterial endocarditis. Table 22–3 lists one recommended workup for dementia. The extent of the workup depends on the patient's age and previous level of function. The laboratory investigation of neurosyphilis includes studies done on the peripheral blood serum and the CSF. Tests done on spinal fluid include a cell count with differential and syphilis serology (RPR and/or FTA-ABS). The characteristic results are shown in Table 22–4. The laboratory similarities between the two types makes these tests of limited use. The physician is dependent on the clinical examination. The colloidal gold curve is quite variable in these causes and is now rarely, if ever, ordered.

TABLE 22–3. DEMENTIA WORKUP

CBC with leukocyte differential	Lumbar puncture
Electrolytes, calcium	Skull x-rays
Liver function tests (AST, ALT, ALP, bilirubin)	CT scan
BUN/Creatinine	Chest x-ray
Thyroxine (T$_4$)	
Vitamin B$_{12}$ and folate	
Urinalysis	
Syphilis serology	
Drug levels (if appropriate)	

MULTIPLE SCLEROSIS

Clinical Features

Multiple sclerosis (MS) is the most common demyelinating disease. The etiology of the disease is not known. The widely varying clinical picture of MS reflects its underlying pathologic changes. There are multiple plaques or islands of demyelination scattered throughout the CNS white matter. The location and number of plaques determine the symptoms and course of the disease.

Laboratory Studies

CSF Electrophoresis

Oligoclonal banding in the gamma globulin region is present in about 80 to 90 percent of patients with MS. This is probably the best single test to detect MS. A negative result is strong evidence against demyelinating disease, but the test is not entirely specific for MS.

IgG Index

The measurement of de novo CNS IgG synthesis is a valuable tool in the diagnosis of MS. De novo synthesis occurs in over 90 percent of patients with clinically definite MS. Because elevated serum gammaglobulin levels can diffuse into the CSF and affect values there, several ratios have been devised to correct for this. One such ratio is the IgG index:

$$\text{IgG index} = \frac{\text{CSF IgG/Serum IgG}}{\text{CSF albumin/Serum albumin}}$$

Values above 0.7 are suggestive of excessive synthesis of IgG in the CNS.

CONVULSIVE DISORDERS

Clinical Features

Seizures occur as a manifestation of a broad spectrum of diseases. They may be merely mild and transient episodes of sensory or psychic changes (psychomotor) or minimal disturbances (petit mal). The severe varieties are characterized by focal sensory or motor disturbances (Jacksonian), or generalized forms which are associated with paroxysms of muscular contractions, incontinence, and loss of consciousness (grand mal).

Any of these variations may be associated with intracranial or extracranial disease. Intracranial causes include idiopathic epilepsy, intracerebral tumor, meningitis, abscess, or posttraumatic brain injury. In intracranial causes focal seizures are probably more common.

Probably the most common extracranial cause of seizures is high fever in young children. Toxic causes include exogenous toxins (ethanol, drugs) or endogenous toxins (uremia, hepatic failure). Other metabolic causes (e.g., hypocalcemia, hypoglycemia) complete the general spectrum of the etiology of convulsive disorders.

TABLE 22–4. SPINAL FLUID FINDINGS IN NEUROSYPHILIS

	Meningovascular–Parenchymetous	Tabes Dorsalis
Cell count/mm³	10–100	10–500
Differential count	Lymphs	Lymphs
Protein (mg/dl)	50–80	50–80
Percent cases with positive serology		
Spinal fluid	90–100	80
Serum	70–90	80

TABLE 22–5. DISEASES OFTEN RECOMMENDED FOR INCLUSION IN NEWBORN SCREENING PROGRAMS

Disease	Incidence	Enzyme Defect	Findings in Blood	Clinical Features
Phenylketonuria	1:12,000	Phenylalanine hydroxylase deficiency	Elevated phenylalanine	Mental retardation Fair hair and skin Eczema Seizures
Galactosemia	1:65,000	Galactose-1-P uridyl trans-ferase	Elevated galactose	Mental retardation Liver dysfunction Renal dysfunction Cataracts
Congenital hypothyroidism	1:6000	—	Depressed T^4 Elevated TSH	Mental retardation Constipation Developmental delays Cretin physical features
Maple syrup urine disease	1:200,000	Branched chain ketoacid decarboxylase	Elevated leucine, isoleucine, and valine	Mental retardation Vomiting Seizures Hypertonia/hypotonia
Tyrosinemia (hereditary)	1:200,000	? Parahydroxy phenylpy-ruvic acid oxidase (liver)	Elevated tyrosine and methionine	Failure to thrive Vomiting Liver cirrhosis Rickets
Homocystinuria	1:200,000	Cystathionine beta-synthase	Elevated methionine and homocystine	Mental retardation Fair hair and skin Dislocated lenses Venous and arterial throm-bosus
Histidinemia	1:17,000	Histidase	Elevated histidine	? Mental retardation ? Speech defects

Laboratory Studies

The clinical examination may quickly uncover the reason for seizures, and the laboratory usually only corroborates this impression. In seizures resulting from unknown cause, the problem is somewhat more difficult. Spinal fluid examination for evidence of hemorrhage, infection, or tumor is important. Laboratory corroboration of hypocalcemia or hypoglycemia may be difficult, and special procedures (e.g., tolbutamide tolerance test, prolonged glucose studies, prolonged fasting) may be necessary to reveal hypoglycemia. The electroencephalogram is diagnostic in idiopathic epilepsy. It also will help establish epilepsy caused by focal brain lesions.

NEUROMETABOLIC DISEASES

There are a number of genetic metabolic disorders associated with brain, liver, or kidney damage. The demonstration of accumulation and excessive excretion of certain metabolites and reduced amounts of others has become an important tool in the early diagnosis of genetic metabolic disorders. Many of these disorders can be successfully treated if discovered early, before irreversible harm to the patient's brain, liver, or kidney has occurred or before the child is blind or has died in an acute metabolic crisis. For example, phenylketonuria (PKU) occurs in one out of every 12,000 live births. It results from a defect in the activity of the enzyme phenylalanine hydroxylase. If unrecognized, it can lead to progressive severe mental retardation, fair hair and skin, eczema, and seizures. If a diet low in phenylalanine is instituted before 3 weeks of age, however, mental and physical retardation is prevented. This implies the necessity of establishing the diagnosis of phenylketonuria very shortly after birth by newborn screening. Most screening tests for PKU detect excess phenylalanine in blood specimens dried on filter paper then subjected to chromatography. Table 22–5 lists the diseases that are often screened for in the newborn.

SUGGESTED READINGS

Alexander E Jr: Lumbar puncture. JAMA 201:316, 1967.
Bakerman S, et al.: Laboratory screening for bacterial meningitis. Lab Mgmt 20:17, 1982.

Bickel H, et al. (eds): Neonatal Screening for Inborn Errors of Metabolism. New York, Springer-Verlag, 1980.

Campbell J: Seeking diseases confused with dementia: "Treatable" dementia. Lab Med 16:414, 1985.

Elkind AH, Friedman AP: Review of headache. NY State J Med 67:255, 1967.

Fishman R: Cerebrospinal Fluid in Disease of the Nervous System. Philadelphia, Saunders, 1980.

Stahlheber P, Peter J: Multiple sclerosis: A clearer path to a complex diagnosis. Diag Med (Jan):43, 1984.

Ward P: Cerebrospinal fluid data: 1. Interpretation in intracranial hemorrhage and meningitis. Postgrad Med 68:181, 1980.

23

THERAPEUTIC DRUG MONITORING AND TOXICOLOGY

GENERAL COMMENTS

This book is primarily oriented toward the presenting signs and symptoms in the patient and thus does not follow an arbitrary and compartmentalized format based on the organization of the hospital laboratory. This chapter departs from the format. The major sections deal with the laboratory tests that corroborate and also quantitate reactions to known therapeutic or toxic agents in patients. For example, in cases of salicylate intoxication, the direct measurement of salicylate levels is both valuable and necessary for the effective care of the patient.

The clinical features and laboratory studies of patients with illness caused by exposure to toxic compounds, overdosage of certain drugs, or idiosyncratic reactions to specific medications have been included in the appropriate sections elsewhere in this book. Hematologic abnormalities caused by certain agents are therefore included in the chapters on anemia and leukemoid reactions (see Chap. 13, 14). Similarly, drugs or chemicals causing jaundice or central nervous system depression are included in the appropriate sections.

Formerly the laboratory confirmation of such reactions consisted of measuring known biochemical or hematologic sequelae of drug exposure. The clinical history usually documented the exposure to the drug or toxic compound. Laboratory studies merely provided indirect evidence for such a reaction. In recent years, with sophisticated instrumentation the direct measurement of the offending agent has been done more frequently.

The following discussions outline a logical approach to the laboratory study of patients who have unwittingly or willfully received toxic quantities of drugs or chemicals. At times this

369

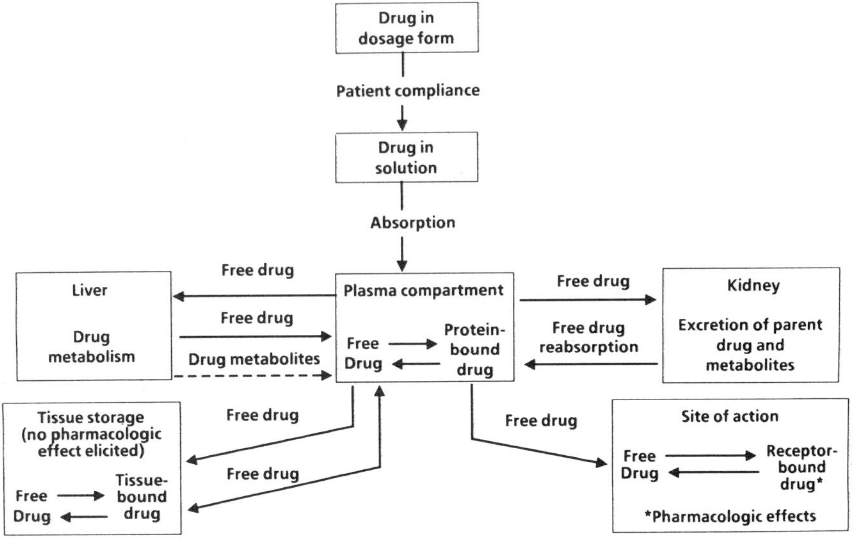

Figure 23–1. Factors affecting plasma drug concentration. *(Adapted from the Syva Monitor, November 1978.)*

exposure will be quite evident, whereas on occasion the possibility may not have been considered by the attending physician.

In these days of widespread use of a great variety of potent drugs as well as potential exposure to a wide variety of toxic chemicals in industry, agriculture, or elsewhere, it is neither appropriate nor possible to give more than a few examples of the approach necessary to study these cases.

Specimen Collection

In patients with known or suspected acute drug toxicity, the attending physician should save all specimens that may con-

TABLE 23–1. CRITERIA FOR THERAPEUTIC MONITORING OF DRUGS

The pharmacokinetics and protein binding of the drug and its metabolites must be known.

The pharmacologic effect must be directly related to the circulating level.

Any toxic effects must be directly related to the circulating level.

The blood levels following the administration of a standard dose must show characteristic variations of absorption, excretion, and metabolism.

The incidence and severity of any toxic effects must be difficult to predict.

A precise, accurate, convenient, and reliable assay must be available.

tain the toxic compound or its breakdown products. Such specimens include blood, urine, and gastric washings. These should be collected in clean specimen containers without added preservatives. Plastic or waxed-lined disposable urine containers are convenient.

Early consultation with the toxicologist or clinical pathologist who will be analyzing these specimens usually is helpful in preventing errors in collections. If there is any possibility that the case may become a medicolegal one, it is mandatory that all specimens be transmitted to the toxicology laboratory by the physician so the chain of evidence is preserved. Appropriate clinical notes, receipts, and records are necessary to ensure this.

Therapeutic Drug Monitoring

With the improvement in instrumentation and methodology for the measurement of various unchanged or metabolic products of drugs, a great amount of data has accumulated regarding the pharmacokinetics of drugs. It has become apparent that the proportion of absorption of drugs from the gut may vary considerably from one patient to the next. In addition, the clearance of the drug may vary depending on the clinical status of the patient and the functional state of the liver and kidneys, the major organs concerned with the metabolism and excretion of drugs. The factors affecting the plasma drug concentration are summarized in Figure 23–1.

If drug levels can vary markedly among patients given apparently equal dosages and if therapeutic success or toxicity is directly related to blood levels of such drugs, it is certainly advantageous to determine such levels if at all possible (Table 23–1).

There are several classes of drugs in which blood levels are measurable. These include cardiac drugs (e.g., digoxin, digitoxin, procainamide, lidocaine, disopyramide, quinidine, and thiocyanate), anticonvulsants (e.g., dilantin, phenobarbital, carbamazepine, valproic acid, primidone, and ethosuximide), aminoglycoside antibiotics, and bronchodilators (theophylline). Other drugs include methotrexate and lithium.

The timing of specimen collection is of utmost importance in drug monitoring. Drug concentrations should be measured at steady state. When a drug is given by continuous infusion or in multiple doses by any route it will accumulate to approximately 97 percent of steady state values by the time five half-lives have passed. Also, drug levels cannot be interpreted unless one knows if they represent a peak or a trough in

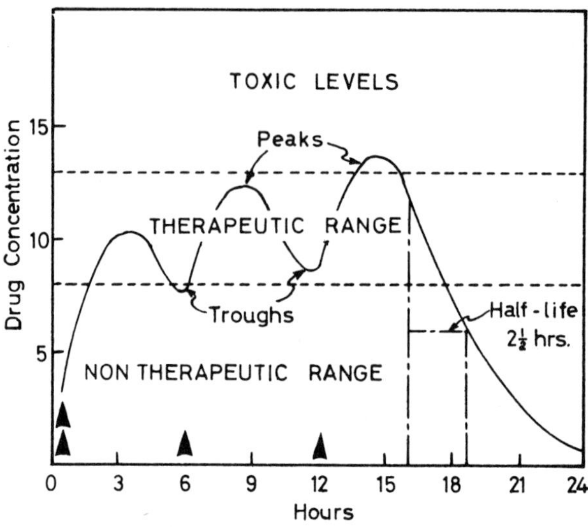

Figure 23–2. Drug concentrations as related to dosage schedule.

relation to the periodic administration of the drug (Fig. 23–2).

An increasing number of therapeutic agents can be measured quickly and accurately in the laboratory. As more drugs fulfill the criteria for therapeutic monitoring (Table 23–1), we can expect to see significant growth in this field of laboratory medicine. Indeed, therapeutic monitoring is probably one of the most important functions of the laboratory service.

A number of drugs that now are frequently monitored are listed in Table 23–2. Additional information about the therapeutic levels, metabolism/excretion, and half-lives can also be found in this table. It should be obvious from the discussions at the beginning of this chapter that the timing of specimen procurement coupled with a knowledge of the pharmacokinetics of the drug in question is vital for the correct interpretation of the result reported by the laboratory.

LABORATORY STUDIES IN SPECIFIC DRUG OVERDOSAGE

There are a variety of techniques available for screening specimens from overdosed patients. They include spectrophotometry, paper chromatography, color tests, thin layer chromatography, gas chromatography, gas chromatography–mass spectrometry, immunoassay, and high performance liquid chromatography. The method a particular laboratory chooses depends on a variety of factors.

TABLE 23–2. PHARMACOKINETIC DATA FOR COMMONLY MONITORED DRUGS

Drug	Significant Plasma Protein Binding	% Excreted Unchanged	Normal Plasma Half-Life (hr)	Recommended Time to Draw Level	Therapeutic Concentration
Amikacin	No	98	2	Peak: 1 hour after start of infusion Trough: JBND	Peak: 20–30 mg/L Trough: 5–10 mg/L
Carbamazepine	Yes (A)	< 5	15	JBND	3–12 mg/L
Chloramphenicol	No	10	3	JBND	10–20 mg/L
Digoxin	No	70	39	JBND > 6 hours after PO dose > 4 hours after IV dose	0.8–2.0 µg/L
Ethosuximide	No	20	60 hours (adults) 30 hours (children)	JBND	40–100 mg/L
Flucytosine	No	75–90	39	3 hours after dose	40–80 mg/L > 100 mg/L potentially toxic
Gentamicin	No	> 90	2	See amikacin	Peak: 4–8 mg/L Trough: < 2 mg/L
Lidocaine	Yes (B)	< 5	2	Suspected toxicity or > 8 hours after starting infusion	2–5 mg/L
Lithium	No	> 95	24	Just before AM dose (> 12 hours after last dose)	0.5–1.5 mEq/L

TABLE 23–2. PHARMACOKINETIC DATA FOR COMMONLY MONITORED DRUGS (Cont.)

Drug	Significant Plasma Protein Binding	% Excreted Unchanged	Normal Plasma Half-Life (hr)	Recommended Time to Draw Level	Therapeutic Concentration
Methotrexate	No	95	8	By protocol	$> 0.1\ \mu M$ for > 48 hours is potentially toxic; maintain folinic acid rescue until MTX $< 0.1\ \mu M$. $> 1\ \mu M$ at 48 hours requires increased folinic acid dose
Phenobarbital	No	25	120	JBND preferred	10–40 mg/L
Phenytoin	Yes (A)	< 5	Plasma concentration dependent	JBND	10–20 mg/L
Primidone	No	40	8	JBND	5–10 mg/L
Procainamide	No	70	7	JBND	4–8 mg/L
N-acetyl-procainamide (NAPA)	No	80	7	—	$^{1}/_{4}$–$^{2}/_{3}$ as active as procainamide
Quinidine	Yes (B)	20	6	JBND	1–4 mg/L
Salicylates	Yes (A)	10 (C)	2–30	JBND	100–300 mg/L
Theophylline	No	10	8	JBND	10–20 mg/L
Tobramycin	No	90	2	See amikacin	See gentamicin
Vancomycin	No	> 90	6	Peak: 1 hour after end of infusion Trough: JBND	Peak: < 50 mg/L Trough: 5–10 mg/L

JBND, just before next dose; A, therapeutic range needs to be decreased for hypoalbuminemia and renal failure; B, therapeutic range needs to be adjusted for a variety of disease states; C, dose and urinary pH dependent.

Reprinted with permission from Winter ME, Fields SM: Essentials of therapeutic drug monitoring. Hosp Phys July 1986, p 26.

ETHYL ALCOHOL

Clinical Features

The clinical manifestations of acute alcoholism are well known and range from almost imperceptible personality changes to coma and death. Although there are notable variations, Table 23–3 correlates alcohol consumption and blood levels with clinical manifestations. A number of assumptions have been in the development of this table, and therefore it provides only general guidelines. But it should be useful in dealing with the problem on a clinical basis. The data are based on the amount of alcohol drunk by a 70-kg person over a period of about 1 hour. One drink is defined as 30 ml (1 oz) of whiskey, 360 ml (12 oz) of beer, or 120 ml (4 oz) of wine. The amount of alcohol should be approximately the same in all three drinks. It is surprising to see the large number of drinks required to produce legal drunkness, i.e., >100 mg/dl alcohol levels (100 mg/dl equals 0.1 percent alcohol levels). The time required for alcohol to disappear is calculated on the basis of the normal disappearance rate of 15 mg/dl/hour.

Laboratory Studies

To measure blood alcohol levels, a whole blood specimen is drawn without the use of alcohol to cleanse the skin. The physician should be aware of local and state laws regarding blood alcohol determinations before obtaining samples, except,

TABLE 23–3. RELATION OF CLINICAL STATUS TO BLOOD ALCOHOL LEVELS

Clinical Reaction	Drinks Consumed	Blood Alcohol (mg/dl)	Time for Alcohol to Disappear (hr)
Subjective warmth, jovial	2	40	2
Slurred speech, euphoria prolonged reaction time	5	100*	6
Responses and coordination severely affected	7	150	10
Stuporous	12	250	16
Comatose	20	400	26

*Legally drunk in most states.

of course, if the life of the patient is in jeopardy. There are three different groups of analytic procedures used for the determination of ethanol: (1) chemical oxidation with acid dichromate; (2) enzymatic oxidation with alcohol dehydrogenase; and (3) gas chromatography. The first two procedures are not specific in that other alcohols such as methanol and isopropanol may give positive results. Therefore, gas chromatography is the reference method.

SALICYLATES

Clinical Features

Because of either prolonged administration of high doses, or more often accidental overdosage in children, toxic levels of

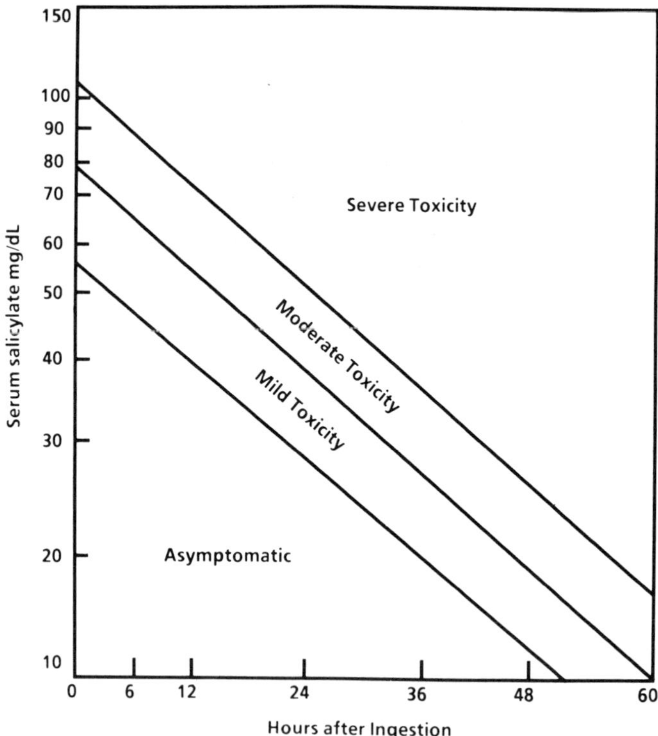

Figure 23–3. Clinical symptoms as related to concentration and time of ingestion of potentially toxic dose of salicylate.

salicylates may occur on occasion. In chronic overdosage, headache, tinnitus, vertigo, and possible nausea and vomiting are common symptoms. The child with accidental overdosage may first exhibit hyperpnea and gastrointestinal disturbances, which may progress from initial respiratory alkalosis to metabolic acidosis. Treatment of salicylate intoxication may include emesis, gastric lavage, forced alkaline diuresis, and dialysis.

Laboratory Studies

Screening Procedures

The addition of a 5 percent ferric chloride solution to an equal quantity of plasma results in a blue color in specimens taken from patients with salicylism, i.e., salicylate intoxication.

Definitive Procedures

The measurement of blood or urine salicylate levels is a widely available and easily performed procedure. The risk of toxicity in salicylate intoxication may be determined from a nomogram comparing the serum salicylate level with the time after ingestion (Fig. 23–3). The blood sample should be obtained at least 6 hours postingestion to allow for complete absorption and peak serum concentration.

Salicylate levels of 15 to 30 mg/dl are necessary for the effective treatment of rheumatoid arthritis.

ACETAMINOPHEN

Clinical Features

Acetaminophen is contained in over 200 formulations in the United States. The early symptoms of acetaminophen toxicity are nonspecific and usually consist of gastrointestinal distress. The most serious toxic effect is hepatic necrosis. Treatment of acetaminophen poisoning should include *N*-acetyl cysteine to reduce the risk of hepatotoxicity.

Laboratory Studies

Acetaminophen Levels

There are a variety of laboratory methods that can be used to measure acetaminophen levels. The method a particular laboratory uses depends on a variety of factors. The risk of hepatic toxicity can be determined from a nomogram comparing the serum acetaminophen level with the time after ingestion (Fig. 23–4). The blood sample should be obtained at least 4 hours postingestion to allow for complete absorption and peak serum concentration. If the time of ingestion is not known with certainty, serial levels can be obtained and the half-life calculated. If the half-life is greater than 4 hours it should be assumed that liver damage has occurred.

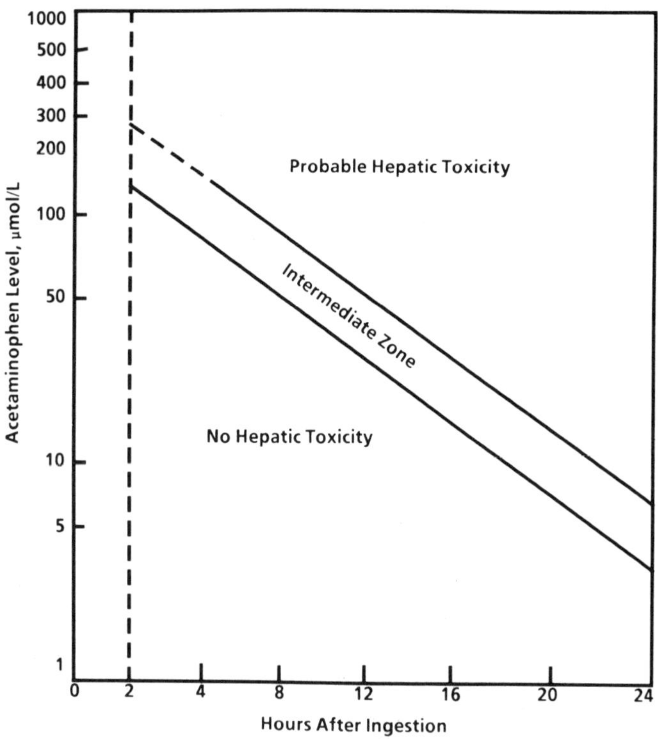

Figure 23–4. Semilogarithmic plot of serum acetaminophen levels versus time. The serum half-life can be estimated using two specimens obtained several hours apart. To convert to μmol/L multiply by 66. *(Modified from Krenzelok EP, Best L, Monoguerra AS: Acetaminophen toxicity. Amer J Hosp Pharm 34:391, 1977.)*

Liver Function Tests

Serum transaminases, bilirubin, and the PT may be determined to assess hepatotoxicity.

BARBITURATE INTOXICATION

Clinical Features

The clinical manifestations of barbiturate overdosage are well known and need not be repeated here. These agents primarily depress the central nervous system and especially the respiratory center.

Laboratory Studies

The measurement of blood barbiturate levels rather than urine or gastric washings is the procedure of choice. Whole blood drawn without anticoagulants is the most suitable specimen. Barbiturate levels can be measured by a wide variety of laboratory methods including gas chromatography, immunoassay, fluorescence polarization, and high-pressure liquid chromatography. Serum barbiturate levels generally correspond to the clinical presentation, although habitual users may tolerate higher doses than persons who are not habitual users. It is important to distinguish between long-acting and intermediate- or short-acting barbiturates because only the long-acting barbiturates can be effectively removed by alkalinization and forced diuresis as a result of their relatively high water solubility and low pKa.

ANTIPSYCHOTIC MAJOR TRANQUILIZERS

Clinical Features

Since the first use of chlorpromazine in the 1950s, a host of medications has become available for the treatment of psychoses, neuroses, and depressions. A wide variety of effects have been noted, including weakness, orthostatic hypotension, palpitations, varying levels of central nervous system depression, hyperreflexia, extrapyramidal signs, and even convulsive seizures.

Laboratory Studies

FPN Test

This is a universal screening test for the phenothiazine drugs. The initials stand for the reagents used in the test. The testing solution is prepared as follows:

FeCl$_3$ (5 percent solution)	5 ml
Perchloric acid (20 percent)	45 ml
Nitric acid (50 percent)	50 ml

To perform the test, mix 1 ml of freshly voided urine with 1 ml of FPN reagent. A positive result is the immediate formation of a pink (1+) ranging to deep purple (6+) color. Any color produced after 10 seconds is disregarded. A 1+ reaction roughly corresponds to a 20- to 70-mg daily dose of phenothiazine drug, and a 6+ reaction roughly indicates a daily dose of 800 to 2000 mg.

HALLUCINOGENS

Clinical Features

Hallucinogen usage has become increasingly prominent in certain segments of the young adult population. A number of drugs are included in this group, including lysergic acid diethylamide (LSD), psilocybin, mescaline, dimethyltryptamine (DMT), diethyltryptamine (DET), marijuana, and phencyclidine (PCP). The effects of many of these drugs are similar. They include nausea, vomiting, hypersensitivity to environmental stimuli, disorientation, anxiety, hallucinations, hypertension, hyperthermia, mydriasis, hyperreflexia, and convulsions.

Laboratory Studies

There are a variety of techniques used to screen for hallucinogens. The method will vary with each laboratory.

HEAVY-METAL POISONING

Clinical Features

Heavy metals associated with either acute or chronic intoxication include arsenic, antimony, mercury, and lead. After acute ingestion the patient may have abdominal pain, vomiting, diarrhea, dehydration, and oliguria. In addition, mercury has particularly striking effects on the kidney, leading to acute tubular necrosis.

Chronic exposure to these metals results in strikingly different clinical pictures. For instance, arsenic exposure usually results in weakness, personality changes, and hyperkeratoic skin lesions. Ingestion of antimony salts results in gastrointestinal disturbances and anorexia. Chronic mercury poisoning is associated with tremors progressing to ataxia and emotional disturbances (the Mad Hatter). Chronic lead poisoning is characterized by gastrointestinal problems (lead colic) and anemia.

Laboratory Studies

Screening Procedures

Reinsch Test. Heavy metals all react positively in the Reinsch test, a reliable semiquantitative procedure. In addition to the metals noted above, the test is also positive for large amounts of bismuth, selenium, tellurium, as well as sulfides. If the results are positive, the heavy metal can be identified as well as quantitated. Lead does not react in this test, and therefore if lead poisoning is suspected other procedures must be requested.

Coproporphyrin. The simplest procedure for chronic lead toxicity is the measurement of urinary coproporphyrin, a substance excreted in increased amounts in lead poisoning (as well as in prophyrias). This test is sensitive and has in recent years become widely available. The measurement of urinary delta-aminolevulinic acid (ALA) has recently been shown to be a more reliable screening procedure for lead intoxication. ALA is another metabolite in the porphyrin synthesis pathway.

Erythrocyte Protoporphyrin. Lead inhibits heme synthetase, the enzyme that incorporates iron into protoporphyrin to form heme. Decreased protoporphyrin conversion leads to increased erythrocyte protoporphyrin. Thus increased levels of erythrocyte protoporphyrin reflect chronic lead exposure. This is becoming the preferred screening test for lead poisoning. It may be increased in disorders other than lead poisoning, including iron deficiency anemia and erythropoietic protoporphyria.

Definitive Procedures

Flameless atomic absorption is the procedure of choice for blood lead levels as well as other heavy metals. This is a very sensitive and specific procedure.

SUGGESTED READINGS

Arena J: Poisoning, 4th ed. Springfield, Ill, C.C. Thomas, 1979.

Cross R, et al.: Therapeutic drug monitoring: A rapid combined system. Lab Mgmt (March) 57, 1982.

Dubowski K: Alcohol determination in the clinical laboratory. Am J Clin Pathol 74:747, 1980.

Gossel T, Bricker J: Principles of Clinical Toxicology. New York, Raven Press, 1984.

Greenblat D, Koch-Weser J: Clinical pharmacokinetics. N Engl J Med 293:702, 1975.

Haddad L, Winchester J: Clinical Management of Poisoning and Drug Overdose. Philadelphia, Saunders, 1983.

McCarron M: The role of the laboratory in treatment of the poisoned patient: Clinical perspective. J Anal Tox 7:142, 1983.

McCarron M: The use of toxicology test in emergency room diagnosis. J Anal Tox 7:131, 1983.

Hanenson I: Quick Reference to Clinical Toxicology. Philadelphia, Lippincott, 1980.

Pippenger C: Therapeutic drug monitoring: Pharmacologic principles. Diag Med (June)28, 1983.

Pippenger C: TDM: What the results mean. Diag Med (June)41, 1983.

Taylor W, Finn A (eds): Individualizing Drug Therapy: Practical Applications of Drug Monitoring. New York, Gross, Townsend Frank, 1981.

Winter ME, Fields SM: Essentials of therapeutic drug monitoring. Hosp Phys July: 22, 1986.

24

LABORATORY PROCEDURES FOR THE WARD OR OFFICE LABORATORY

BASIC INFORMATION

Choosing Appropriate Procedures

Although many laboratory determinations require complicated instrumentation and technical expertise, there are a number of determinations that should be mastered by the student or house officer because he or she may on occasion be called on to perform them. Also, these procedures can be considered to be a nucleus of procedures that can be conveniently and satisfactorily done in the physician's office laboratory. A moderate investment in instruments and equipment as well as glassware, culture media, and stains is required. Major equipment includes the following:

- Microscope with mechanical stage, oil immersion lens, and adequate substage light source
- Spectrophotometer (for hemoglobin) or microhematocrit centrifuge (for microhematocrit)
- Bacteriology incubator (37C)

Simplified instructions for key procedures are found on the next sections. Those tests that are notoriously poorly done or are much too complex and time-consuming to be worthwhile for the medical student or general physician to master have been omitted.

A list of laboratory studies that should be familiar to students and physicians are noted in Table 24–1.

Specimen Collection

The laboratory determination can be only as good as the specimen. If attention is paid to the details of the collection proce-

TABLE 24–1. PROCEDURES FOR THE WARD OR OFFICE LABORATORY

Hematology
  Hemoglobin and hematocrit
  Wright stain of blood film
  Differential leukocyte count
  Hemocytometer white blood cell
    count
  Reticulocyte preparation
  Marrow aspiration and biopsy

Coagulation Studies
  Estimation of platelets on stained
    film
  Activated coagulation time
  Skin bleeding time

Urinalysis
  Routine, including microscopic

Microbiology
  Gram or Wayson stain
  Inoculation of agar plates
  Inoculation of liquid culture media
  Inoculation of blood culture
    bottles

Miscellaneous
  Cytologic examination
  Tissue biopsy
  Lumbar puncture

dure, the amount of inaccurate or artifactually altered laboratory data is minimized. There are several potentially troublesome areas to be considered:

1. Time of collection. Obtain a fasting specimen when indicated, or a timed. specimen, e.g., in glucose tolerance testing.
2. Site of collection. Avoid veins proximal to intravenous infusions. Proper antiseptic preparation of venipuncture site is mandatory.
3. Venipuncture. Make a clean stick with prompt flow of blood. Traumatic venipuncture will, for instance, generate significant amounts of tissue thromboplastin and thereby invalidate certain coagulation procedures by initiating blood coagulation.

TABLE 24–2. VACUUM TUBE SPECIMEN TUBES

Stopper Color	Volume Draw (ml)	Additive	General Use
Red	10	None	Routine chemistry
Green	10	Heparin	Chemistry (pH, NH_3)
Lavender	7	EDTA	Hematology
Blue	4.5	Sodium citrate (0.105 M, 3.2%)	Coagulation studies
Gray	2	Siliceous earth (12 mg)	Activated coagulation time
Gray	7	Sodium fluoride	Blood glucose

4. Anticoagulants or preservatives. Use the proper anticoagulant or preservative for the test desired (Table 24–2). Completely expend the vacuum in the tubes when vacuum tubes are used.
5. Complete collections. Make sure that the 24-hour urine specimens or other timed collections are accurately timed and completely collected. This is a most formidable task.
6. Identification. Properly label the specimen. This is especially important for transfusion service specimens. Fill out the laboratory request form completely, including a working diagnosis.
7. Avoid sample delay. Promptly deliver the specimen in the laboratory.

Important Variables in Specimen Collection

Collection Tubes. The vacuum tube system is excellent for routine specimen collection. The appropriate tubes for use in some major classes of laboratory tests are given in Table 24–2. Vacuum tubes are also supplied for many special uses with a great variety of anticoagulants or preservatives, or both. The vacuum tubes contain sufficient material for proper anticoagulation of a filled container. Less than complete filling of the tube (i.e., incomplete expending of the vacuum) can result in artifactual changes in red blood cell volume as well as in certain chemical determinations. Underfilling or overfilling of the specimen tube may invalidate the hematocrit and blood film evaluation as well as CO_2, pH, and NH_3 values. Coagulation studies such as the PT and PTT can be markedly changed if clotting is initiated before the sample is mixed with the anticoagulant. Smaller collection tubes should be used if less blood is available.

Fasting. A patient who has not eaten for 8 hours or more is considered to be fasting, except for lipid studies for which a 12-hour fast is required. The patient may have had water, but not coffee, which is said to influence blood uric acid levels. Of the routine parameters measured, only glucose and phosphorus levels are significantly altered between the fasting and nonfasting state. If there is appreciable lipemia, however, many methods require special extraction procedures. Therefore, only in special cases are procedures done on such specimens because if lipemia is present it is usually more convenient to draw another truly fasting specimen. Most hematology specimens can be drawn without regard to the dietary status of the patient.

Sample Delay. All procedures are preferably done on fresh specimens. For this reason all blood drawn should be sent to the laboratory as soon as possible. This is of special importance in coagulation testing.

Transfusion Sevice Specimens. Blood specimens or crossmatch procedure must be labeled at the bedside or in the operating room with the patient's full name, hospital number, and date. Some hospitals use special wristband identification systems. The procedures must be followed to the letter to prevent identification errors.

Venipuncture. The venipuncture is a technique that should be mastered by all medical students and practitioners. It is only through experience and the confidence developed therefrom that the physician becomes proficient with this technique. The following hints may be helpful:

1. Always use sharp and preferably disposable needles. The venipuncture will be easier, and the patient will be most grateful.
2. After cleaning the venipuncture site with alcohol, pass the needle, bevel up, through the skin. If the vein is very superficial it may be entered on the initial puncture; otherwise it is entered with a second thrust of the needle.
3. In the more obese patient a wider tourniquet or blood pressure cuff may help to increase venous distension. In very difficult cases, leaving the arm dependent for several minutes or warming it with hot wet towels may be of help.
4. "Rolling veins" can be better controlled by fixing them between the thumb and index finger of one hand while controlling the needle with the other hand.
5. If a hematoma begins to form, loosen the tourniquet immediately and apply pressure to the site. Go to another site for specimen collection.
6. After completing the venipuncture, place a small dressing over the site.

Arterial Puncture. Arterial puncture has become a common and important technique used in the care of critically ill patients. As with the venipuncture, the technique should be mastered by all medical practitioners who work in clinical care units. The following hints regarding the procedure should be useful.

1. A 5-ml glass syringe with Luer lock is most suitable. It is fitted with a 22-gauge, 4-cm (1.5-inch) needle.
2. The inside of the syringe and needle is coated with heparin by aseptically aspirating a few milliliters of sodium heparin solution (1,000 or 10,000 USP units/ml) into the syringe. The entire internal surface is wetted by rotation of the plunger. All bubbles are expelled, but the needle is filled with heparin.
3. After informing the patient about the procedure, begin the search for a suitable artery on either the arms or the legs. Use three fingers simultaneously although two fingers may suffice in thin patients. Identify the artery by its pulsation.
4. The puncture site is not anesthetized, but cleaning with an antiseptic solution is required.
5. Anchor the artery by exerting digital pressure on the vessel. Holding the syringe and needle at 45 to 90 degrees, like a pencil, pierce the artery with a firm movement.
6. The syringe will be self-filling when the systolic blood pressure is above 110 mm Hg. If the patient is hypotensive, gentle aspiration will be required.
7. When sufficient sample is obtained (usually within about 1 minute), withdraw the needle and syringe, seal the syringe, and ice the specimen. Send or take the specimen to the laboratory promptly.
8. A sterile pledget is placed over the puncture site. Apply firm pressure to the puncture site for a full 5 minutes to prevent hematoma formation.

HEMATOLOGY PROCEDURES

In practice either a hemoglobin or a hematocrit will give adequate information for initial screening or emergency care. There is no need to routinely do both procedures, except as a check on the other. Present methods make even this consideration of more theoretical than practical importance.

Hematocrit or Packed Cell Volume

Equipment

- Microhematocrit centrifuge (12,000 rpm)
- Microhematocrit reader

Materials

- Heparinized microhematocrit capillary tubes
- Clay or plasticine sealer

Method

1. Thoroughly mix the tube of anticoagulated blood (EDTA or heparin) by gentle inversion for at least 1 minute. Longer mixing time is required for a specimen that has sedimented prior to the determination.
2. Open the blood tube, incline it toward the horizontal, and dip two capillary tubes into the blood, allowing them to almost fill by capillary action.
3. Carefully close the clean ends of the capillary tubes with the index finger and wipe away any blood with a sponge or absorbent paper. Remove the index finger from the end (to avoid injury if the capillary tube breaks) and press the capillary tube into the plastic sealer material by holding it firmly between the fingers and the thumb.
4. Place the sealed capillary tubes into the microhematocrit centrifuge, close the covers, and centrifuge for 4 to 5 minutes. Shortening the centrifugation time will artefactually increase the hematocrit level. Read the hematocrits on the microhematocrit reader and average the two readings. Also note the size of buffy coat (increased in leukocytosis and leukemia) as well as the color (jaundice?, hemolysis?) and character (lipemia?) of the supernatant plasma.

The reproducibility of the procedure at normal ranges is ±0.025 (±2 SD). A significant change in hematocrit is therefore an increase or decrease greater than 0.037 hematocrit units (>3 SD).

Hemoglobin

Equipment

- Spectrophotometer or colorimeter
- Micropipettes: Sahli 0.02 ml (± 1 percent tolerance)

Reagent

- Drabkin's solution: potassium ferricyanide–potassium cyanide solution. This reagent is most conveniently and accurately prepared by purchasing commercial pre-weighed powder. Prepare according to the manufacturer's directions.

Standard Curve

- Prepare according to the manufacturer's directions using standards certified by the International Committee for Standards in Haematology.

Method

1. Into exactly 5.0 ml of Drabkin's solution in a cuvette add exactly 0.02 ml of well-mixed blood (see hematocrit procedure above) by using a Sahli pipette with attached aspirating tube. Be sure to clean the pipette tip before introducing blood into the Drabkin's solution. Rinse the pipette several times by alternately aspirating and expressing the solution so as to completely clear the pipette of any residual blood.
2. After waiting several minutes, read the optical density of the unknown against a Drabkin's reagent blank at 540 nm (nanometers).
3. Determine the hemoglobin concentration by reference to the current standard curve.
4. If the blood–Drabkin's solution mixture fails to become crystal clear within a minute or so, it may indicate abnormal erythrocytes, which fail to lyse normally. Such cells may be noted in sickle cell anemia or trait, thalassemia major or minor, or other hemoglobiniopathies. Also, plasma abnormalities such as hyperlipemia or hyperglobulinemia may cause turbidity in this determination.

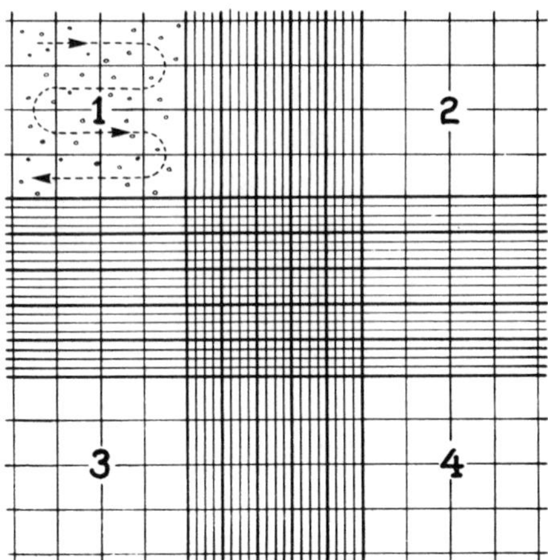

Figure 24–1. Hemocytometer grid. The white blood cells in the numbered areas (each with 16 smaller squares) are counted for the white count determination. See the text for calculations.

The reproducibility of this procedure at nearly normal values is ±0.6 g/dl (±2 SD). A significant change in hemoglobin would be a change greater than 0.9 g/dl (>3 SD).

White Blood Cell Count

Although semiautomated particle counters are found in most large laboratories, usually such equipment is not available for student use. Such counters, however, are frequently found in the physician's office or small laboratories.

The hemocytometer white count is adequate in many cases and, therefore, should be one of the procedures that the student or general physician can readily perform.

Equipment

- White cell counting pipette (clean, dry)
- Hemocytometer with chamber cover glass
- Microscope with mechanical stage
- Vibrating mixer

Materials

- White cell diluting fluid:
    Glacial acetic acid, 15 ml
    Distilled water, 475 ml

Methods

1. Fill the white blood cell pipette with fingerstick blood or well-mixed anticoagulated blood to the 0.5 mark, wipe the tip, and then fill the pipette to the 11 mark with diluting fluid (1:20 dilution).
2. Mix on a vibrating mixer for 3 minutes.
3. Expel the first several drops of fluid from the pipette and then carefully fill the hemocytometer.
4. Count the cells in the four large corner squares and the central square of the hemocytometer (Fig. 24–1). Count only those cells touching the top or left borders. Each square measures 1 by 1 by 0.1 mm and therefore contains 0.1 mm^3. Average the five counts. Refill and recount the chamber if there is a variation greater than 20 percent between the individual counts.
5. The white blood cell count $\times$ 10^6/L is the average count per 0.1 mm^3 $\times$ 10 $\times$ 20 (dilution factor).

The reproducibility of the procedure varies widely, depending on the skill and experience of the student or the technologist. A good technologist should be able to reproduce a hemocytometer white count in the normal range within ± 0.6 $\times$ 10^6/L. A significant change of white count is, therefore, greater than ± 0.9 $\times$ 10^6/L ($>$3.9 SD).

Preparation of Wright Stained Blood Film

Materials

Wright Stain. Commercially prepared Wright stain is available, but it is not always completely satisfactory. The following recipe has been satisfactory in our laboratory:

1. All containers must be absolutely dry before being used.
2. Place 0.3 g of powdered Wright stain (Harleco No. 376) in a mortar and add 3 ml of glycerin.
3. Grind thoroughly in a mortar with a pestle until a smooth paste is formed.
4. In small portions add 100 ml of acetone-free methyl alcohol from a newly opened bottle. Previously opened alcohol invariably absorbs water from the atmosphere. This water spoils the prepared stains.
5. Stopper the bottle tightly and let stand with occasional shaking for at least 1 week.
6. Filter before using.

Wright Stain Buffer (pH 6.4)

Potassium phosphate, monobasic (KH_2PO_4)	6.63g
Sodium phosphate, dibasic (anhydrous Na_2HPO_4)	2.56g
Distilled water	qs 1000 ml

Method

1. On a firm working surface make a "pulled" blood film by placing a small drop of fingertip, earlobe, or anti-coagulated blood near one end of a clean (preferably alcohol-washed) glass microscope slide. Immediately spread the blood with a second slide (held at about a 30-degree angle) that has been first "backed onto" the drop of blood. Hesitate a second or two while the blood spreads in the trough formed by the slides and then with a firm unwavering motion pull the blood film out toward the far end of the slide. A well-prepared slide should present a symmetric "feather-edge."
2. Air-dry the slide. Then fix it for a few seconds with just enough drops of absolute methyl alcohol to cover the film. This fixation avoids many troublesome and confusing erythrocyte artifacts. Dry the slide in air. With a lead pencil label the thick (unusable) end of the film with the patient's name and date.
3. Cover the entire slide with Wright stain for several minutes. The exact time varies from one batch of stain to another.
4. Add dropwise an equal amount of buffer to the Wright stain and mix by gently blowing over the slide several times. A golden-green sheen will form on the surface.
5. After several minutes (dependent again on the batch of stain used) wash the slide with tap water and allow it to drain dry.
6. Examine the slide by using the procedures outlined in the chapters on anemia and leukemia and leukemoid reactions.

Reticulocyte Count

Materials

New methylene blue stain

New methylene blue powder	1.0 g
Sodium chloride	8.9 g
Distilled water	qs 100 ml

Test tube or microhematocrit tube

Method

1. Mix together equal amounts of stain and whole blood in a test tube or in a microhematocrit tube. Mix by inverting the capillary several times.
2. Allow to stand at room temperature for 1 to 2 minutes.
3. Prepare a very thin film using a second slide as a spreader.
4. Allow the film to dry and then determine the number of reticulocytes per 1000 erythrocytes. The reticulin in reticulocytes stains a sharp dark blue, whereas the erythrocytes stain a pale green. No fixation or counterstain is required. Heinz bodies stain as medium blue bodies on the edge of the cells.
5. The number of reticulocytes per 1000 red blood cells divided by 10 equals the percentage of reticulocytes.

COAGULATION PROCEDURES

Prothrombin time determinations to monitor coumarin anticoagulation are sometimes performed in office laboratories. However, they are not done in ward or student laboratories and therefore have not been included in this chapter. Careful attention to specimen collection and the technical aspects of coagulation testing is required if they are performed in the above setting.

Estimation of Platelets from a Stained Film

In many situations the platelet count estimated by a well-trained technologist is as useful as an actual count. In emergency situations it is a fast and entirely adequate method for assessing the platelet count. But a well-prepared blood film is mandatory. No clumping of the platelets must be present, and an even distribution of the cells and platelets is required. Count the platelets in 10 separate oil immersion fields and average the counts. To estimate the platelet count use the following formula:

One platelet/oil immersion field $= 10 \times 10^9$/L (10,000/mm^3)

This rule of thumb may vary depending on the size of the field for the individual microscope used.

Activated Clotting Time

There are many variants, some important, in the estimation of clotting (coagulation) time. The most important point is that the procedure be standardized so that it is comparable from one estimation to the next in the same patient, if, for example, he or she is on heparin anticoagulation. The activated clotting time is especially sensitive to intrinsic coagulation defects such as hemophilia.

Method

1. Prewarm (37C) a special vacuum tube (BD Vacutainer 3865) that contains siliceous earth as an activator.
2. After first clearing the needle with another vacuum tube, fill the special tube with blood.
3. Begin timing as soon as the blood enters the tube.
4. After the tube is filled, invert it three times to mix the contents completely.
5. Incubate the tube at 37C in a water bath or heating block.
6. At 1 minute and at 5-second intervals thereafter, check the tube for the formation of a film clot. Note the time.

Reference of Normal Values

Normally blood clots within 2 minutes and 15 seconds when this procedure is used. Any elevation is significant. Hemophiliacs usually clot in 3 to 6 minutes. Patients on heparin therapy are maintained at about a 3- or 4-minute clotting time.

Skin Bleeding Time

One of the best tests of platelet function is the skin bleeding time. Congenital and acquired platelet disorders may have a prolonged bleeding time. The bleeding time, however, will also be lengthened in thrombocytopenia ($<55 \times 10^9/L$) and therefore may not be interpretable in such patients.

Materials

- Sterile disposable bleeding time device (e.g., Simplate-II or Surgicutt)
- Blood pressure cuff
- Stopwatch

Method

1. With the patient comfortably seated or lying down select a site on the volar surface of the forearm about 5 to 10 cm distal to the antecubital fossa. Avoid an area with superficial vessels, scars, and bruises.
2. Clean the chosen surface with alcohol and allow to completely dry.
3. Place a blood pressure cuff on the upper arm and inflate to 40 mm Hg.
4. After 30 to 60 seconds place one of the disposable bleeding time devices firmly, but without excessive pressure, perpendicular to the arm on the preselected and cleansed site.
5. Depress the trigger and simultaneously start the timer. Remove the device.
6. At 30-second intervals touch a piece of filter paper close to the edge but take care not to touch the wound.
7. Stop the timer when blood no longer stains the filter paper.
8. Remove the cuff and apply a small bandage to the wound.

URINALYSIS

The complete array of dipstick techniques has made the chemical portion of this procedure simple as well as accurate. Certain points must be remembered (e.g., the specificity of glucose oxidase versus the range of sugars that react with Clintest tablets) so gross errors are not made. Timing of the reading of the reagent pads is important and must be closely observed.

The microscopic examination of the sediment still requires considerable skill and experience. An aliquot (12 ml) of well-mixed urine is centrifuged for 5 minutes, and the supernatant is decanted. The packed sediment is shaken and a drop is placed on a clean microscope slide. A cover glass is placed on top of the drop of sediment. New disposable plastic slides have made this a more standardized method.

The sediment is thoroughly examined for cellular elements, various types of casts and formed elements, crystals, and any other unusual features. The relative quantities of

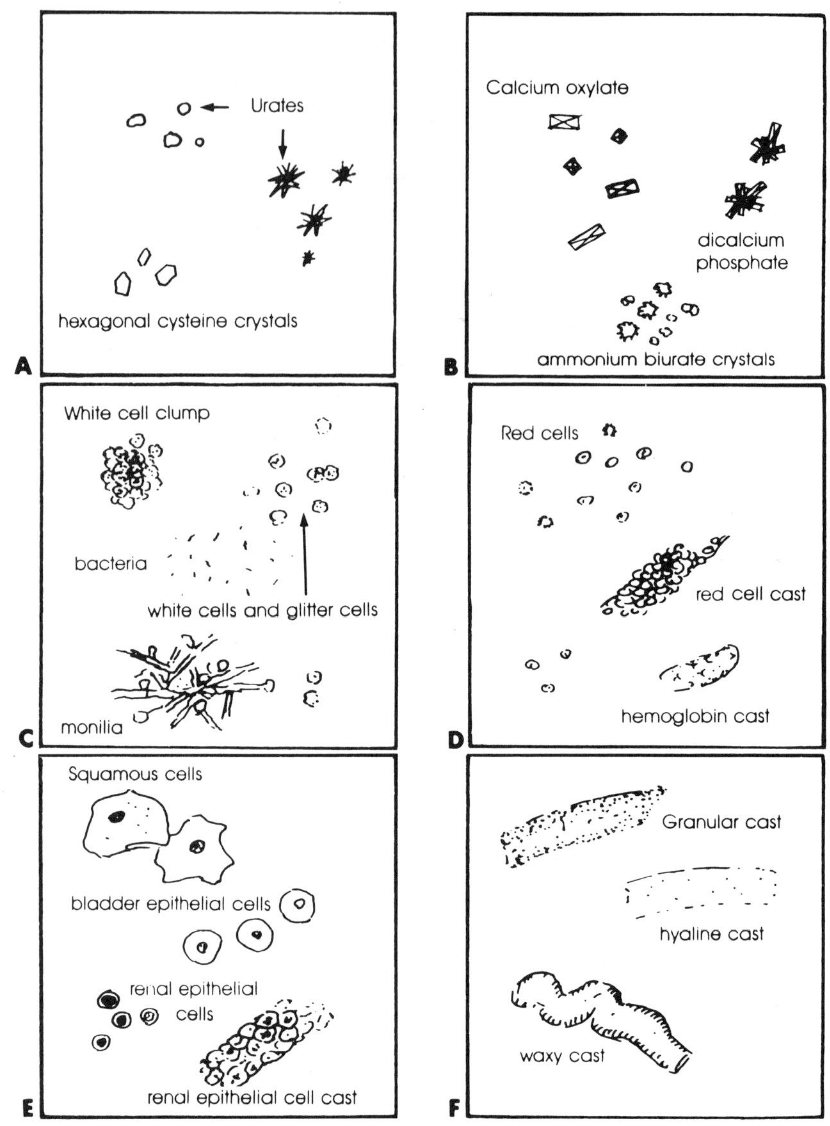

Figure 24–2. A. Urine crystalline sediment in acid urine. Urates and hexagonal cysteine crystals. **B.** Urine crystalline sediment in neutral or alkaline urines. Calcium oxylate, dicalcium phosphate, and ammonium biurate crystals. **C.** Urine sediments in cystitis and pyelonephritis. White cell clump, white cells and glitter cells, bacteria, and monilia. **D.** Red cells in urine sediments. Red cells, red cell cast, and hemoglobin cast. **E.** Epithelial cells in urine sediments. Squamous cells, bladder epithelial cells, renal epithelial cells, and renal epithelial cell cast. **F.** Casts in urine sediments. Granular cast, hyaline cast, and waxy cast.

these materials is reported semiquantitatively as the number per low-power or high-power field.

Line drawings of the more common elements are found in Figure 24–2.

MICROBIOLOGY

Quite often one can and must make at least a tentative diagnosis in cases of infectious and, it is hoped, treatable disease. Many times the medical student or house officer has the first chance to make these diagnoses. Usually this is done by the discovery of pathogenic organisms in spinal fluids, secretions, sputa, or other body fluids. The first step toward a definitive diagnosis is the preparation of a Gram-stained smear or its equivalent. After examination and correlating this information with the patient's clinical picture, appropriate initial inoculations of culture media are done.

The Gram-stained smears and all specimen fluids (spinal, joint, pleural, or abdominal) should be properly labeled and retained for review and any additional studies later deemed necessary.

Gram Stain

Staining Solutions

1. Crystal violet
   Solution A:

Crystal violet (90 percent dye content),	20 g
Ethyl alcohol (95 percent v/v)	20 ml

   Solution B:

Ammonium oxalate	8 g
Distilled water	800 ml

   Mix solutions A and B. Store for 24 hours before use. The resulting stain is stable.
2. Iodine solution

Potassium iodide	8 g
Iodine crystals	4 g
Distilled water	800 ml
3. Safranin counterstain (stock solution):

Safranin O (certified)	2.5 g
Ethyl alcohol (95 percent v/v)	100 ml

   For use, add 10 ml of stock solution to 90 ml of distilled water.
4. Decolorizing solution, 45 percent ethyl alcohol

Staining Procedure

1. Fix the slide by heating over a bunsen flame.
2. On a staining rack, stain the film for 1 minute with crystal violet stain.
3. Wash briefly in water.
4. Rinse off the water with iodine solution and let stand on the slide for 1 minute.
5. Wash with water but do not blot dry.
6. Decolorize several times with 45 percent ethyl alcohol for 30 seconds.
7. Wash for 5 seconds and then counterstain for 10 seconds with safranin.
8. Wash a final time for 5 seconds, dry and examine.

Wayson Stain

This is a simple staining procedure that is useful because of its simplicity and speed. Both gram-positive and gram-negative organisms stain blue, however.

Staining Solutions

1. Solution A:

Basic fuchsin	0.2 g
Methylene blue	0.75 g
Ethyl alcohol (absolute)	200 ml

2. Solution B:

Phenol crystals	10 g
Distilled water	200 ml

3. Dissolve the fuchsin and methylene blue in the absolute alcohol (solution A). Add the phenol to the distilled water (solution B). Then add solution A to solution B.

Staining Procedure

After heat-fixing the slide, cover the slide with stain and immediately wash with water. Blot dry and examine.

Acid-fast Stain

As the method is rather difficult, it is usually best to refer this procedure to those experienced with it. But, because at times this may not be possible, the method is included.

TABLE 24–3. PRIMARY EXAMINATION AND PLATING MEDIA FOR BACTERIOLOGY SPECIMENS

Specimen	Use of Preliminary Direct Smear	Routine Media for Inoculation
Blood	No	Commercial blood culture bottles, aerobic and anaerobic
Urine	Occasionaly	BA, EA
Sputum	Yes	BA, EA, Choc
CSF	Yes	BA, Choc, EB
Throat	No	BA, SAGP
Pericardial, pleural or peritoneal fluid	Yes	BA, EA, Choc, PRAS, EB
Joint fluid	Yes	BA, A, Choc, EB
Urethra	Occasionally	TM
Deep wound (open)	Yes	BA, EA, PRAS, EB
Feces	Occasionally	EA, ESA, EEB

BA, blood agar; EA, enteric agar (e.g., MacConkey or EMB); choc, chocolate blood agar; EB, enrichment broth; SAGP, selective agars for streptococci and staphylococci; PRAS, anaerobic agars; TM, Thayer-Martin; ESA, selective agars for enteric; EEB, enteric enrichment broth.

Staining Solutions

1. Phenol solution (6 percent):
   Phenol crystals   6 g
   (Instead of phenol crystals, 6.0 ml of melted
   phenol or 6.6 ml of carbolic acid liquid may
   be used)
   Distilled water   94 ml
2. Basic fuchsin solution:
   Saturated alcoholic solution of
   basic fuchsin (5 g/100 ml)   25 ml
   Phenol solution 6 percent   75 ml
   Before use, add 3 to 4 drops of Tergitol no. 7
3. Acid–alcohol solution:
   HCl, concentrated   3 ml
   Alcohol (95 percent or 70 percent alcohol)   97 ml
4. Methylene blue counterstain:
   Methylene blue (1 percent in 95
   percent alcohol)   30 ml
   KOH (0.01 percent in distilled water)   100 ml
   Before use, dilute 1:20 with distilled water

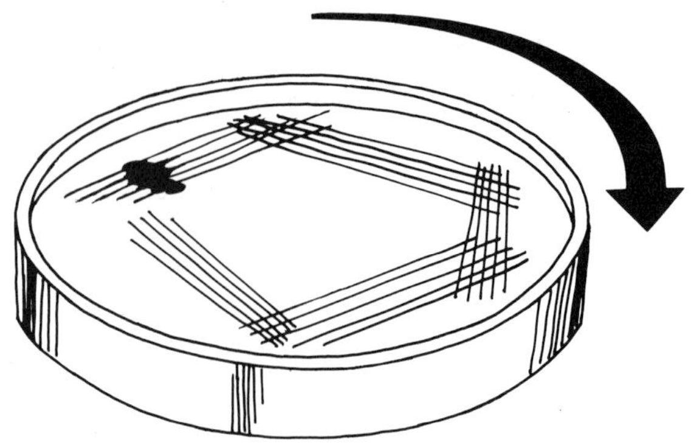

Figure 24–3. Inoculation of an agar plate. The diagram shows a five-stage streaking of the inoculum. The loop is flamed between each stage.

Staining Procedure

1. Heat fix the smears.
2. Stain with basic fuchsin solution for 3 to 5 minutes.
3. Wash in tap water.
4. Decolorize with the acid–alcohol solution.
5. Wash thoroughly with tap water.
6. Counterstain with diluted methylene blue solution for 1 minute.
7. Wash in tap water.
8. Dry in air or blot dry and examine for organisms.

Inoculation Guide for Initial Isolators

The number and types of media for primary inoculation of specimens must be determined individually within each laboratory, and they are influenced by the specimen, the patient type, the geographic location, and the laboratory budget. The media used for primary isolation must include types that provide the proper growth conditions for microorganisms potentially present in a particular specimen type. Table 24–3 lists the media that should be used routinely for a specific type of specimen. In many cases, additional selective media may improve the isolation of certain bacteria or decrease the time necessary for identification.

Figure 24–3 illustrates one technique used to inoculate an agar plate. Cultures should be incubated at an optimal temperature (usually 35C) and in an optimal atmosphere. Most facultative anaerobic and obligate aerobic bacteria grow well in the presence of CO_2 gas, and there are certain bacteria that require CO_2 for growth. Thus, a CO_2 environment is generally used in most incubators. The use of candle jars is an inexpensive and yet reasonably effective method to insure a CO_2 atmosphere for small numbers of bacteriologic plates. The incubator should also have a humidity of about 70 percent.

STOOL FOR OCCULT BLOOD

The time honored guaiac test for examination of stools and other specimens for occult blood has been effectively replaced by more efficient and convenient methods. The urine dipsticks are very sensitive and specific for the presence of hemoglobin, either free or as intact red cells.

Convenient commercial tests for occult blood in the stool are also widely available and are being promoted as effective screening for gastrointestinal malignancies. The package inserts give detailed instructions for the use of these methods.

BONE MARROW ASPIRATION

Bone marrow aspiration is a traumatic experience for most patients, and the physician should do everything possible to relieve the psychic and physical discomfort.

Two sites are frequently aspirated: the sternum at about the level of the third or fourth rib and the posterior spine of the iliac crest. The iliac crest is the preferred site because a biopsy can also be obtained as part of the procedure. It is also less painful for the patient. After the site of aspiration is located, it is cleansed and antiseptic solutions are applied. A long-acting local anesthetic (lidocaine) is carefully infiltrated into the skin and also into the periosteum. The intervening subcutaneous tissue is relatively insensitive. After a 4- or 5-minute wait for the anesthetic to act, a small nick is made in the skin with a scalpel to allow the large bore needle to be advanced easily. The needle is directed with a twisting motion to and through the outer table of bone (a slight "give" will be felt) until it is held firmly in place in the cancellous bone.

The patient is then cautioned to expect a sharp pain if the marrow is aspirated from the sternum. The obturator is removed, and marrow is aspirated with a 10-ml glass syringe with a tightly fitting plunger. No more than one-half of a milliliter of material (preferably one-half to one-third of a milliliter) is aspirated from the marrow cavity. Larger amounts result in a specimen unnecessarily diluted with sinusoidal blood.

Approximately six (or more if desired) films are prepared on clean glass slides or coverslips. The remainder of the aspirate is allowed to clot in the syringe, the physician pulling back the plunger about halfway while the marrow is still fluid. As soon as the aspirate has coagulated, excess blood is removed by gently rolling the clot over filter paper. The specimen is placed into a tissue paper and then into a specimen jar containing 10 percent formalin. Histologic slides are prepared from this material. An alternate procedure is to collect the aspirate in EDTA solution, filter it through fine lens paper, and place the button of marrow fragments and overfolded lens paper into the formalin.

After it is determined that the aspirate is satisfactory, withdraw the needle with the obturator in place. A second site (that uses the same skin incision) is then used for obtaining of the biopsy. Several different devices are available and the specific methods differ somewhat.

When the procedures are completed, apply an adhesive dressing to the wound. Requisition forms are appropriately labeled and submitted with the specimen for examination. If microbiology cultures are also required, the appropriate tubes of media are inoculated at the time the marrow is aspirated.

ADMINISTRATION OF BLOOD

Blood transfusion is to be initiated only by, or under the supervision of, a physician after all identification numbers and names on blood units and forms are rechecked. After the antiseptic solutions, tape, clamps, tourniquet, necessary needles or intracaths (16- to 18-gauge), and infusion set (with filter) are assembled, the patient's arm is prepared for the venipuncture. The selected site is cleansed and wiped with alcohol. Preliminary application of the tourniquet will usually indicate an adequate vein on the forearm, avoiding the antecubital fossa and the hand. An air vent is not necessary because bags require only one entry port. The infusion set is then filled with blood from the unit.

The tourniquet is reapplied, and the venipuncture is made. The less experienced transfusionist may find it easier to insert the 16- or 18-gauge needle if it is attached to a small syringe. After a good flow of blood is obtained, the syringe is removed and the infusion line is attached. More experienced operators usually insert the needle while attached to the infusion set, so that no transfer of equipment is necessary. The needle is held in place by several strips of tape. Occasionally an arm board may be of use.

The blood recipient is kept under constant surveillance by a physician, medical student, or professional nurse during the first 15 minutes of the transfusion so that any transfusion reactions will be discovered at the earliest possible moment. Frequent observation is required until the transfusion has been completed.

Upon completion of the transfusion, the needles are withdrawn and a small dressing is applied to the venipuncture site.

LUMBAR PUNCTURE

The lumbar puncture is not an innocuous procedure and due caution is necessary to avoid serious and possibly fatal complications. The prior examination of the eyegrounds for evidence of papilledema is mandatory to rule out the possibility of increased intracranial pressure, and possible supratentorial herniation and sudden death.

The lumbar tap can be done with the patient lying on the side and the back flexed as much as possible to open up the interspinous spaces. More conveniently and somewhat easier to perform is the lumbar puncture done with the patient in a sitting position, straddling the back of a straight-back chair.

The site of puncture (third or fourth lumbar vertebral interspace) is marked, and the skin is sterilized. The skin and underlying tissue is anesthetized with local anesthetic (1 percent procaine or 0.5 percent lidocaine). The lumbar puncture needle, with stylet in place, is pushed through the skin and then is aimed in a slightly cephalad direction, always in a midline position. The needle is advanced slowly and when in about 2 to 3 cm, the stylet is frequently removed to check for the flow of spinal fluid. Before it is advanced farther, the stylet is always returned in place. If bone is encountered, withdraw and redirect the needle away from the bone. If the patient complains of one-sided pain, the needle is presumably wandering off the midline and is appropriately redirected away from the nerve roots. A "give" may be noted when the needle passes through the ligamentum flavum as well as the dura.

When the spinal fluid begins to flow, a manometric reading is taken (opening pressure). Then three tubes, each filled with 2 to 3 ml of fluid, are collected. One is for chemical determinations, one for cell count and differential count as well as serology, and a third for microbiology, if indicated.

If the tap is bloody, 2 or 3 ml of fluid is allowed to drain. If it clears, a small vessel was ruptured in the puncture and specimens of clear fluid are then collected. If it continues to be bloodly, it may indicate an acute cerebrovascular accident and invalidate most laboratory studies.

After all specimens are obtained, the stylet is replaced and the needle withdrawn. A small dressing is applied. The patient is asked to remain flat in bed for several hours following the procedure.

EXFOLIATIVE CYTOLOGIC EXAMINATIONS

Cellular material from cervical or vaginal areas should be thinly spread on slides and the slides immersed immediately in fixative (95 percent ethanol) before drying occurs. If drying occurs, undesirable artifacts are introduced that usually render the specimen worthless.

Information concerning hormone or irradiation therapy is extremely important in the evaluation of cytologic specimens. Indicate the date of the last menstrual period, whether the patient is pregnant, or whether any lesion is present. Failure to indicate the foregoing may result in an invalid interpretation.

Materials such as bronchial washings, urine, and fluids from serous cavities should be collected in a clean, dry, glass container and brought to the cytology laboratory for fixation and processing immediately following collection.

Buccal smears for sex chromatin evaluation are made by using a tongue blade scraped over the buccal mucous membrane. Thin films are made and immediately fixed in 95 percent ethanol.

TISSUE BIOPSY

It is beyond the scope of this book to describe techniques for biopsy other than those that are ordinarily performed by medical students or house officers. Tissue biopsies, however, require "tender, loving care". In this context the student or resident is important in ensuring that the specimen is handled in an optimal manner.

Presently, diagnostic biopsies are obtained on many different tissues including lymph nodes, liver, kidney, skin, and muscle. Other biopsy sites include lung, brain, and bone marrow. Thin needle aspiration has become quite popular in the last several years.

Prior to the procedure, the exact site to be biopsied and the tissue to be obtained should be carefully planned. The studies deemed appropriate should be decided on and appropriate arrangements made for their accomplishment. For example, if microbiological cultures (bacteriologic, mycobacteriologic, and fungal) are required, sterility in the technique of tissue handling must be guaranteed and necessary culture media must be available.

The operator must treat the tissue as gently as possible, taking care to avoid crush artifact or other tissue destruction. An adequate biopsy should be taken if at all possible.

After the specimen is obtained it should be divided appropriately for the various studies required. Routine tissue sections require prompt formalin fixation, electron microscopy requires glutaraldehyde fixation, and immunofluorescent studies require prompt delivery to the laboratory.

RECOMMENDED SOURCES OUTLINING STANDARD LABORATORY PROCEDURE METHODOLOGY

Cartwright GE: Diagnostic Laboratory Hematology, 4th ed. New York, Grune and Stratton, 1968.

Cooper OV: Arterial puncture simplified. Res Staff Phys, April 1972.

Engley FB Jr: Pocket Reference Guide to Medical Microbiology. Boston, Little Brown, 1963.

Fischer PM, Addison LA, Curtis P, Mitchell JM: The Office Laboratory. East Norwalk, Conn, Appleton-Century-Crofts, 1983.

Henry J (ed): Clinical Diagnosis and Management by Laboratory Methods. Philadelphia, Saunders, 1984.

Kark RM: A Primer of Urinalysis, 2nd ed. New York, Hoeber, 1963.

Koneman E, et al.: Color Atlas and Textbook of Diagnostic Microbiology. Philadelphia, Lippincott, 1983.

Miale JB: Laboratory Medicine-Hematology, 6th ed. Saint Louis, C.V. Mosby, 1982.

Petito F, Plum F: The lumbar puncture. N Eng J Med 290:225, 1974.

Urine Under the Microscope. Nutley, NJ, Rocom Press, 1973.

Widmann F: Technical Manual. Arlington, Va, American Association of Blood Banks, 1985.

When you hear hoofbeats,
think of horses, not zebras.

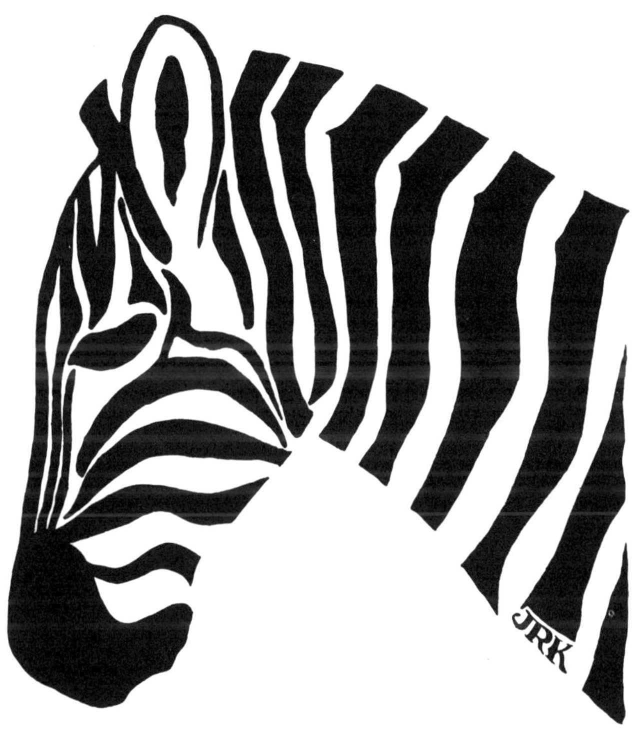

INDEX